CURRENT TECHNIQUES IN

Ophthalmic Laser Surgery

CURRENT TECHNIQUES IN
Ophthalmic Laser Surgery

EDITED BY

William E. Benson
Director, Retina Service
Wills Eye Hospital
Professor of Ophthalmology
Thomas Jefferson Medical College
Philadelphia, PA, USA

Gabriel Coscas
Professor and Chairman
Eye University Clinic of Créteil
University of Paris XII
Créteil, France

L. Jay Katz
Attending Surgeon
Wills Eye Hospital
Assistant Professor of Ophthalmology
Thomas Jefferson Medical College
Philadelphia, PA, USA

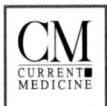

CM
CURRENT
MEDICINE

1994
Philadelphia

Current Medicine

Managing editor: **Chris Baumle**

Developmental editor: **Rachel Delp**

Art director: **Paul Fennessy**

Designer: **Patrick Whelan**

Illustration director: **Larry Ward**

Illustrators: **Gary Welch, Marie Dean, and Ann Saydlowski**

Production: **David Myers and Wendy Feinstein**

Typesetting director: **Jayne Walko**

ISBN: 1-878132-57-1

ISSN: 1062-4813

Printed in Kong Kong by Paramount Printing Group Limited

5 4 3 2 1

Preface

The authors of the chapters in this book are widely recognized, not only as leading clinicians, but also as innovative researchers in their fields. Their thorough understanding of current and past ophthalmic therapy is combined with a desire to push forward toward more safe and effective treatments. Their extensive personal experience and thorough review of the world's literature allows them to place the latest advances in laser therapy in proper context with what is currently accepted. We, the co-editors for this volume, have been fortunate that such an outstanding group has agreed to take the time necessary to contribute to our efforts to update our knowledge of laser treatment. We believe that the reader will find a wealth of useful information.

The latest lasers, such as the diode, holium-yttrium aluminum garnet (Ho:YAG), potassium titanyl phosphate-yttrium aluminum garnet (KTP:YAG), and neodymium-yttrium lithium fluoride (Nd:YLF) are discussed. These lasers and new delivery systems, such as the laser indirect ophthalmoscope, have made possible more cost-effective, and often better, means of treating various ophthalmic conditions. For example, the diode indirect laser will probably become the treatment of choice for retinal conditions, such as retinopathy of prematurity. Another new and exciting development is pretreatment of the target tissue with drugs. Early evidence indicates that because indocyanine green absorbs light best at almost exactly the wavelength emitted by the diode laser, safer obliteration of choroidal neovascular membranes will be possible. Similarly, clinical and laboratory testing of the newest generation of photosensitizing agents suggests that photodynamic therapy may become a standard form of therapy for intraocular tumors and neovascularization. Finally, new lasers may replace or complement the way we perform iridotomy, trabeculoplasty, and ab interno sclerostomy.

For cataract surgeons, yttrium aluminum garnet (YAG) capsulotomy is discussed in detail, including pretreatment evaluation, treatment techniques for anterior capsulorhexis syndrome and pigment lysis, and complications. For those interested in photorefractive keratectomy and phototherapeutic keratectomy using the excimer laser, there is a state of the art presentation of equipment indications, technique, and complications. Ironically, although excimer laser therapy is being perfected, others are developing and testing other, less expensive lasers to perform intrastromal keratoablation, avoiding damage to Bowman's membrane. The latest in oculoplastic laser therapy is presented, including endonasal and intracanalicular laser techniques for no-incision dacryocystorhinostomy. Selective argon laser ablation of individual eyelash follicles may replace cryotherapy in the treatment of trichiasis, and the tunable pulsed dye laser may eliminate the need for local and systemic steroid therapy in the treatment of capillary hemangiomas.

After more than 20 years of use, laser photocoagulation of retinal disorders remains one of our more efficient therapeutic approaches in our daily practice. Laser surgery is considered by patients and by ophthalmologists less invasive than instrumental endocular surgery. Laser use in ophthalmology is now very diversified, with a laser treatment for refractive disorders, glaucoma management, and cataract surgery. Lasers appear to many patients as the "magic response" to ocular diseases.

The retinal indications of laser surgery are very precisely codified in ocular practice, particularly in many important diseases, (eg, diabetic retinopathy or well-defined choroidal new-vessels complicating age-related maculopathy) thanks to different randomized clinical trials. However, the field of use of this retinal laser surgery appears wider than ever. The technical progresses allow photocoagulation with the help of a slit lamp, but also with indirect ophthalmoscopy and with different probes during vitrectomy, using the endolaser devices. New indications also appear, such as photocoagulation of pigmented intraocular tumors.

The following chapters synthesize our knowledge of these indications in both common and less common diseases. The experience of many experts was required for the redaction of these chapters. We hope that the reader will find guidelines for laser treatment in retinal diseases and information about new technology—new wavelengths, new devices, and new technology of retinal laser surgery.

The diversity of laser application for glaucoma management has rapidly developed to such a magnitude that this edition of *Current Techniques in Ophthalmic Laser Surgery* contains seven chapters on the subject. These chapters are devoted to various laser methods used to treat glaucoma using a staggering array of different types of lasers including argon, diode, YAG, holmium, and excimer.

Laser trabeculoplasty has been commonly performed for the past 15 years, but the indications and technique are continually evolving. The role of argon laser trabeculoplasty before medical therapy and its usefulness in repeated applications are discussed, and recent studies examining the long-term effectiveness of laser trabeculoplasty are reviewed.

For pupillary block, laser peripheral iridotomy and iridoplasty have been described, and the controversial issue of performing a peripheral iridotomy for pigmentary glaucoma where a postulated "reverse pupillary block" may exist is explored.

Guarded glaucoma filtering surgery has been the surgical mainstay for patients who have failed medical and angle laser therapy. New techniques are rapidly emerging using ab externo and ab interno approaches to deliver laser energy at the limbus to create new outflow pathways from the anterior chamber into the subconjunctival space. The ab interno approaches that have been used are listed, and insight using the holmium laser, which has rapidly become the dominant laser for performing sclerostomy in the United States, has been provided. Interesting work using an excimer laser, which is best known for keratorefractive use, as a nonpenetrating filtration procedure has been presented, and the different methods whereby failing filtration blebs can be revived by laser techniques are explained.

These methods include cutting scleral flaps and sutures for relief of external obstructions and reopening closed internal sclerostomies.

Ciliary destruction has been increasingly performed by laser cilioablation using the YAG laser and, more recently diode lasers, with contact and non-contact methods. Cyclocryotherapy may gradually be replaced, and a great deal of practical insight into laser cyclophotocoagulation is provided.

Why have lasers become so popular in treating patients with glaucoma? There are a variety of reasons, but simplicity and a relatively low complication rate are major determinants. Effectiveness of argon laser trabeculoplasty of holmium laser sclerostomy may not compare favorably with a surgical trabeculectomy. However, the demand for quicker, cost-effective, and less hazardous procedures with a reasonable chance of success has driven the development of the present laser procedures. With future experience and modification, it would be expected that many of these laser techniques will evolve into techniques with success rates comparable or even more favorable than our scalpel surgery.

William E. Benson, MD
Gabriel Coscas, MD
L. Jay Katz, MD

Contributors

Richard L. Anderson, MD
University of Utah
Salt Lake City, Utah

Francesco Bandello, MD
Istituto Scientifico Ospedale S. Raffaele
Universitá di Milano
Milano, Italy

Howard Barnebey, MD
Glaucoma Consultation and Microsurgery
Seattle, Washington

Rosario Brancato, MD
Istituto Scientifico Ospedale S. Raffaele
Universitá di Milano
Milano, Italy

Massimo Corazza, MD
Clinica Oculistica dell'Universita
di Genova
Genova, Italy

Gabriel Coscas, MD
Eye University Clinic of Créteil
Créteil, France

J. William Doyle, MD
University of Florida
Gainesville, Florida

Daniel Finkelstein, MD
Wilmer Ophthalmological Institute
Johns Hopkins Hospital
Baltimore, Maryland

Patrick Flaharty, MD
Eye Centers of Florida
Fort Myers, Florida

Evangelos S. Gragoudas, MD
Massachusetts Eye and Ear Infirmary
Boston, Massachusetts

David R. Guyer, MD
Manhattan Eye, Ear, and Throat Hospital
New York, New York

Robert Haimovici, MD
Maassachusetts Eye and Ear Infirmary
Boston, Massachusetts

Pamela R. Henderson, MD
WK Kellogg Eye Center
Ann Arbor, Michigan

Luke Herbert, BSc, MB, BS
Royal Postgraduate Medical School
Hammersmith Hospital
London, UK

Eve J. Higginbotham, MD
WK Kellogg Eye Center
Ann Arbor, Michigan

Allen C. Ho, MD
Manhattan Eye, Ear, and Throat Hospital
New York, New York

Darmakusuma Ie, MD
The Retina Institute of Maryland
Baltimore, Maryland

Eva M. Kohner, MD, FRCP, FRCOphth
Royal Postgraduate Medical School
Hammersmith Hospital
London, UK

Joel M. Krauss, MD
Manhattan Eye, Ear, and Throat Hospital
New York, New York

Peter R. Laibson, MD
Wills Eye Hospital
Philadelphia, Pennsylvania

Kwang J. Lee, MD
Louisiana State University
New Orleans, Louisiana

Jeffrey Liebmann, MD
New York Eye and Ear Infirmary
New York, New York

Joan Miller, MD
Massachusetts Eye and Ear Infirmary
Boston, Massachusetts

Dominic McHugh, MD, FRCS, FRCOphth
Moorfields Eye Hospital
Hammersmith Hospital
London, UK

Ugo Murialdo, MD
Clinica Oculistica dell'Universita di Genova
Genova, Italy

Robert P. Murphy, MD
The Retina Institute of Maryland
Baltimore, Maryland

Younghyun G. Oh, MD
Loma Linda University
Loma Linda, California

Stephen S. Pappas, MD
The Retina Institute of Maryland
Baltimore, Maryland

Bhupendra K. Patel, MD
University of Utah
Salt Lake City, Utah

Gholam A. Peyman, MD
Louisiana State University
New Orleans, Louisiana

Seth D. Potash, MD
New York Eye and Ear Infirmary
New York, New York

Christopher J. Rapuano, MD
Wills Eye Hospital
Philadelphia, Pennsylvania

Robert Ritch, MD
New York Eye and Ear Infirmary
New York, New York

M. Bruce Shields, MD
Duke University
Durham, North Carolina

Mary Fran Smith, MD
University of Florida
Gainesville, Florida

Gisèle Soubrane, MD
Eye University Clinic of Créteil
Créteil, France

Richard L. Tipperman, MD
Wills Eye Hospital
Philadelphia, Pennsylvania

Giuseppe Trabucchi, MD
Istituto Scientifico Ospedale S. Raffaele
Universitá di Milano
Milano, Italy

Carlo Traverso, MD
Clinica Oculistica dell'Universita di Genova
Genova, Italy

Leonidas Zografos, MD
Jules Gonin University Eye Clinic
Lausanne, Switzerland

Contents

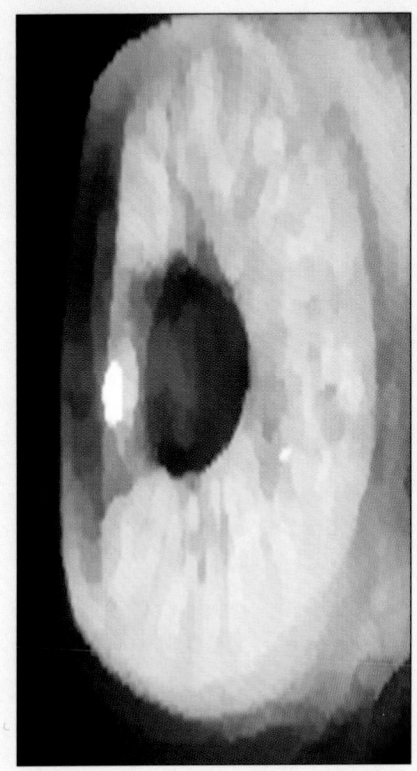

CHAPTER 1

LASERS FOR THE CATARACT SURGEON

RICHARD TIPPERMAN

One of the greatest advances in the evolution of cataract surgery was the shift to extracapsular surgery, which preserved the posterior capsule and allowed placement of an intraocular lens (IOL) within the posterior chamber; however, with preservation of the posterior capsule came the problem of delayed opacification of the posterior capsule. This complication ultimately led to the development of the neodymium-yttrium aluminum garnet (Nd:YAG) laser for posterior capsulotomy. Although the Nd:YAG laser has been widely used in ophthalmic procedures, new techniques and information regarding complications with the laser are constantly evolving. In the past year, several studies have evaluated new techniques and complications associated with Nd:YAG laser.

In this chapter we will evaluate these developments in three sections: new techniques for the preoperative evaluation of patients undergoing Nd:YAG capsulotomy, new techniques and uses for the Nd:YAG laser, and, finally, complications associated with the use of the Nd:YAG laser.

PREOPERATIVE EVALUATION OF PATIENTS UNDERGOING NEODYMIUM-YTTRIUM ALUMINUM GARNET CAPSULOTOMY

Potential visual acuity testing

Determining a patient's potential visual acuity before performing an Nd:YAG capsulotomy can be helpful, just as it can be helpful at times to determine a patient's potential visual acuity before performing cataract surgery when there is another ophthalmic problem (eg, retinal disease or glaucoma) associated with the cataract. Strong [1•] evaluated the accuracy of the Haag-Streit (Lotmar) white-light laser interferometer, the Rodenstock laser interferometer, and the Site white-light machine in predicting visual acuity after Nd:YAG laser capsulotomy. In 93% of the cases the Rodenstock laser interferometer predicted a final visual acuity with one line of that actually achieved. The Haag-Streit interferometer did not perform as well and predicted to within one line of final visual acuity in 64% of the cases. The accuracy of the Site unit was 77%.

The differences in performance among the different instruments was greatest in patients with the poorest preoperative visual acuity. After Nd:YAG laser capsulotomy all three units obtained a visual acuity similar to the post-laser Snellen visual acuity. The differences in predictive accuracy between the three units was attributed to capsular thickening, which produces a greater degree of optical degrada-

tion of the image produced by a white-light interferometer than by a laser interferometer.

Glare testing

Because of the low but definite complications associated with Nd:YAG laser capsulotomy, this procedure should only be undertaken when patients are manifesting visual symptoms. At times, however, patients will describe increasing difficulty with visual function and will appear to have only minimal changes to the posterior capsule. Sunderraj and coworkers [2] demonstrated that many of these patients have diminished vision when tested under glare conditions. In their study, Snellen visual acuity was measured under standard and glare conditions both before and after Nd:YAG capsulotomy. All patients had a best corrected vision of at least 20/40 but also experienced progressive difficulty with visual function. All patients had clinically observable posterior capsule opacification without other known causes of glare disability (eg, malpositioned IOL). After Nd:YAG capsulotomy 65% of patients had an improvement in Snellen visual acuity under standard conditions and 97% had an improvement under glare conditions. Of 46 patients, there were 16 whose standard Snellen visual acuity did not improve after capsulotomy but in 14 of these patients there was an improvement in Snellen acuity under glare conditions. The authors concluded that glare testing was clinically useful in evaluating pseudophakes with posterior capsular opacification who complain of progressive visual difficulty despite good Snellen visual acuity under standard testing conditions.

NEW TECHNIQUES AND INDICATIONS FOR THE NEODYMIUM-YTTRIUM ALUMINUM GARNET LASER

Anterior capsulorhexis contraction syndrome

The shift toward small-incision cataract surgery and small-incision implants has produced a corresponding shift in capsulotomy techniques. Small-incision IOLs require capsular bag placement with small anterior capsular openings to assure long-term IOL centration. These changes in both IOL style and capsulorhexis construction have created new problems and uses for the Nd:YAG laser.

With IOL optic diameters of 5.5 and 6.0 mm the anterior circular capsulorhexis is often attempted to be sized at 5 mm. Occasionally, there can be a progressive contraction of the anterior capsule down to a diameter as small as 1 to 2 mm, a complication that can severely reduce a patient's visual acuity (Fig. 1-1).

The Nd:YAG laser can be used to open this constricted ring; however, at times an Nd:YAG laser capsulotomy can require significantly elevated energies than will a standard capsulotomy. One approach toward solving this problem is to attempt to break the ring in two sections 180 degrees apart from each other (Fig. 1-2). If this procedure does not work then additional openings in the ring can be made at 90-degree intervals to the initial openings. Because opening the ring can become more difficult once the anterior leaflets become fibrotic, patients with suspected anterior capsular ring contraction should be monitored periodically, and if the diameter of the anterior capsule starts to constrict then consideration should be given to performing Nd:YAG anterior capsulotomy.

Hurvitz [3•] described using the Nd:YAG laser to perform anterior capsulotomy and lysis of posterior synechiae in nine patients. Three separate techniques were used depending on the presence or absence of posterior synechiae and the relationship and alignment of the constricted anterior capsular ring to the pupil (Fig. 1-3). In the first technique the anterior capsular opening is enlarged by removing an ellipse of anterior capsule superior to the anterior capsular opening. In the second technique, "relaxing incisions" in the form of radial openings in anterior capsular ring are made, and in the third technique a circular opening is made. In all patients the energy settings of the laser were less than 2 mJ although a "significant" number of applications were described as being necessary. All patients developed bleeding from the iris adjacent to the areas where the capsule was treated even though no direct laser applications were

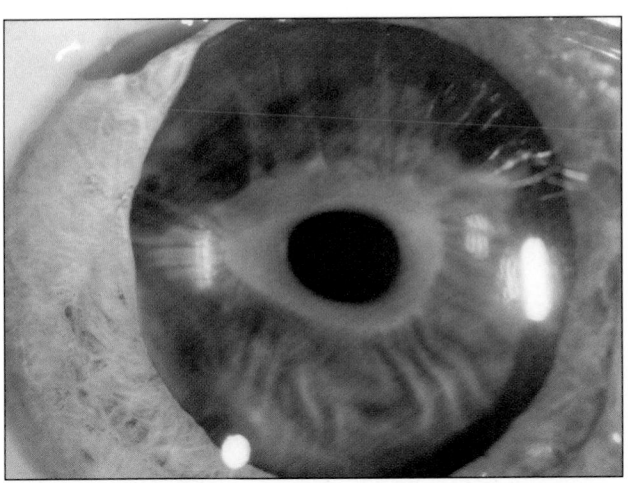

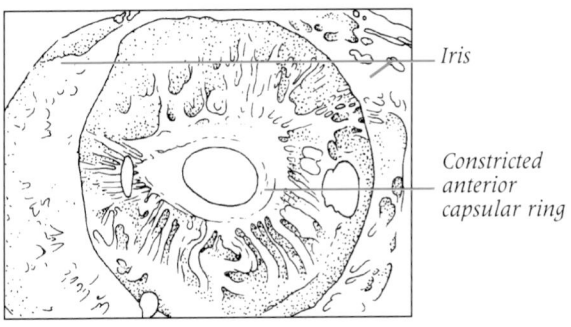

Iris

Constricted anterior capsular ring

FIGURE 1-1 Patient is 6 months status-post posterior chamber intraocular lens implantation "in the bag" with an intact

anterior capsulorhexis. Note how the anterior capsulorhexis has severely constricted.

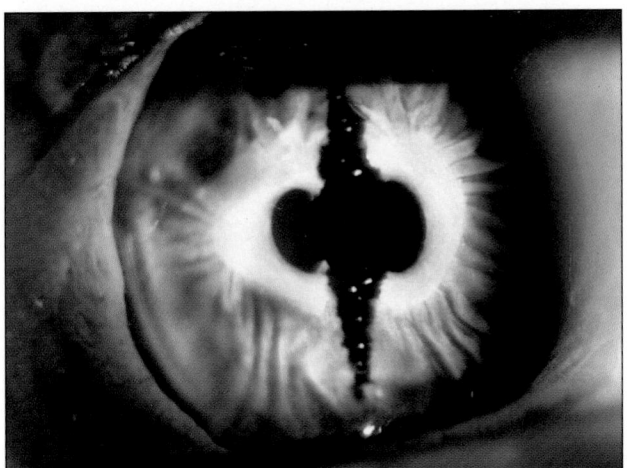

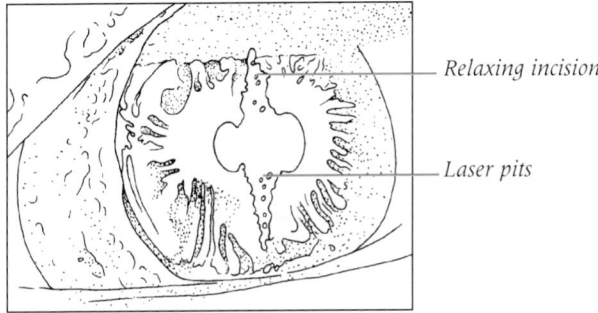

Relaxing incision

Laser pits

FIGURE 1-2 Constricted anterior capsular ring following placement of "relaxing incisions" with neodymium-yttrium

aluminum garnet laser. Laser pit marks are shown on the anterior optic surface.

applied to the iris. Pitting of the anterior optic surface was described in "almost all cases" although none were in the visual axis.

Laser pigment lysis

Occasionally, patients will have pigmented deposits form on the anterior surface of the IOL optic. Usually, this development does not have any consequences on vision; however, rarely, the pigment deposits will be so dense that there will actually be a decrease in the patient's visual acuity (Fig. 1-4). If these patients are examined closely with the slit lamp a diaphanous membrane can often be seen extending between the different islands of pigment precipitates.

The Nd:YAG laser can be used to debride these precipitates and membrane from the surface of the optic (Fig. 1-5). To remove the precipitates the aiming beam should be focused directly on one of the pigmented deposits. Retrofocusing, which is commonly used for posterior capsulotomies, should not be used because the energy from the optical breakdown of the laser moves anteriorly from the point of focus. Most laser bursts will disperse the precipitates off the optic and as the precipitates move forward the diaphanous membrane between them will become more apparent. Typ-

ically, a very low power (0.6 mJ) is used initially and increased in 0.2-mJ increments as needed. Patients are given topical corticosteroid treatment for at least 1 week to help decrease any inflammation that might lead to reformation of the pigment precipitates..

Anterior capsulotomy

At one time the Nd:YAG laser was used to perform anterior capsulotomies before performing conventional surgery. Aron-Rosa and Aron [4•] reported that this practice led to a markedly reduced rate of capsular opacification. The authors no longer use, nor do they recommend, preoperative laser anterior capsulorhexis because of problems such as increased inflammation. However, the markedly decreased incidence of posterior capsular opacification in this group of patients is an intriguing finding.

Aron-Rosa and Aron reported using a picosecond laser to perform anterior capsulotomy 12 to 20 hours before cataract surgery in one eye and a standard manual capsulotomy in the other eye at the time of surgery. Between 1980 and 1981, 122 patients were treated in this manner. At reevaluation 10 years later, only 4 (3.27%) of the eyes treated with the laser capsulorhexis had developed opacified posterior capsules,

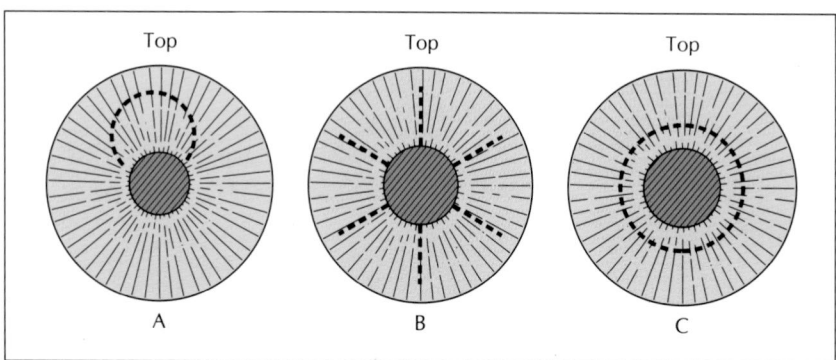

FIGURE 1-3 Three separate methods of enlarging a constricted anterior capsular ring. (*From* Hurvitz [4]; with permission.)

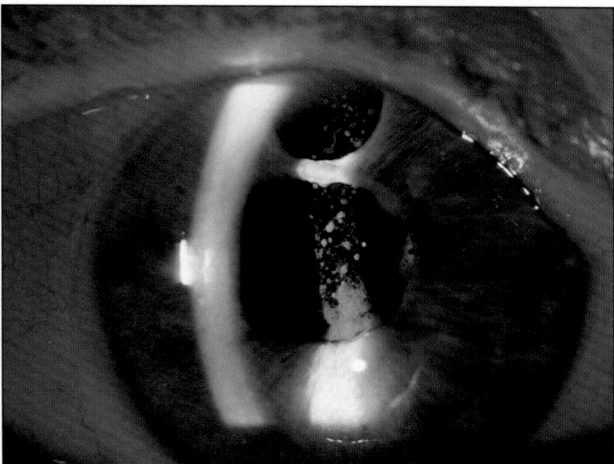

FIGURE 1-4 Silicone lens with numerous pigmented precipitates. Area of diaphanous membrane is shown.

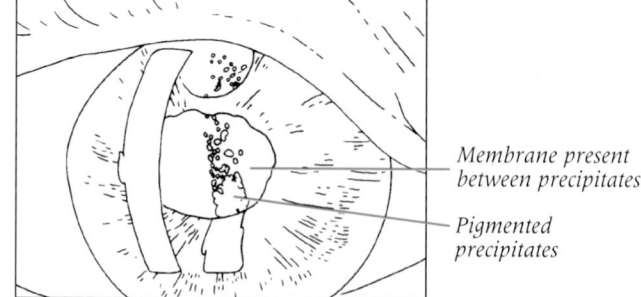

Membrane present between precipitates

Pigmented precipitates

whereas 61 (50%) of the eyes treated by manual capsulotomy had developed opacified capsules that had to be treated with Nd:YAG capsulotomy.

Bilateral persistent pupillary membranes

Ramakrishnan and coworkers [5] reported using the Nd:YAG laser to treat two patients with extensive persistent pupillary membranes (Figs. 1-6 and 1-7). Neither patient's vision had improved preoperatively with dilation. One patient was 50 years of age and had a best corrected vision of 20/80 in both eyes, which improved to 20/20 in one eye and 20/30 in the other postoperatively. The other patient was 18 years of age and had a best corrected vision of 20/120 in both eyes, which improved to 20/30 in each eye after laser surgery. The pupils of the eyes of both patients were covered with an extensive network of heavily pigmented uveal tissue before the laser procedure was initiated.

The Nd:YAG laser was used in single-pulse mode, with energies ranging from 0.8 to 1.8 mJ. The laser energy was directed at the attachment of the membrane to the iris collarette. Patients were given a regimen of prednisolone acetate, 1%, cyclopentalate, 1%, and acetazolamide, 250 mg twice daily, after the procedures.

COMPLICATIONS ASSOCIATED WITH THE NEODYMIUM-YTTRIUM ALUMINUM GARNET LASER

Retinal detachment after neodymium-yttrium aluminum garnet capsulotomy

Retinal detachment has been reported to occur at a frequency of between 0.17% and 3.6% after Nd:YAG posterior capsulotomy. In an article that received a great

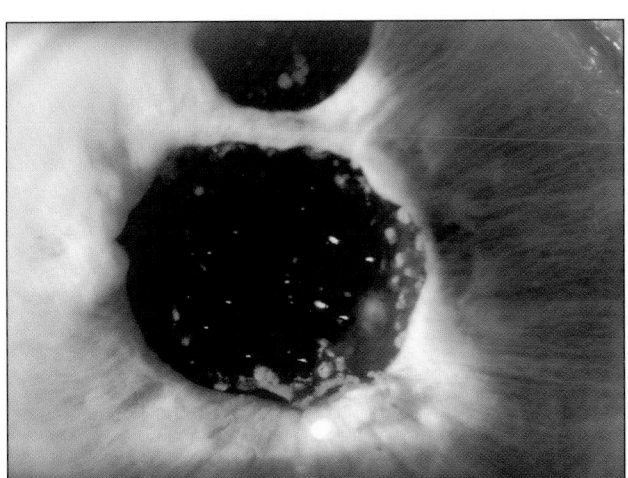

FIGURE 1-5 Same patient as in Figure 1-4 after neodymium-yttrium aluminum garnet laser capsulotomy to remove precipitates.

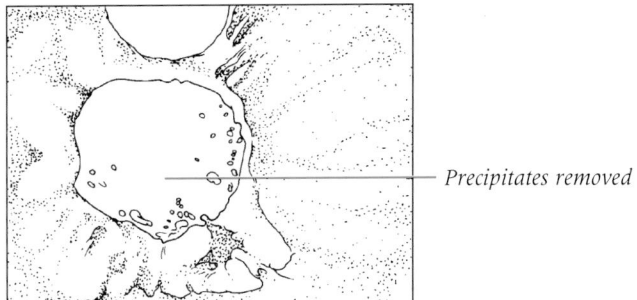

Precipitates removed

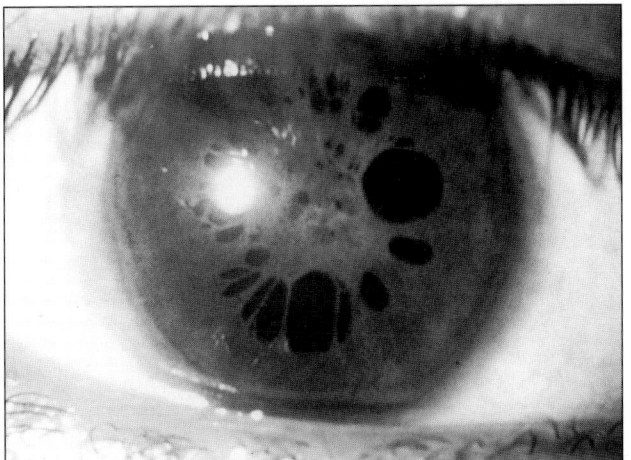

FIGURE 1-6 Patient with extensive persistent pupillary membrane before neodymium-yttrium aluminum garnet treatment. (*From* Ramakrishnan *et al.* [5]; with permission.)

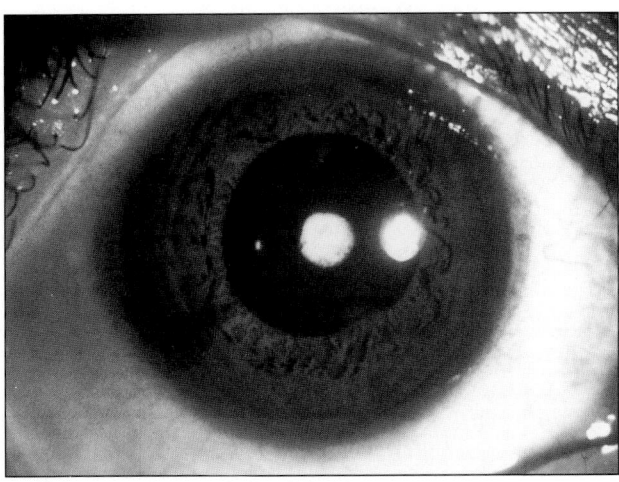

FIGURE 1-7 Same patient as in Figure 1-6 after treatment.

deal of media attention, Javitt and coworkers [6••] reported a 3.9-fold increase in the risk for retinal detachment or retinal tear in those patients who had undergone cataract surgery followed by Nd:YAG capsulotomy. With the aid of the Medicare database the authors reviewed the cases of 57,003 patients who had undergone extracapsular cataract surgery between 1986 and 1987. The patients were identified through claims submitted to Medicare that were followed through to 1988. Patients with histories of cataract surgery, posterior capsulotomy, and retinal detachment were identified by using diagnostic codes from physician bills and hospital discharge records.

Of the original 57,003 patients, 13,709 had undergone Nd:YAG capsulotomy during the period of 1986 to 1988. Of these patients, 337 had developed an aphakic or pseudophakic retinal detachment and an additional 194 patients required repair of a retinal tear without detachment. Younger age, male sex, and white race were also associated with an increased risk for retinal complication following laser capsulotomy.

There have been several criticisms of this study by Javitt and coworkers [6••]. Because the authors used the Medicare database rather than individual charts, they could not verify that all retinal complications had occurred in the same eye that had been subjected to capsulotomy. In addition, it was not noted whether any of the patients had also had difficult or complicated surgery. Although patients were excluded from the study if a vitrectomy was coded at the time of cataract surgery, it is likely that the incidence of vitreous loss and anterior vitrectomy is underreported.

It is likely that the patients who underwent more difficult surgery would be likely to have more posterior segment complications. Many patients with posterior capsular rupture end up with residual retained cortex and a fibrotic remnant of posterior capsule that still requires Nd:YAG laser treatment to clear the visual axis. Steinert and coworkers [7••] reviewed the cases of a series of patients who had developed retinal detachment following Nd:YAG capsulotomy. In this series, three of the six patients who had ultimately developed a retinal detachment after capsulotomy and also had complicated surgery. Two of the patients had an anterior chamber lens and the third had an iris fixated lens. Although the retinal detachment in these cases may be attributed to the Nd:YAG laser capsulotomy, it is clear that these patients did not have "routine" uncomplicated surgery.

Another criticism was that no attempt was made to determine whether the IOLs were fixated within the capsular bag with a continuous capsulorhexis or whether there were multiple radial tears in the anterior capsule. There is some evidence to suggest that the type of implant fixation may play a role in the inci-

dence of retinal detachment that occurs after Nd:YAG capsulotomy. Van Westenbrugge and coworkers [8••] reported an incidence of 1% retinal detachment after capsulotomy in patients with a continuous circular capsulorhexis and in-the-bag IOL placement. They reviewed cases of a series of 218 consecutive Nd:YAG capsulotomies performed from 1982 to 1989 and found that the median time between cataract extraction and laser capsulotomy was 24.8 months. Retinal detachment in their two patients occurred at 15 and 17 months postcapsulotomy. The authors propose that in-the-bag placement of the IOL can decrease the incidence of retinal complications that occur after Nd:YAG capsulotomy by providing greater stability for the implant and anterior vitreous.

Finally, although not a criticism, Hoffer [9] commented on the timing of the Nd:YAG laser capsulotomies as reported by Javitt and coworkers (Fig. 1-8). Approximately 15% of the capsulotomies performed were done less than 3 months after the initial cataract surgery and 29% were done less than 6 months postoperatively. Fifty-five percent of patients had had Nd:YAG capsulotomy performed before a full year had elapsed since their surgery. Hoffer reported that his ultimate long-term rates for capsulotomy were the same as those in the Javitt series; however, the timing of the procedure was markedly different. In the past 10 years, Hoffer has reported performing only four capsulotomies within 1 year of having performed cataract surgery.

Besides differences in the timing of Nd:YAG capsulotomy, the study by Javitt and coworkers demonstrated

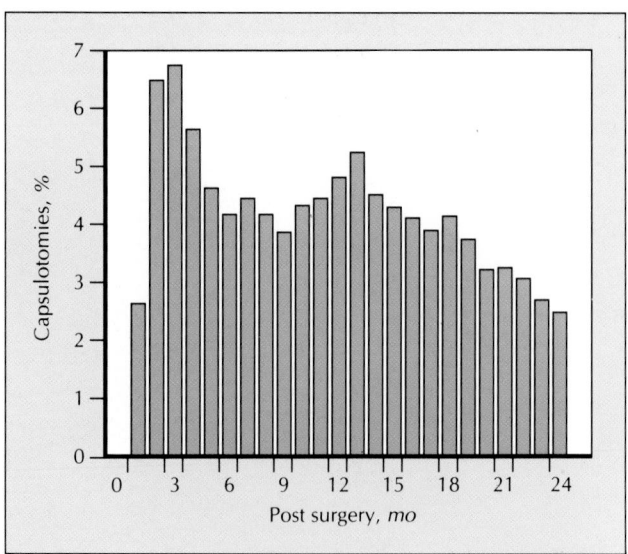

FIGURE 1-8 Frequency histogram of the percentage of cases of neodymium-yttrium aluminum garnet capsulotomy being performed within 2 years of cataract surgery. Note that 50% of all capsulotomies were performed within 1 year of surgery. (*From* Javitt *et al.* [6]; with permission.)

a tremendous variation in the rate of capsulotomy per person-year of presumed pseudophakia depending on where in the United States the patient lived (Fig. 1-9). The highest rate was in Nevada (27%) and the lowest rate in Wyoming (2.5%).

All these data demonstrate that, although Nd:YAG laser capsulotomy is a common procedure, there certainly is a great deal of variability in the way in which it is used and in the presumed risk for retinal complications associated with its use.

Elevated intraocular pressure and neodymium-yttrium aluminum garnet capsulotomy

Increases in intraocular pressure (IOP) after the performance of Nd:YAG capsulotomy have been well documented. Elevations in IOP occurring after capsulotomy have been described as early as 1 hour after and up to 24 hours after completion of the procedure. Altamirano and coworkers [10••] prospectively studied the effect of Nd:YAG capsulotomy on IOP and inflammation (as measured by a laser flare-cell meter). Thirty-four percent of patients were found to have a significant flare rise over precapsulotomy values. The degree of aqueous particles increased at 6 hours and was followed by a peak in flare at 18 hours postcapsulotomy. Acute intraocular hypertension defined as a rise in IOP of greater than 7 mm Hg was noted between 3 and 6 hours after laser capsulotomy in 19% of patients. Elevation of IOP positively correlated with both an increase in aqueous particles and flare.

Silverstone and coworkers [11••] prospectively studied the effect of apraclonidine hydrochloride,

1%, in controlling elevations in IOP after laser capsulotomy. A double-blind clinical trial was used, which demonstrated an incidence of raised IOP (defined as greater than 5 mm Hg) of 7% in the apraclonidine-treated group and 39% in the placebo-treated group. In addition, the mean maximal IOP rise in the apraclonidine-treated group was actually a 1.3 mm Hg decrease, whereas for the placebo-treated group it was a 5.3 mm Hg increase. Although apraclonidine is not always used routinely for laser capsulotomy, its clinical effectiveness can make it beneficial when treating patients with glaucoma who require capsulotomy.

CONCLUSIONS

The Nd:YAG laser capsulotomy is one of the most successful and commonly performed procedures in ophthalmology despite the potential risks associated with its use. Although controversy may exist regarding the exact increase in risks, such as elevated IOP or retinal complications, no one would argue that the procedure should only be performed when the patient's visual symptoms are significant enough to warrant the intervention.

In addition to treating opacification of the posterior capsule successfully, the Nd:YAG laser can also be used to treat a number of other problems that the anterior-segment surgeon may encounter, including postoperative constriction of the anterior capsule, pigment deposition on the IOL optic, vitreous strands incarcerated in the incision, and persistent pupillary membranes.

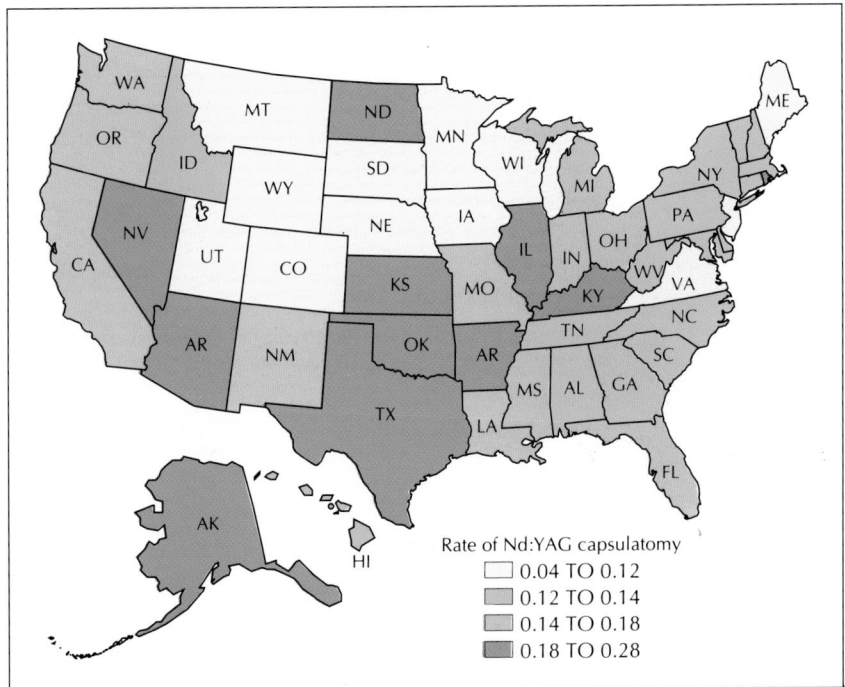

FIGURE 1-9 This map demonstrates the tremendous variability between states in the likelihood of posterior capsulotomy being performed after cataract extraction per person-year of observation. (*From* Javitt *et al.* [6]; with permission.)

Rate of Nd:YAG capsulatomy
☐ 0.04 TO 0.12
☐ 0.12 TO 0.14
☐ 0.14 TO 0.18
☐ 0.18 TO 0.28

REFERENCES AND RECOMMENDED READING

Recently published papers of particular interest have been highlighted as:
• Of interest
•• Of outstanding interest

1.• Strong N: Interferometer assessment of potential visual acuity before YAG capsulotomy: relative performance of three instruments. *Graefes Arch Clin Exp Ophthalmol* 1992, 230:42–46.

Reviews the different instruments used to evaluate potential visual acuity before performing Nd:YAG capsulotomy.

2. Sunderraj P, Villada JR, Joyce PW, *et al.*: Glare testing in pseudophakes with posterior capsule opacification. *Eye* 1992, 6:411–413.

3.• Hurvitz LM: YAG anterior capsulotomy and lysis of posterior synechiae after cataract surgery. *Ophthalmic Surg* 1992, 23:103–107.

Describes a series of patients who developed progressive constriction of the anterior capsulorhexis, which resulted in decreased vision. The methods in which the Nd:YAG laser was used to enlarge the openings are described.

4.• Aron-Rosa DS, Aron JJ: Effect of preoperative YAG laser anterior capsulotomy on the incidence of posterior capsule opacification: ten year follow-up. *J Cataract Refract Surg* 1992, 18:559–561.

A fascinating study wherein the authors demonstrate that patients who had a capsulorhexis performed preoperatively with an Nd:YAG laser in one eye and by surgery in the other eye had a significantly low incidence of posterior capsular opacification in the eye that had the laser capsulotomy performed.

5. Ramakrishnan R, Natchiar G, Michon J, *et al.*: Bilateral extensive persistent pupillary membranes treated with the neodymium-YAG laser. *Arch Ophthalmol* 1993, 111:28.

6.•• Javitt JC, Tielsch JM, Canner JK, *et al.*: National outcomes of cataract extraction: increased risk of retinal complications associated with Nd:YAG laser capsulotomy: the cataract patient outcomes research team. *Ophthalmology* 1992, 99:1487–1497.

This study uses the Medicare database to evaluate retinal complications following Nd:YAG capsulotomy. Most major newspapers cited the study and published headlines such as "Common laser procedure can damage the retina." As a result of this media coverage, most ophthalmologists can recall at least one patient who called concerned regarding possible complications of the laser use. The strength of the study is that by using the Medicare database a large patient base was analyzed (more than 53,000); however, this is also the weakness in that individual charts were not examined.

7.•• Steinert RF, Puliafito CA, Kumar SR, *et al.*: Cystoid macular edema, retinal detachment, and glaucoma after Nd:YAG laser posterior capsulotomy. *Am J Ophthalmol* 1991, 112:373–380.

An excellent review of some of the more common complications following Nd:YAG capsulotomy. Individual patient charts are reviewed, and although the number of patients evaluated is not nearly as large as in the series by Javitt and coworkers [6], this study is helpful in analyzing some aspects of Nd:YAG complications that are lost when examining only the Medicare database.

8.• Van Westenbrugge JA, Gimbel HV, Souchek J, *et al.*: Incidence of retinal detachment following Nd:YAG capsulotomy after cataract surgery. *J Cataract Refract Surg* 1992, 18:352–355.

This series evaluates the incidence of retinal detachment following Nd:YAG capsulotomy in patients who have had phacoemulsification and continuous tear capsulotomy performed. It raises the question as to whether these techniques might predispose to a lower incidence of retinal complications.

9. Hoffer KJ: Risk of retinal detachment after YAG capsulotomy [Letter]. *Ophthalmology* 1993, 100:582–583.

10.•• Altamirano D, Mermoud A, Pittet N, *et al.*: Aqueous humor analysis after Nd:YAG laser capsulotomy with the laser flare-cell meter. *J Cataract Refract Surg* 1992, 18:554–558.

A rise in IOP after Nd:YAG capsulotomy is mirrored by a rise in anterior chamber inflammation as measured by the laser flare-cell meter. The authors hypothesize that this inflammation alters trabecular meshwork filtration and leads to the pressure rises.

11.•• Silverstone DE, Brint SF, Olander KW, *et al.*: Prophylactic use of apraclonidine for intraocular pressure increase after Nd:YAG capsulotomies. *Am J Ophthalmol* 1992, 113:401–405.

A large prospective double-blind multicenter study that demonstrates that efficacy of apraclonidine in controlling the IOP rise that occurs after Nd:YAG capsulotomy.

SELECT BIBLIOGRAPHY

March E: *Ophthalmic Lasers: A Second Generation.* Thorofare, NJ: Slack Inc.; 1990

Ophthalmic procedures assessment: Nd:YAG photodisruptors. *Ophthalmology* 1993, 100(suppl 11):1736–1740.

Trokel S: *YAG Laser Ophthalmic Microsurgery.* Norwalk, CT: Appelton Century Crofts; 1983.

Weingart T, Sneed: *Laser Surgery in Ophthalmology: Practical Applications.* Norwalk, CT: Appleton and Lange; 1992.

CHAPTER 2

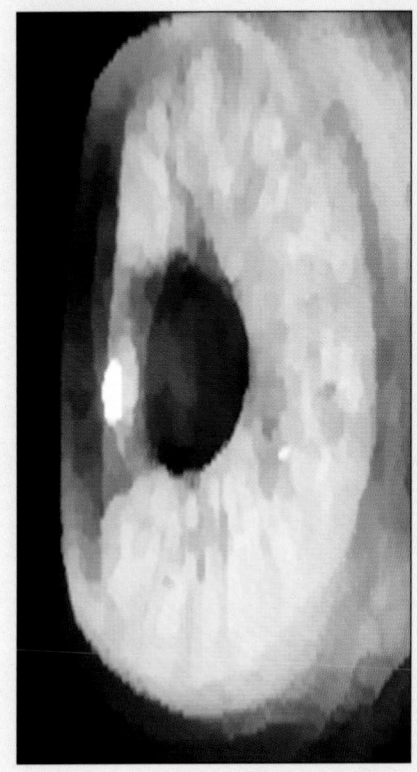

LASERS IN CORNEAL SURGERY

CHRISTOPHER J. RAPUANO
PETER R. LAIBSON

As the 1980s were frequently called the decade of vitreoretinal surgery in ophthalmologic circles, the 1990s are often dubbed the decade of the cornea. The major advances in corneal surgery continue to involve refractive lasers—primarily the excimer laser. Curiously, medical and lay press interest in the excimer laser has been a factor in the resurgence of older forms of keratorefractive surgery, especially radial and astigmatic keratotomy. Along with newer and better refractive surgical techniques and instrumentation have come significantly improved methods with which to evaluate corneal curvature. Computerized corneal topography not only enhances the surgeon's ability to better select candidates for keratorefractive procedures, but greatly improves his or her capability to evaluate the effects of numerous types of surgery on corneal curvature. New techniques using the excimer laser, along with novel ways to evaluate the effects of surgery will also lead to ongoing improvements in this area of refractive surgery. In addition, advances in the treatment of pathologic corneal conditions with the excimer and other lasers continue to be made.

EXCIMER LASER

New developments

VISX, Inc. (Sunnyvale, CA), which merged with Taunton Technologies (Monroe, CT) in 1991, and Summit Technology (Waltham, MA) are the only two excimer laser delivery system companies currently involved with United States Food and Drug Administration (FDA) trials (beyond Phase I, which deals with safety). As of this writing, the FDA has not yet approved the excimer laser for photorefractive keratectomy (PRK) or phototherapeutic keratectomy (PTK).

Although only relatively few patients continue to be treated as part of the FDA trials in the United States, far more patients are being treated in other countries. As more and more patients are treated, improvements in hardware, software, and laser techniques continue to be made. For example, originally, VISX excimer lasers used a nitrogen gas flow across the surface of the cornea during photoablation. This gas flow was used to remove the plume of ablated material from over the cornea so as not to interfere with subsequent laser pulses. It was later discovered that eyes that were subjected to PRK with nitrogen gas flow had, on average, more subepithelial haze and poorer refractive results than did eyes in which the surgery was performed without nitrogen gas flow. Campos and coworkers [1•] performed PRK on rabbit corneas with and without nitrogen gas flow. They found both longer times to reepithelialization and greater amounts of corneal haze in the nitrogen-flow group. Consequently, investigators using VISX machines were instructed to eliminate completely or to reduce significantly the nitrogen gas flow over the cornea during photoablation.

Another change in the past year involves the mode of movement of the iris diaphragm, which regulates the diameter of the excimer laser ablation zone. The VISX company started off using a contracting iris diaphragm, meaning that the diaphragm started out open to the selected ablation zone (eg, 6.0 mm) and then closed in a slow stepwise fashion during the ablation. Summit Technology uses an expanding iris diaphragm. Sinbawy and coworkers [2] performed photoablations on human eye bank eyes and pig eyes, using both contracting and expanding iris diaphragms, and compared the corneas histopathologically. They found that the use of an expanding iris diaphragm resulted in a pseudomembrane with fewer discontinuities compared with a contracting diaphragm. The authors concluded that the use of an expanding iris diaphragm might be preferable as it may result in a more uniform surface. The VISX company then changed its machines from contracting to expanding iris diaphragms. Expanding iris diaphragms were also found to be somewhat more "patient friendly." Smaller ablation zones create much softer "popping" sounds than do larger ablation zones, and it is much easier on the patient for the treatment to start off with fainter ablation "pops" and slowly build up to louder "pops" than vice versa. A later study from the same institution did not demonstrate any significant clinical difference in epithelial healing or degree of anterior stromal haze between contracting and expanding iris diaphragms in rabbits [3]. Even so, VISX still uses an expanding iris diaphragm.

A recent change in excimer laser ablation technique has been in the fixation of the globe during photoablation. Some of the early work used peribulbar anesthesia and fixation of the globe by the surgeon [4]. Later, topical anesthesia was used but globe fixation was still performed by the surgeon with the use of fixation forceps or a suction fixation ring [5,6•]. More recently, many investigators have decided that topical anesthesia and patient self-fixation on a coaxial target is the best method to use for ocular fixation. It has been found that patients can accurately fixate on a target for the duration of the photoablation, which may last several minutes; therefore, self-fixation may be more accurate than fixation provided by the surgeon. In addition, suction fixation rings have been shown experimentally to change ocular dynamics. Pico and coworkers [7] applied limbal-scleral suction fixation rings to rabbit eyes and found significantly elevated intraocular pressures, significant induced corneal flattening and astigmatism, and a 14% increase in corneal thickness. Although rabbit and human eyes are different, this study suggests that suction fixation rings may unknowingly change the structure and curvature of the cornea just before photoablation is performed. These potential corneal changes are another reason for patient self-fixation.

Differences also exist in the technique of epithelial removal. Photorefractive and most phototherapeutic applications of the excimer laser depend on ablation of Bowman's membrane and anterior stroma. To reach these layers the epithelium needs to be removed, and this can be performed with the excimer laser or by mechanical débridement. Advantages to removing the epithelium with the laser include its ease of use, speed, and no mechanical damage to the cornea. An important disadvantage is that the thickness of the patient's epithelial layer is unknown. For example, if the surgeon predicts the epithelium to be 50 μm deep and the photorefractive treatment requires a 50-μm Bowman's and stromal ablation centrally, then the laser is set for a 100-μm depth ablation centrally. However, if the epithelium is really only 30 μm thick, then 70 μm of stroma is ablated centrally, resulting in a potential overcorrection. Conversely, an undercorrection might result if the epithelial layer really measures 70 μm. With mechanical epithelial débridement, this unknown is eliminated. Mechanical débridement is more time consuming, however, and may create irregularities in Bowman's membrane. Surgeons who perform mechanical epithelial débridement use either a sharp or a dull instrument. Campos and coworkers [8] compared these two methods of mechanical epithelial débridement histopathologically using human eye bank eyes. They found a slightly rougher surface with occasional linear scratches in the eyes débrided by the sharp instrument, but more residual epithelial cells and basement membrane in the eyes debrided by the dull instrument. Overall, it is unclear which of these three methods of epithelial débridement is superior and all three continue to be used.

Postoperative treatment has also been an area of controversy and change in the past few years. Because of the large epithelial defect and damage to the highly sensitive corneal nerves, pain after excimer laser photokeratectomy can be severe. Standard postoperative regimens at many centers as recently as 1992 included the use of topical antibiotics, cycloplegics, and pressure patching until the epithelial defect was healed. Most patients endured a moderate to severe amount of pain for 24 to 48 hours, which usually resolved by 72 to 96 hours postoperatively. More recently, postoperative regimens have changed to the use of topical antibiotics, nonsteroidal anti-inflammatory agents (*eg*, diclofenac or ketorolac), possibly a cycloplegic agent, and a bandage soft contact lens. Although a few patients still have significant degrees of pain, on average the pain is markedly less than with the pressure-patching regimen. Sur-

geons should be cautioned to use the nonsteroidal anti-inflammatory drops only as frequently as directed (typically, every 6 hours) and to monitor patients using bandage soft contact lenses very closely. The bandage soft contact lens is typically removed on postoperative day 1, 2, or 3. Rarely is the lens required for longer periods, in which case it should be replaced frequently.

Either immediately postoperatively or as soon as the epithelial defect is healed, topical steroids have been used by most investigators in attempts to reduce corneal inflammation and subsequent corneal haze, scarring, and refractive regression. Gartry and coworkers [9••] performed a prospective, double-blind, randomized trial comparing dexamethasone (0.1%, five times a day, tapered over 3 months) with placebo in 113 patients after PRK. They found significantly more refractive effect in the steroid-treated group at 6 weeks, but not at 3 months. They did not find a statistically significant effect of steroids on anterior stromal haze at any stage. Because of the minimal apparent effect of steroids after PRK and their potential side effects, the authors suggested that these agents not be used after PRK.

Because the use of excimer laser technology on humans is essentially limited to the FDA protocols in the United States, and the fact that these protocols are difficult to alter midstream, most US investigators continue to use postoperative steroids. Other investigators around the world heeded the advice of Gartry and coworkers [9••]. Tengroth and coworkers [10•] were one such group of investigators who subsequently reported two retrospective studies comparing the use of postoperative steroids (dexamethasone, 0.1%, five times a day, tapered over 3 months) and no steroids after PRK. They found significantly better refractive results at 3 months in the steroid-treated group and did not comment on corneal haze. The authors concluded that steroids are "active and necessary during the healing phase" after PRK. The postoperative steroid controversy goes on.

Surgical techniques

Photorefractive keratectomy and PTK techniques differ from surgeon to surgeon and are still evolving. Given that preface, the following are descriptions of standard PRK and PTK procedures at our institution. PRK procedures, whether for "normal" myopes or unusual or postoperative refractive errors, are relatively straightforward. After careful centering, calibration, and testing of the laser delivery system, the patient is placed in the operating chair. Proparacaine drops are given bilaterally and the uninvolved eye is patched. The patient is positioned under the operating microscope with a Vac-Pac head rest (Olympic Medical, Seattle, WA) to stabilize the head. Care is taken to make certain the eye is well centered under the microscope and the head is level. Additional tetracaine and an eyelid speculum are placed in the eye undergoing to the procedure. A 6.0- or 7.0-mm circular optical zone marker is centered over the pupil and the epithelium is marked using a relatively low light source. A specially prepared 6.0-mm diameter circular disc of filter paper is soaked in lidocaine, 4%, and placed within the epithelial mark for 90 seconds. The epithelium is then mechanically débrided with either blunt or sharp instrumentation. Special care is necessary to assure that Bowman's membrane appears smooth and without residual epithelium before photoablation is performed. Occasionally, additional tetracaine or Tears Naturale II (Alcon Ophthalmics, Fort Worth, TX) are placed on the cornea and smoothed with a surgical spear (Merocel Corporation, Mystic, CT), but, typically, fluid is not needed after epithelial removal.

The computer had been previously programmed with the patient's ablation parameters and rechecked by the surgeon. The patient is told to stare at the fixation target and the ablation is performed centered on the pupil. In higher myopes, multiple ablation zones may be used to decrease the depth of the ablation centrally. Once the ablation has been completed, cyclopentolate, 1%; tobramycin; and diclofenac or ketorolac drops are placed in the eye along with a low-power disposable soft contact lens. Oral narcotics (eg, acetaminophen with codeine) are also given. Patients are followed every 24 to 48 hours, with the antibiotic and nonsteroidal anti-inflammatory drop administered every 6 hours until the epithelial defect is healed, which typically requires 3 to 5 days. The contact lens is usually removed or replaced on postoperative day 2.

Although pain is common, severe pain is rare with this regimen. Once the epithelial defect is healed, the antibiotic therapy is stopped, the nonsteroidal anti-inflammatory drop is tapered over several days, and fluorometholone, 0.1%, is started four times a day,

and tapered over 4 months. Very good to excellent vision is typically achieved between 2 and 6 weeks postoperatively, but it may take up to several months. Anterior stromal corneal haze is typically first noted within 4 to 6 weeks, peaks by 3 to 6 months, and then slowly fades (Fig. 2-1).

Assuming the laser delivery system is programmed correctly and is working as expected, the two most important aspects of PRK are epithelial removal and ablation centration. Centration of keratorefractive procedures has been a topic of controversy for many years. Most surgeons are now centering keratorefractive procedures on the center of the entrance pupil when the patient and surgeon are fixating coaxially as has been described and well discussed in an article by Uozato and Guyton [11]. Another issue is whether to constrict the pupil artificially before selecting its center. Fay and coworkers [12•] discovered significant movement (up to 0.5 mm) of the center of the pupil when it was constricted pharmacologically as opposed to its being in its natural state. It may be best to determine the center of the pupil under relatively normal light conditions before increasing illumination or adding constricting drops.

Ease and accuracy of determining the success of centration of PRK have improved dramatically in the past year or two. New software for computerized corneal video topography systems can now determine the edges and center of the pupil in relation to the ablation zone. Consequently, the centers of the pupil and ablation zone can be accurately compared. Several studies have evaluated the centration of PRK procedures [13,14•,15,16]. Most investigators have found centration to be good, but not perfect, in most patients. Cavanaugh and coworkers [13] found that mean uncorrected Snellen visual acuity was 20/20 for decentrations of up to 1.0 mm, but fell to 20/30 for deviations of greater than 1.0 mm. They also found a

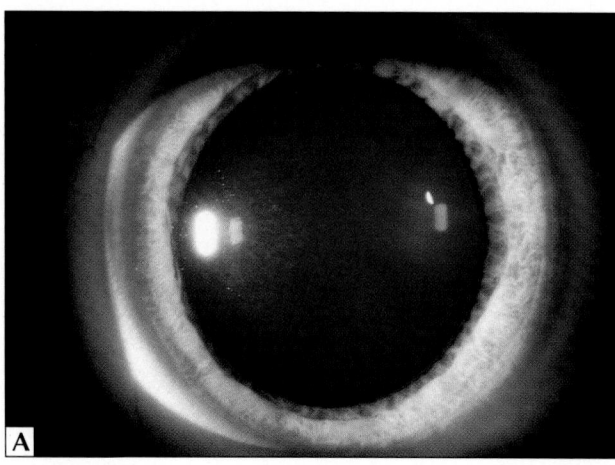

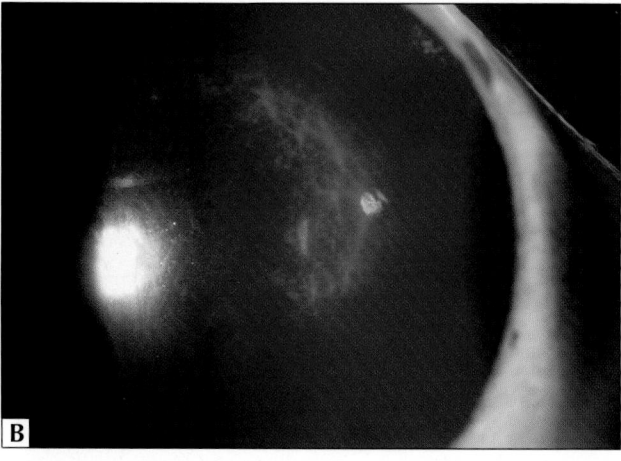

FIGURE 2-1 Corneal haze after excimer laser photorefractive keratectomy (PRK). **A**, Faint circular anterior stromal haze 1 month after PRK. **B**, Sectorial reticular haze 9 months after PRK in another patient.

decline in best corrected visual acuity with decentrations of more than 1.0 mm. Because centration is so important and the actual location of laser ablation is difficult to determine intraoperatively, we check the centration of the laser ablation before every patient undergoes the procedure.

The PTK procedure for corneal abnormalities can be very different from PRK. In fact, PTK procedures vary greatly depending on the particular cornea being treated [17•,18]. In general, the objective of PTK is to remove or reduce anterior corneal opacity, smooth the anterior corneal surface, or both. The use of PTK to treat recurrent erosions, which works very well, and to treat corneal infections, which works less well, are separate issues. When a cornea is smooth but has an anterior corneal opacity, such as a scar or dystrophy, then the epithelial surface is not removed mechanically, but is instead ablated with the excimer laser. The epithelium, in effect, acts as a smoothing agent over a potentially irregular stromal surface. The ablation is continued until the stromal abnormality is adequately removed. To determine the effect of treatment during the laser session, the patient is evaluated at a slit lamp many times during the procedure. Typically, a plano ablation is performed (as deep peripherally as centrally); however, if the patient has myopia or astigmatism, a refractive ablation can also be used.

When the corneal surface is irregular, the technique used depends on the type of irregularity. Epithelium is removed from well-defined elevated areas of pathologic tissue and a small-diameter ablation spot is used to "chip away" at these elevated areas. A masking fluid, as previously mentioned, can be used to protect surrounding tissue. Kornmehl and coworkers [19] found that corneas ablated with Tears Naturale II as the masking agent had fewer surface irregularities than did corneas ablated with other masking agents. If the surrounding tissue is clear and smooth, then only the elevated area needs to be treated (Fig. 2-2).

However, if there are numerous areas of irregular tissue, or if the irregular areas are not discrete enough to treat individually, then the epithelium over the affected areas should be removed mechanically. The entire area of pathologic tissue can then be treated by

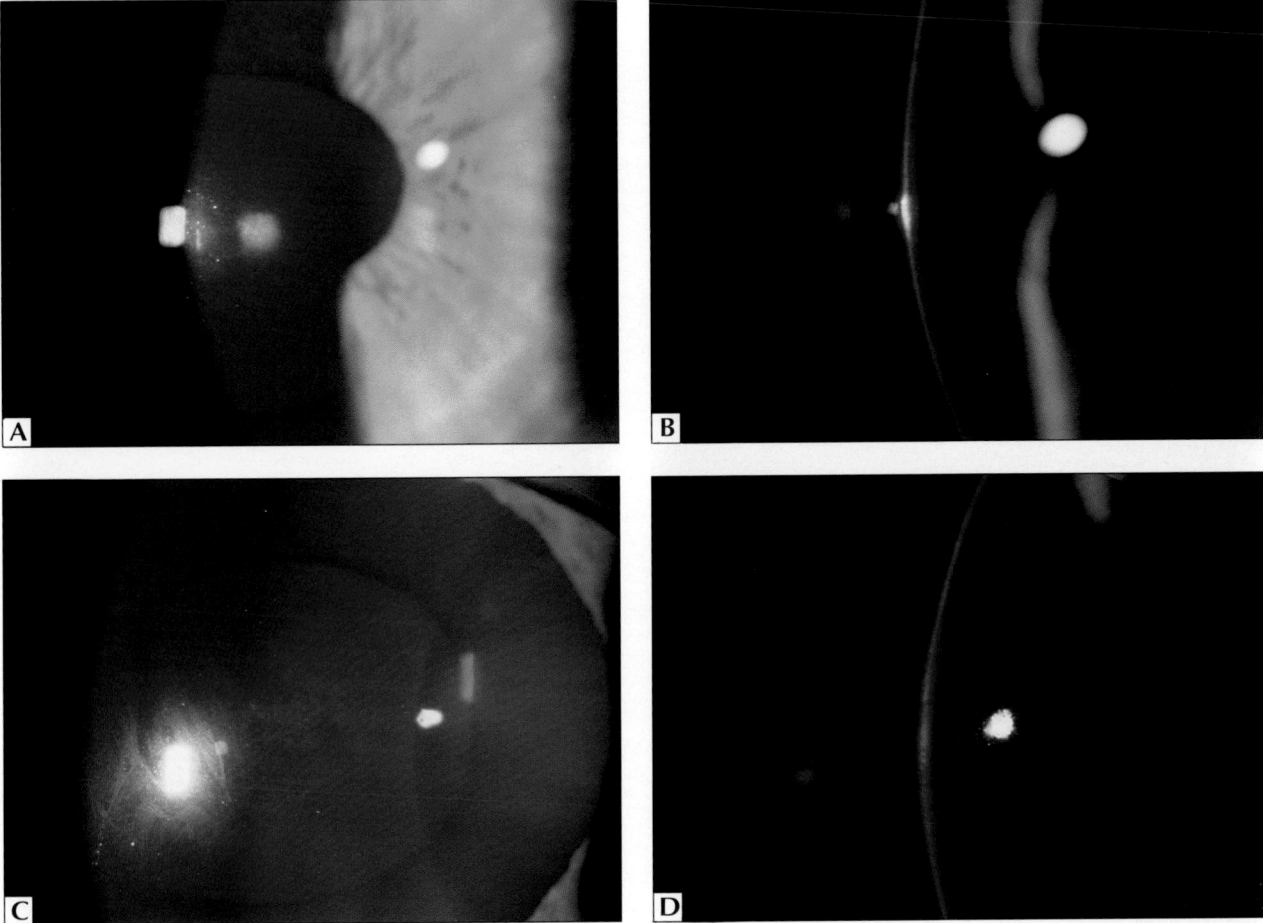

FIGURE 2-2 Elevated corneal nodule in a patient with keratoconus inhibiting contact lens wear. **A** and **B**, Preoperative excimer laser phototherapeutic keratectomy (PTK). **C** and **D**, One month after PTK. Note elimination of the opacity, which has left a smooth surface with minimal underlying scarring and no damage to adjacent tissue.

using a masking agent to protect areas of depression (Fig. 2-3). The goal is a smooth clear surface (Fig. 2-4).

Recurrent erosions can be treated with the excimer laser when surgical intervention is necessary. We still prefer to use an anterior stromal puncture for areas of abnormality outside the visual axis. However, for anterior stromal puncture failures and for areas involving the visual axis, excimer laser PTK can work very well. We débride the epithelium mechanically in the involved area. Five to 10 µm of tissue are ablated, which should reach into Bowman's membrane but not stroma. This treatment tends to cause minimal to no anterior stromal haze nor refractive effect, and we have noted no recurrences of erosions in the treated areas.

The greatest problem with PTK is induced refractive effect, especially hyperopia, but astigmatism in asymmetric ablations also occurs. Theoretically, PTK smooths elevated areas to the level of the rest of the cornea, removes a plano disc of tissue, or both. Ideally, neither of these procedures should change refractive error. However, PTK, especially removal of central corneal stromal abnormalities, tends to flatten the central cornea and induce hyperopia. The deeper the ablation, the more extensive the corneal flattening.

There are several theories regarding this hyperopic shift. Subsequent epithelial hyperplasia may be greater at the peripheral edge of the ablation, where there is a significant drop-off, and less prominent centrally, creating a flatter central cornea (Fig. 2-5) [20•]. Liu [20•] also suggested that masking agents may creep up the wall of deeper central ablations while the laser is firing, thus causing a deeper ablation centrally and subsequent corneal flattening. Because of the curvature of the cornea there may be less effective ablation peripherally because the excimer laser beam is interacting with the cornea at an oblique angle in the periphery and not perpendicular to the cornea as it is centrally. This nonperpendicular peripheral ablation will not be as deep toward the center of the eye as the perpendicular central ablation (Fig. 2-6) [21••]. Gartry and coworkers [22,23] also proposed that corneal lamellae could undergo centrifugal differential contraction with central flattening. In any case, this potential untoward side effect needs to be understood and addressed before PTK becomes a good reliable alternative to mechanical

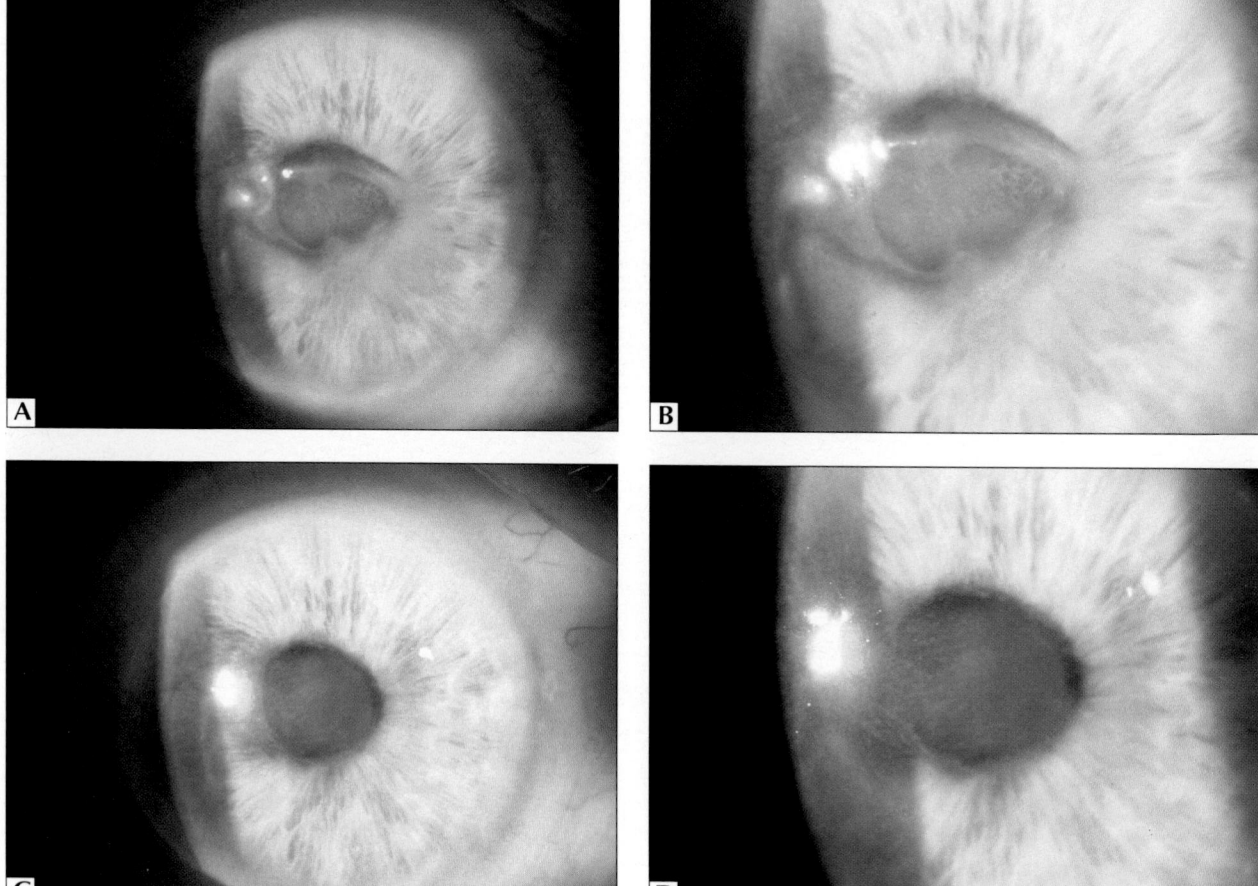

FIGURE 2-3 Large central irregular corneal scar from a chemical injury 40 years previously. **A** and **B**, Preoperative excimer laser phototherapeutic keratectomy (PTK), low and high magnification. **C** and **D**, One month after PTK, low and high magnification. The central cornea is significantly clearer and smoother, and the corneal light reflex is much more regular.

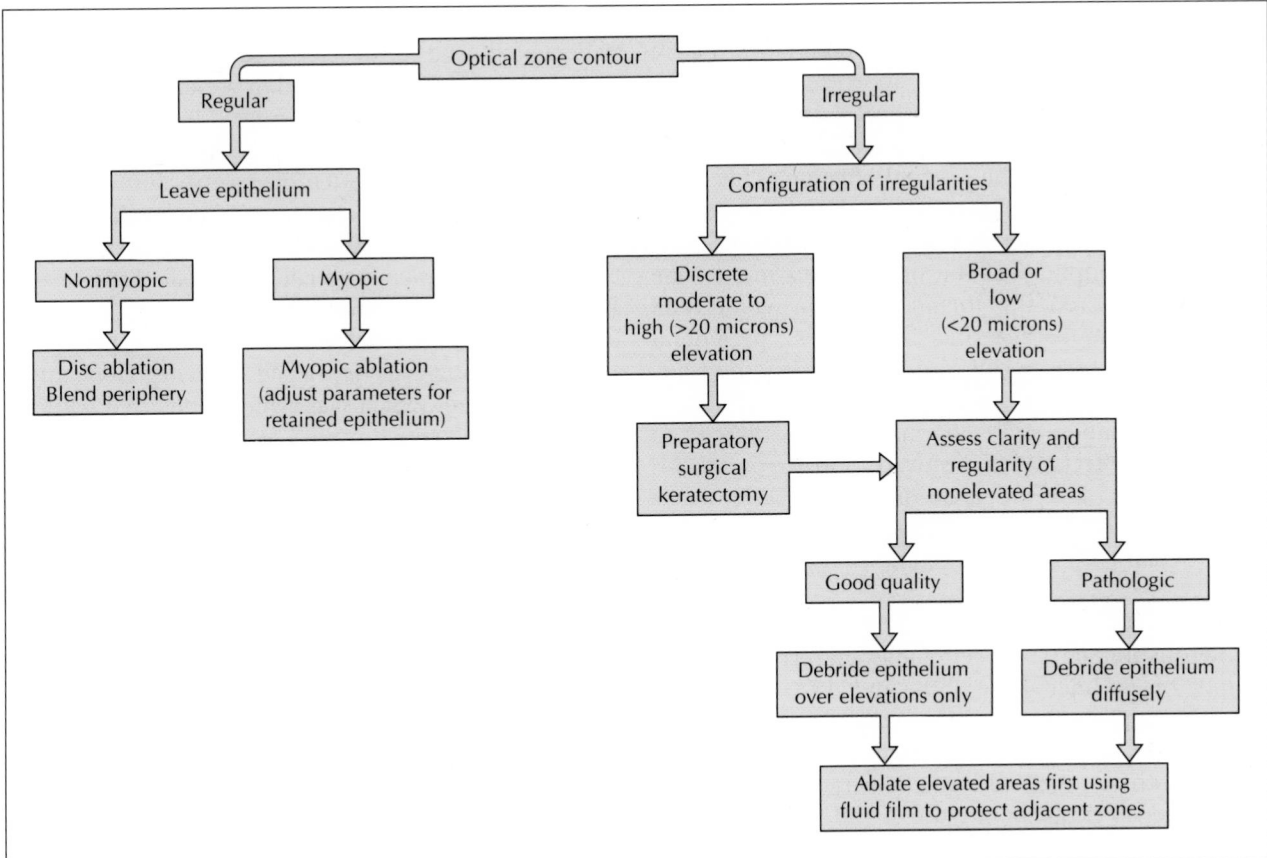

FIGURE 2-4 Treatment strategy for excimer laser phototherapeutic keratectomy of superficial corneal opacities and irregularities. (*From* Talamo *et al.* [17•]; with permission.)

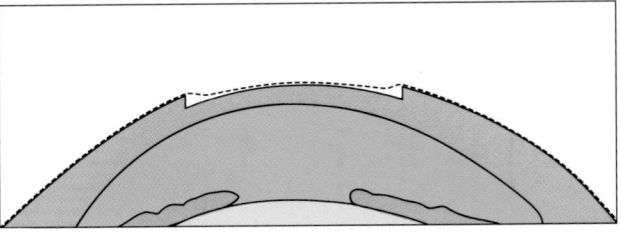

FIGURE 2-5 Epithelial hyperplasia may occur in the periphery of an excimer phototherapeutic keratectomy, which will result in central corneal flattening and induced hyperopia.

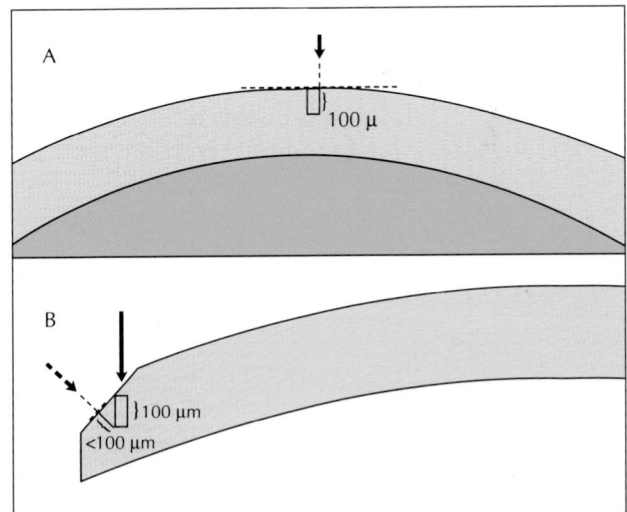

FIGURE 2-6 **A**, Central perpendicular excimer laser photoablations penetrate deeper into the corneal stroma. **B**, Peripheral excimer laser photoablations remove tissue at an oblique angle, resulting in a shallower ablation. Deeper central and more shallow peripheral ablations tend to cause corneal flattening and induced hyperopia.

lamellar keratectomy. To combat this induced corneal flattening, Stark and coworkers [21••] performed a modified taper in an attempt to correct hyperopia. After the central ablation of corneal pathologic tissue, they used a 2.0-mm-diameter circular ablation to treat the circumference of the original ablation. This additional ablation straddled the original treatment to taper the edge of unablated tissue and create a deeper ablation in the periphery of the original treatment zone (Fig. 2-7). Theoretically, this modification would tend to steepen the cornea and induce less peripheral epithelial hyperplasia. Unfortunately, there is no standard manner in which to perform this additional peripheral ablation and, consequently, it is difficult to evaluate its effect. When software and hardware for the correction of hyperopia become more widely available, this type of peripheral ablation should become easier to standardize, perform, and evaluate.

Clinical results

Numerous studies have been published recently on the results of excimer laser PRK and PTK. Sher and coworkers [24] reported the results of PRK with Taunton Technologies machines on 31 eyes followed for 6 months. Attempted corrections ranged from -4 to -12 diopters. Peribulbar anesthesia and 5.2-to 6.0-mm-diameter ablation zones were used. The authors found that 68% of eyes were corrected to within 2 diopters and 55% to within 1 diopter of attempted correction. Salz and coworkers [6] reported the 1-year data from 12 eyes of 12 patients after -1.75 to -5.0 diopter PRK using a VISX unit. Topical anesthesia and a 5.0-mm-diameter ablation zone were used. Eleven of 12 eyes achieved 20/30 uncorrected Snellen visual acuity and were within 0.50 diopters of attempted correction. One eye was moderately undercorrected with 20/70 uncorrected Snellen acuity.

Gartry and coworkers [25•] reviewed the results of PRK using a Summit Technology machine for -2 to -7

diopters of attempted correction in 120 eyes of 120 patients followed for at least 1 year. Topical anesthesia and a 4.0-mm-diameter ablation zone were used. The authors reported that 95% of eyes undergoing -2 diopter and 70% of eyes undergoing -3 diopter corrections were within 1.0 diopter of attempted correction. However, only 40% of eyes undergoing -6 diopter and 20% of eyes undergoing -7 diopter corrections were within 1.0 diopter of attempted correction. Overall, 11% of eyes lost one or two lines of best corrected Snellen visual acuity. Refractions were stable by 3 to 6 months postoperatively. Almost all eyes developed some degree of anterior stromal haze, which was typically detected within 1 month, was maximal around 5 to 6 months, and then gradually faded. Although most patients noted a halo effect, only 10% considered it enough of a problem to prevent treatment of the other eye.

Tengroth and coworkers [26•], using a Summit Technology unit, reported the results of PRK on 420 eyes with a minimum of 1 year of follow-up. Attempted corrections ranged from -1.25 to -7.50 diopters. Topical anesthesia and ablation zones of 4.3 to 4.5 mm were used. At 1 year postoperatively, 86% of eyes were within 1.0 diopter of attempted correction and 91% had uncorrected Snellen visual acuity of 20/40 or better (Fig. 2-8). The authors found, as did Gartry and coworkers [25•], significantly better results for lower degrees than higher degrees of myopia.

Overall, PRK results are good to excellent and appear to be improving with modifications in technol-

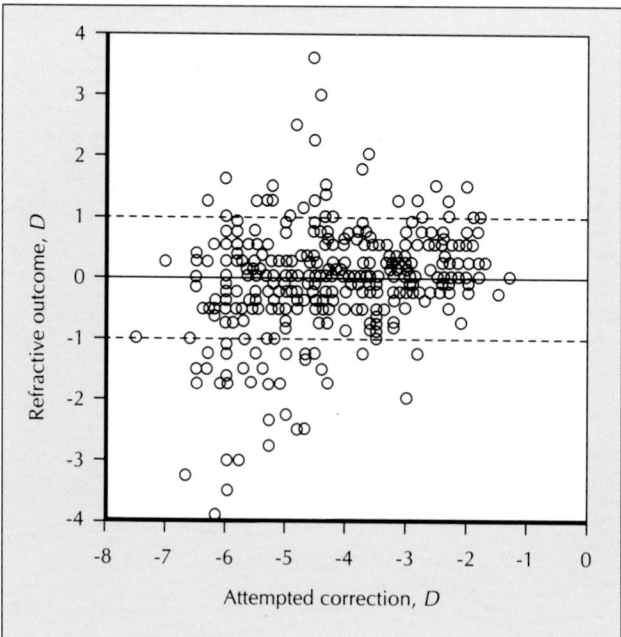

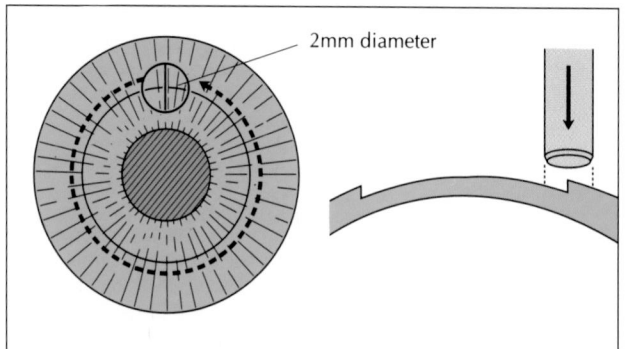

FIGURE 2-7 Modified peripheral excimer laser taper after phototherapeutic keratectomy (PTK). After the central PTK ablation, a 2.0-mm-diameter circular ablation is used to treat the circumference of the original ablation in an attempt to correct hyperopia.

FIGURE 2-8 Scattergram demonstrating refraction (spherical equivalent) 12 months after excimer laser photorefractive keratectomy in 420 eyes; 86% of the eyes were within 1.0 diopter of attempted correction. (*From* Tengroth *et al.* [26•]; with permission.)

ogy and technique. Kahle and coworkers [27] investigated the satisfaction of 26 patients 1 year after PRK for up to -6 diopters of myopia. Twenty patients had their other eye treated at least 3 months after the first eye was treated. The other six patients did not undergo second eye treatment because of preoperative anisometropia. The authors found extremely high satisfaction with PRK, and all patients would decide again to undergo PRK for myopia.

Two studies have recently reported the results of excimer laser PRK in higher degrees of myopia. Sher and coworkers [28•] described the results of surgery in 16 eyes with between -8.62 and -14.50 diopters of myopia with a follow-up of at least 6 months, performed at three centers using Taunton Technologies units. Eyes were treated with 5.5-, 5.6-, or 6.0-mm-diameter single ablation zones. All eight patients treated at one center with a 6.0-mm ablation zone achieved refractions within 2 diopters of attempted correction. Five of the eight eyes treated with smaller ablation zones at the other two centers were undercorrected by more than 2 diopters. Overall, 11 of 16 eyes achieved refractions within 2 diopters of attempted correction. Best corrected Snellen visual acuity in all but two patients returned to within one line of preoperative visual acuity by 6 months; one patient lost two, and another patient lost four lines.

Ehlers and Hjortdal [29] reported results of PRK in 22 eyes of 13 patients with attempted corrections of -5 to -8 diopters and in 18 eyes of 11 patients with attempted corrections of -9 to -12 diopters. They used an Aesculap-Meditec (Heroldsberg, Germany) excimer laser, a 5.0-mm-diameter single ablation zone and followed patients for at least 6 months. Although all eyes achieved improved uncorrected vision, best corrected Snellen visual acuity decreased significantly in six eyes. In the -5 to -8 diopter group, 90% of the eyes achieved within 2.5 diopters of attempted correction, whereas only 50% of the eyes in the -9 to -12 diopter group achieved the same results. One eye was overcorrected by 3 diopters. They found no difference in endothelial cell counts in the 12 patients tested before and 6 months after PRK for these high degrees of myopia.

Excimer laser PRK has also been used to treat severe postkeratoplasty astigmatism. Campos and coworkers [30] used a VISX laser to treat 12 eyes with between 2.25 and 12 diopters of attempted cylinder correction. The mean preoperative refractive cylinder was 7.0 diopters, which decreased to 3.1 diopters at 1 month and 4.3 diopters at last follow-up between 6 and 14 months postoperatively. Full astigmatism correction was not attempted in every patient, however. The mean spherical equivalent decreased from -7.4 to -3.3 diopters. The authors concluded that excimer laser PRK for postkeratoplasty astigmatism was safe, although there was often substantial regression. At our

institution we have also found significant undercorrection in the treatment of astigmatism after corneal transplantation.

Dausch and coworkers [31•] used an Aesculap-Meditec unit to treat 23 eyes with hyperopia. Fifteen eyes had between +2.0 and +7.5 diopters of hyperopia and eight eyes were aphakic, with between +11.0 and +16.0 diopters of hyperopia. All patients were followed for 1 year. A specialized eye mask with a spiral aperture was placed in a suction fixation ring and rotated to create an ablation peripherally but not centrally to induce central steepening (Fig. 2-9). The authors reported that 12 of the 15 eyes in the less hyperopic group were corrected to within 1 diopter of intended correction. Only three of the eight aphakic eyes achieved the same result. In addition, the refractions were more stable in the less hyperopic group. They concluded that PRK can work well for lower amounts of hyperopia, but not for aphakia, possibly because a slight amount of decentration in aphakic eyes can lead to a very poor refractive result.

Radial keratotomy undercorrections have also been treated with excimer laser PRK. Seiler and Jean [32] described the results of PRK in five eyes of four patients at least 15 months after radial keratotomy. A Summit Technology unit with a 5.0-mm-diameter ablation zone was used and patients were followed for 6 to 12 months. Pre-PRK spherical equivalent refractions ranged from -1.25 to -2.75 diopters. The most recent refractions on all of these patients were within 1 diopter of emmetropia and all patients had uncorrected Snellen visual acuities of 20/30 or better. Frangie and coworkers [33] reported similar PRK results in six eyes of five patients 5 to 77 months after radial keratotomy using a VISX unit and 5.0- and 5.5-mm ablation

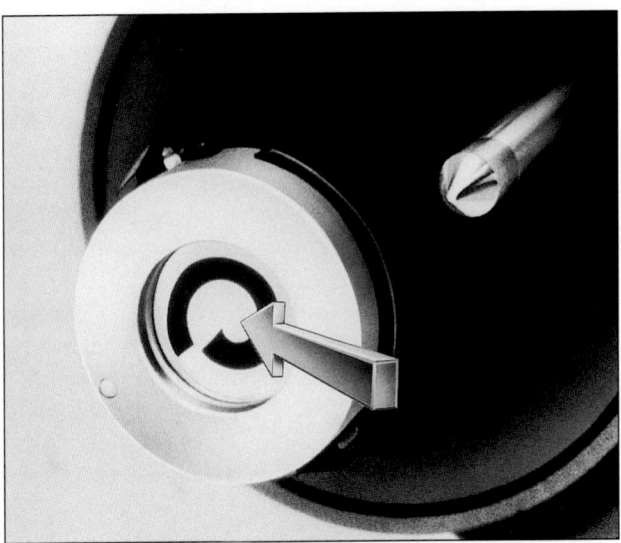

FIGURE 2-9 Specialized eye mask with a spiral aperture for the correction of hyperopia with the excimer laser. (*From* Dausch *et al.* [31•]; with permission.)

zones. The mean spherical equivalent decreased from -2.40 to -0.48 diopters, with uncorrected Snellen visual acuities ranging from 20/20 to 20/80 1 to 12 months postoperatively.

Although it is usually not necessary, PRK can be repeated. Seiler and coworkers [34•] performed repeat PRK on 30 eyes of 30 patients at least 6 months after the first PRK, using a Summit Technology system. Indications for re-treatment were corneal scarring and undercorrection. Patients were followed for at least 6 months after the second PRK. Only 1 eye demonstrated scar formation after the second treatment. Nineteen of 30 patients (63%) achieved a refraction within 1 diopter of attempted correction. The authors concluded that repeat PRK can be highly successful when required.

Phototherapeutic keratectomy results for the treatment of corneal opacities have been very promising. Stark and coworkers [21••] reported results with a VISX unit in 27 eyes followed for 3 to 24 months after PTK. Preoperative diagnoses included primary and recurrent lattice and granular dystrophies, corneal scars, and other dystrophies and degenerations. The authors reported functional improvement in vision in 21 of 27 (78%) eyes. As previously discussed, induced hyperopia can be a problem after PTK. Stark and coworkers [21••] found a high correlation between the depth of ablation and the amount of induced hyperopia. Although the numbers were too small to detect a significant difference, they did find a trend in reducing the amount of induced hyperopia by using the modified peripheral taper described earlier.

Campos and coworkers [35•] reported PTK results with a VISX laser used to treat 18 eyes with corneal scars, dystrophies, and calcific degeneration in patients who were followed for 3 to 18 months. They found improved corneal clarity in 14 of 18 eyes. The three patients with calcific degeneration and one patient with a dense postinfection scar did not improve. Best corrected vision improved in 11 patients, remained stable in five patients (including the four previously mentioned failures), and worsened in two patients, most likely from irregular astigmatism. A hyperopic shift, occasionally as high as 10 to 20 diopters, was noted in 10 of 18 patients.

We have reported our results of PTK with a VISX system in 10 patients with corneal opacities and in one patient with recurrent erosions who had 2 weeks to 7 months of follow-up [36•]. We were careful not to ablate more than was absolutely necessary in order to minimize induced hyperopia. Some patients received a modified peripheral taper to achieve the same effect. We found visual improvement of at least two Snellen lines in six of the 10 patients with corneal opacities (one patient's vision did not improve after PTK because of a dense cataract, but subsequently improved after cataract

surgery). Keratometric corneal flattening and induced refractive hyperopia were much less pronounced than in previous reports, but more follow-up is necessary to determine long-term results. The vision of the one patient with recurrent erosion remained 20/20 and he has not had any recurrent erosions in the 18 months since the laser surgery.

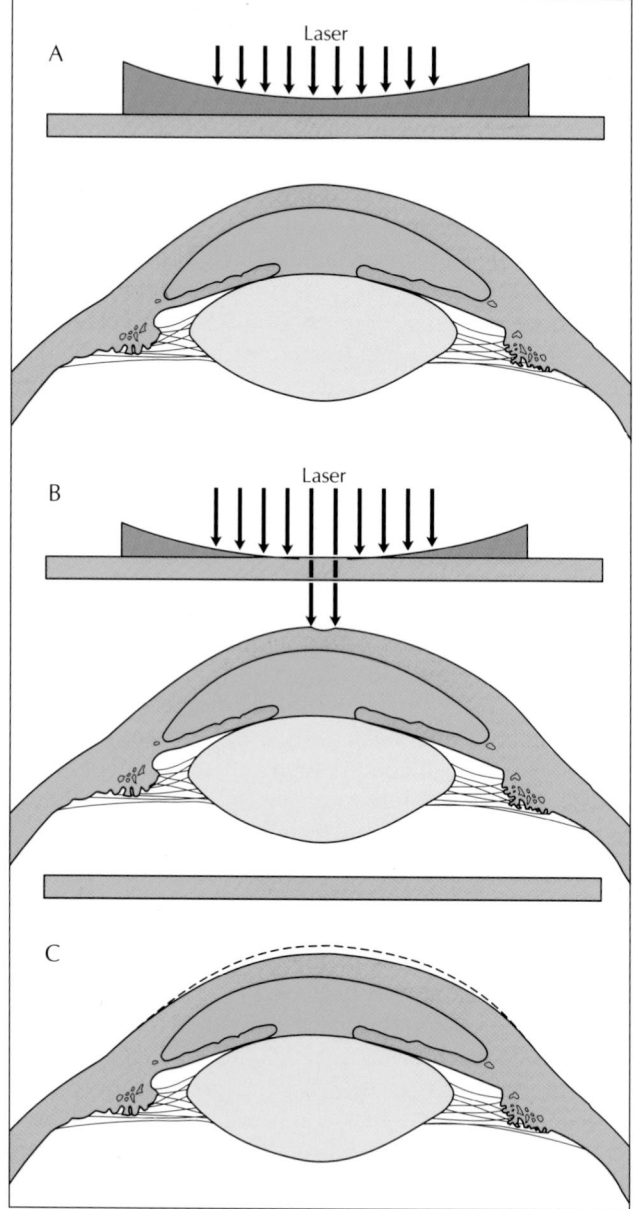

FIGURE 2-10 Erodible mask delivery system. **A,** A mask made of erodible material is placed between the excimer laser and the eye. **B,** The laser ablates through the thinnest part of the mask first, and begins removing corneal tissue. The shape of the mask governs the correction achieved. Illustrated is a mask designed for myopic correction; the laser ablates through the center of the mask first, so more tissue is removed from the central cornea than the peripheral cornea, resulting in corneal flattening. **C,** Intuitively, the shape of the mask is transferred onto the corneal surface. (*From Maloney et al.* [40••]; *with permission.*)

One indication for excimer laser PTK is corneal scarring from herpes simplex virus (HSV) keratitis. Vrabec and coworkers [37] reported recurrent HSV keratitis in two patients 3 months after PTK. It is unclear whether the excimer laser treatment precipitated these recurrences or whether it was the natural course of the disease. Pepose and coworkers [38] reported that excimer laser photoablation may induce reactivation of latent HSV type 1 in a mouse model. Prophylactic antiviral agents may therefore be beneficial after excimer laser photokeratectomy in patients with HSV. HSV scar density, treatment depth, and ablation rates vary greatly. It is probably best to be conservative with treatment depth in patients with HSV because the scar may ablate more quickly than expected.

Future developments

Two disadvantages to the use of PRK are the large epithelial defect, with its accompanying pain, and the destruction of Bowman's membrane. Buratto and coworkers [39•] reported their findings in 30 eyes of 22 patients with severe myopia who underwent keratomileusis combined with excimer laser photokeratectomy and were followed for 6 months. This procedure involved using a microkeratome to shave off a cap of the anterior cornea, including epithelium and Bowman's membrane. A Summit Technology excimer laser was then used to ablate either the underside of the excised cap (28 of 30 eyes) or the corneal bed (two of 30 eyes, when the cap thickness was less than 250 μm). A running suture was used to secure the cap back on the cornea. Mean preoperative myopia decreased from -17.9 to -2.1 diopters. No significant induced regular astigmatism and minimal intrastromal corneal haze were found. Best corrected Snellen visual acuity worsened in three (10%) eyes because of irregular astigmatism. The authors concluded that excimer laser photokeratectomy can be very useful in conjunction with keratomileusis, and may offer better results than standard PRK in the correction of moderate and severe myopia.

The current method by which more tissue is ablated centrally than peripherally in PRK procedures for myopia is through the movement of an iris diaphragm. Such diaphragms move in discrete steps, resulting in a stepped ablation on the corneal surface. By increasing the number of steps, a smooth ablation can be approximated. Currently, iris diaphragms are unable to produce hyperopic corrections. Maloney and coworkers [40••] developed an erodible mask delivery system for the excimer laser that can theoretically be used to correct hyperopia, astigmatism, and myopia. A mask was created and placed between the laser beam and the cornea. The laser beam ablated the mask first and then the cornea. In this fashion, the shape of the mask was transferred to the corneal surface. For example, thinner areas of the mask will be completely ablated first, allowing the laser beam to reach the cornea earlier in those areas and consequently resulting in deeper ablations in those areas as well (Fig. 2-10).

Maloney and coworkers also reported their results using erodible masks to correct myopia and hyperopia in rabbit eyes. They found their technique worked well for myopic corrections of -2.5 diopters but resulted in undercorrections when -5 diopter ablations were attempted. They also reported paradoxical myopic corrections using the hyperopic masks. Corneas ablated with the masks appeared clearer with smoother beds than did corneas ablated with iris diaphragms. Although still in the developmental stages, this technique has the potential to improve results and expand indications for excimer laser PRK.

Another interesting technique is the use of a collagen gel mold applied to the cornea to act as a refractive template or a smoothing agent. Englanoff and coworkers [41••] placed a bovine type 1 collagen suspension on pig eyes. As the suspension polymerized into a gel a rigid contact lens was placed on the gel to mold it to a specific curvature. Similarly, collagen gel was placed on irregular corneal surfaces to fill in depressions and a rigid contact lens was used to smooth the surface. The contact lens is then removed. After ablation with the excimer laser, the corneal curvature was altered according to the base curve of the rigid contact lens used (Fig. 2-11). The authors found the ablation rate of

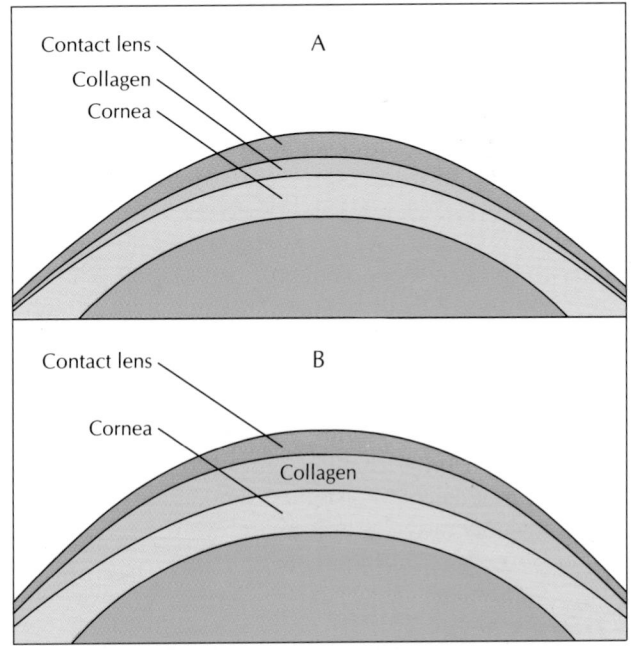

FIGURE 2-11 The relationship between the cornea, collagen gel, a flat (35-diopter) rigid contact lens (*panel A*), and a steep (52-diopter) contact lens (*panel B*). Steeper contact lenses are associated with greater central thickness of collagen. (*From* Englanoff *et al.* [41••]; with permission.)

the gel to be the same as for the cornea, so when the gel was applied to an irregular corneal surface, shaped with a rigid contact lens, and ablated, a smooth surface resulted. This type of gel not only has the potential of the erodible mask to correct myopia, hyperopia, and astigmatism, but also the ability to correct irregular astigmatism and corneal surface abnormalities.

Occasionally, corneas after PRK have an unintentional multifocal effect with good uncorrected distance and near vision. Moreira and coworkers [42] attempted to create a multifocal effect with the excimer laser on plastic spheres, blocks, and rabbit corneas. They found they could intentionally produce a multifocal effect, but it was unclear how much the image might be degraded. Although this procedure may become a useful technique in the future, it might be technically very difficult to perfect because accurate centration is thought to be even more critical to maintain than in routine PRK.

Other future developments include improved evaluation of the effects of excimer and other laser surgeries. Seiler and coworkers [43] described the use of the Scheimpflug camera to measure both corneal curvature and corneal haze objectively. Lohmann and coworkers [44] developed a digital video system for the objective measurement of corneal light scattering and found it to be more sensitive and reproducible than subjective or lensometer methods. Allemann and coworkers [45] used a high-frequency ultrasound unit (requiring waterbath immersion) to evaluate corneal clarity after PRK in rabbits. They found this technique to be a good noninvasive method of quantifying corneal scarring. It was also used to calculate light backscatter ratios, which appear to correlate with visual performance.

Another exciting innovation in the area of corneal evaluation is the PAR Corneal Topography System (PAR Microsystems Corporation, New Hartford, NY) [46••]. This system uses close-range raster photogrammetry to create a topographic corneal map (Fig. 2-12). An important advantage over current video keratoscopy is that the PAR system does not require an excellent light reflex. In fact, it can be used on deepithelialized tissue. The system can also be integrated into laser delivery systems and can theoretically be used during a photoablation procedure. With such a system it may become possible to modify a PRK treatment intraoperatively based on evaluation of the corneal curvature during the laser surgery.

OTHER LASERS

Although not as glamorous, perhaps, nonexcimer lasers are also used to treat corneal abnormalities. Baer and Foster [47•] used a 577-nm yellow dye laser to treat corneal neovascularization in 25 eyes of 23 patients. Patients were classified in four groups:

1) those who had active graft rejection, 2) those who had precorneal transplants, 3) those who had lipid keratopathy with opacity or edema threatening the visual axis, and 4) those with extensive corneal neovascularization who were not candidates for corneal grafts. Patients underwent between one and five laser sessions with between 60 and 7881 total laser spots. Patients in groups 1 and 3 enjoyed a statistically significant reduction in the area of corneal neovascularization. The areas of neovascularization decreased in size in four of five patients in group 2, but overall the decrease was not statistically significant. Patients in group 4 responded poorly. Nirankari and coworkers [48•] used a 577-nm yellow dye laser to treat rabbits with experimentally induced corneal neovascularization. They found this laser surgery to be effective at reducing corneal stromal vascularization in their rabbit model for at least 6 months without damaging deeper stroma or endothelium.

Goto [49] used a Q-switched neodymium-yttrium aluminum garnet laser to treat nine eyes of nine patients with corneal neovascularization from HSV keratitis. He found a significant reduction in the amount of corneal neovascularization and corneal opacity in eight of nine patients, with between 3 and 36 months of follow-up (mean, 17 months). Two of the patients had failures of previous argon laser treatments to the areas of neovascularization. Specular microscopic evaluation of the five transparent corneas before and after laser treatment revealed no significant change to the corneal endothelium. Corneal stromal neovascularization is often associated with decreased vision and also with corneal graft rejection and failure. Such laser

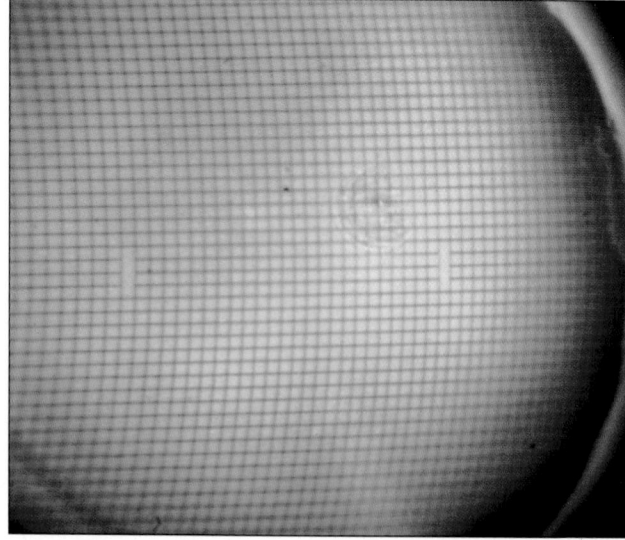

FIGURE 2-12 Close-range raster photogram showing a grid pattern projected onto a fluorescein-stained cornea. The two vertically oriented rectangles are used in centering the grid. A small photoablation is shown slightly below and central to the left aiming rectangle. (*From* Belin [46••]; with permission.)

treatments may be very beneficial in preventing visual loss in patients with clear central corneas and corneal transplants or even in improving vision when the central cornea is already affected.

CONCLUSIONS

As we reach into the middle of the "decade of the cornea," laser corneal surgery is fastly coming into its own. Rapid improvements in excimer laser hardware, software, and techniques continue to occur, and new and different treatment and evaluation modalities are around every corner. In practically every month's ophthalmology journals an intriguing new development is reported in the ever-growing field of laser corneal surgery. The next few years are certain to be just as exciting as the last several have been as we build on our knowledge and experience.

REFERENCES AND RECOMMENDED READING

1.• Campos M, Cuevas K, Garbus J, *et al.*: Corneal wound healing after excimer laser ablation: effects of nitrogen gas blower. *Ophthalmology* 1992, 99:893–897.

The authors found longer time to reepithelialization and more corneal haze in rabbit corneas treated with nitrogen gas flow over the cornea during PRK than without.

2. Sinbawy A, McDonnell PJ, Moreira H: Surface ultrastructure after excimer laser ablation. Expanding vs contracting apertures. *Arch Ophthalmol* 1991, 109:1531–1533.

3. Campos M, Cuevas K, Shieh E, *et al.*: Corneal wound healing after excimer laser ablation in rabbits: expanding versus contracting apertures. *Refract Corneal Surg* 1992, 8:378–381.

4. Zabel RW, Sher NA, Ostrov CS, *et al.*: Myopic excimer laser keratectomy: a preliminary report. *Refract Corneal Surg* 1990, 6:329–334.

5. McDonald MB, Frantz JM, Klyce SD, *et al.*: Central photorefractive keratectomy for myopia: the blind eye study. *Arch Ophthalmol* 1990, 108:799–808.

6.• Salz JJ, Maguen E, Macy JI, *et al.*: One-year results of excimer laser photorefractive keratectomy for myopia. *Refract Corneal Surg* 1992, 8:269–273.

Eleven of 12 eyes with between -1.75 and -5.0 diopters of myopia achieved 20/30 or better uncorrected visual acuity and were within 0.5 diopters of attempted correction at 1 year. One patient was moderately undercorrected, with 20/70 visual acuity.

7. Pico JF, Stamper RL, McMenemy M: Intraocular pressure and corneal curvature changes on application of limbal-scleral suction fixation ring in rabbits. *Cornea* 1993, 12:25–28.

8. Campos M, Hertzog L, Wang XW, *et al.*: Corneal surface after deepithelialization using a sharp and a dull instrument. *Ophthalmic Surg* 1992, 23:618–621.

9.•• Gartry DS, Kerr Muir MG, Lohmann CP, *et al.*: The effect of topical corticosteroids on refractive outcome and corneal haze after photorefractive keratectomy: a prospective, randomized, double-blind trial. *Arch Ophthalmol* 1992, 110:944–952.

Findings from a study of 113 patients who were randomly assigned to receive either dexamethasone, 0.1%, tapered over 3 months, or placebo after PRK. They found significantly greater refractive change at 6 weeks in the steroid-treated group, but this difference disappeared by 3 months. They did not find a statistically significant difference in corneal haze at any stage in the study. This study prompted many centers to stop using steroids after PRK.

10.• Tengroth B, Fagerholm P, Soderberg P, *et al.*: Effect of corticosteroids in postoperative care following photorefractive keratectomies. *Refract Corneal Surg* 1993, 9(suppl):S61–S64.

A retrospective study that concluded the use of steroids did significantly affect refractive results 3 months after PRK.

11. Uozato H, Guyton DL: Centering corneal surgical procedures. *Am J Ophthalmol* 1987, 103:264–275.

12.• Fay AM, Trokel SL, Myers JA: Pupil diameter and the principal ray. *J Cataract Refract Surg* 1992, 18:348–351.

A small but interesting study demonstrating that pharmacologic constriction of the pupil can significantly affect its center.

13. Cavanaugh TB, Durrie DS, Riedel SM, *et al.*: Topographical analysis of the centration of excimer laser photorefractive keratectomy. *J Cataract Refract Surg* 1993, 19:136–143.

14.• Cavanaugh TB, Durrie DS, Riedel SM, *et al.*: Centration of excimer laser photorefractive keratectomy relative to the pupil. *J Cataract Refract Surg* 1993, 19:144–148.

New corneal topography software allowed the authors to compare the center of the ablated zone (which was aimed at the center of the pupil) and the center of the pupil to assess the accuracy of the aiming technique. Good, but not perfect, centration was found.

15. Klyce SD, Smolek MK: Corneal topography of excimer laser photorefractive keratectomy. *J Cataract Refract Surg* 1993, 19:122–130.

16. Lin DTC, Sutton HF, Berman M: Corneal topography following excimer laser photorefractive keratectomy for myopia. *J Cataract Refract Surg* 1993, 19:149–154.

17.• Talamo JH, Steinert RF, Puliafito CA: Clinical strategies for excimer laser therapeutic keratectomy. *Refract Corneal Surg* 1992, 8:319–324.

The authors discuss different techniques for treating a variety of anterior corneal abnormalities. They include clinical examples and a flow chart describing their treatment guidelines.

18. Hersh PS, Spinak A, Garrana, *et al.*: Phototherapeutic keratectomy: strategies and results in 12 eyes. *Refract Corneal Surg* 1993, 9(suppl):S90–S95.

19. Kornmehl EW, Steinert RF, Puliafito CA: A comparative study of masking fluids for excimer laser phototherapeutic keratectomy. *Arch Ophthalmol* 1991, 109:860–863.

20.• Liu C: Hyperopic shift and the use of masking agents in excimer laser superficial keratectomy [Letter]. *Br J Ophthalmol* 1992, 76:62–63.

A very interesting letter describing several possible causes of the disturbing hyperopic shift often noted after PTK.

21.•• Stark WJ, Chamon W, Kamp MT, *et al.*: Clinical follow-up of 193-nm ArF excimer laser photokeratectomy. *Ophthalmology* 1992, 99:805–812.

The authors report findings on 27 eyes with anterior corneal abnormalities (group 1) and four eyes with refractive errors after penetrating keratoplasty (group 2) followed for 3 to 24 months after PTK. Visual function improved in 21 of 27 eyes in group 1 and in two of four eyes in group 2. The authors noted a significant hyperopic shift in many patients and discuss possible causes. They also describe a peripheral ablation taper that attempts to avoid the occurrence of induced hyperopia.

22.   Gartry D, Kerr Muir M, Marshall J: Excimer laser treatment of corneal surface pathology: a laboratory and clinical study. *Br J Ophthalmol* 1991, 75:258–269.

23.   Gartry D, Kerr Muir M, Marshall J: Hyperopic shift and the use of masking agents in excimer laser superficial keratectomy [Letter]. *Br J Ophthalmol* 1992, 76:63.

24.   Sher NA, Chen V, Bowers RA, *et al.*: The use of the 193-nm excimer laser for myopic photorefractive keratectomy in sighted eyes: a multicenter study. *Arch Ophthalmol* 1991, 109:1525–1530.

25.• Gartry DS, Kerr Muir MG, Marshall J: Excimer laser photorefractive keratectomy: 18-month follow-up. *Ophthalmology* 1992, 99:1209–1219.

Fair overall refractive results in 120 patients followed for 12 to 22 months. Results were very good in the -2.0 to -3.0 diopter correction range but poor in the -6.0 to -7.0 diopter range.

26.• Tengroth B, Epstein D, Fagerholm P, *et al.*: Excimer laser photorefractive keratectomy for myopia: clinical results in sighted eyes. *Ophthalmology* 1993, 100:739–745.

Very good refractive results in 420 eyes that had between -1.25 and -7.50 diopters of myopia and were followed for 12 to 15 months. Eyes with up to -4.9 diopters of myopia achieved significantly better results than did eyes with -5.0 to -7.5 diopters of myopia.

27.   Kahle G, Seiler T, Wollensak J: Report on psychosocial findings and satisfaction among patients 1 year after excimer laser photorefractive keratectomy. *Refract Corneal Surg* 1992, 8:286–289.

28.• Sher NA, Barak M, Daya S, *et al.*: Excimer laser photorefractive keratectomy in high myopia: a multicenter study. *Arch Ophthalmol* 1992, 110:935–943.

The authors describe reasonably good results in this study of single-ablation-zone high myopia. The results when using a 6.0-mm-diameter ablation zone at one center were better than those in the 5.5- or 5.6-mm-diameter ablation zones at the other two centers.

29.   Ehlers N, Hjortdal JO: Excimer laser refractive keratectomy for high myopia: 6-month follow-up of patients treated bilaterally. *Acta Ophthalmol* 1992, 70:578–586.

30.   Campos M, Hertzog L, Garbus J, *et al.*: Photorefractive keratectomy for severe postkeratoplasty astigmatism. *Am J Ophthalmol* 1992, 114:429–436.

31.• Dausch D, Klein R, Schroder E: Excimer laser photorefractive keratectomy for hyperopia. *Refract Corneal Surg* 1993, 9:20–28.

The authors treated 15 patients with +2.0 to +7.5 diopters and eight aphakic patients with between +11.0 and +16.0 diopters of hyperopia and followed them for 1 year. They found good results for the lower hyperopia group, but poor results for the aphakic group.

32.   Seiler T, Jean B: Photorefractive keratectomy as a second attempt to correct myopia after radial keratotomy. *Refract Corneal Surg* 1992, 8:211–214.

33.   Frangie JP, Park SB, Kim J, *et al.*: Excimer laser keratectomy after radial keratotomy. *Am J Ophthalmol* 1993, 115:634–639.

34.• Seiler T, Derse M, Pham T: Repeated excimer laser treatment after photorefractive keratectomy. *Arch Ophthalmol* 1992, 110:1230–1233.

Good results after repeat PRK in 30 eyes with scarring, undercorrection, or both, followed for at least 6 months after the second PRK.

35.• Campos M, Nielsen S, Szerenyi K, *et al.*: Clinical follow-up of phototherapeutic keratectomy for treatment of corneal opacities. *Am J Ophthalmol* 1993, 115:433–440.

Corneal clarity improved in 14 of 18 eyes, but vision improved in only 11 of 18 and decreased in two eyes. The authors noted significant hyperopic shift in 10 of 18 eyes.

36.• Rapuano CJ, Laibson PR: Excimer laser phototherapeutic keratectomy. *CLAO J* 1993, 19:235–240.

The authors report good results in 11 patients with anterior corneal abnormalities and fair results in four patients with postoperative refractive error.

37.   Vrabec MP, Durrie DS, Chase DS: Recurrence of herpes simplex after excimer laser keratectomy [Letter]. *Am J Ophthalmol* 1992, 114:96–97.

38.   Pepose JS, Laycock KA, Kelvin Miller J, *et al.*: Reactivation of latent herpes simplex virus by excimer laser photokeratectomy. *Am J Ophthalmol* 1992, 114:45–50.

39.• Buratto L, Ferrari M, Rama P: Excimer laser intrastromal keratomileusis. *Am J Ophthalmol* 1992, 113:291–295.

The authors performed PRK on the corneal cap or the corneal bed after keratomileusis in 30 eyes of 22 patients with high myopia. The mean spherical equivalent decreased from -17.9 to -2.1 diopters at 6 months. Four eyes developed irregular astigmatism, one severe enough to require surgery.

40.•• Maloney RK, Friedman M, Harmon T, *et al.*: A prototype erodible mask delivery system for the excimer laser. *Ophthalmology* 1993, 100:542–549.

Currently, excimer laser photoablation is typically controlled by an iris diaphragm, which creates a stepped ablation on the cornea. The authors describe preliminary results using an erodible mask to treat myopia and hyperopia in rabbit eyes. Although the refractive results were only fair, this technique has potential to correct myopia, hyperopia, and astigmatism.

41.•• Englanoff JS, Kolahdouz-Isfahani AH, Moreira H, *et al.*: In situ collagen gel mold as an aid in excimer laser superficial keratectomy. *Ophthalmology* 1992, 99:1201–1208.

The authors describe a fascinating innovation that may be useful in treating routine refractive errors such as myopia, hyperopia, and astigmatism, but also irregular astigmatism and superficial corneal irregularities. The procedure involves placing a collagen suspension on the cornea over which a rigid contact lens of known base curve is placed. The suspension polymerizes into a gel that has the same excimer laser ablation rate as does corneal tissue, after which the contact lens is removed. When the authors ablated pig corneas using this technique, a smooth corneal surface resulted that had the shape of the rigid contact lens.

42. Moreira H, Garbus JJ, Fasano A, *et al.*: Multifocal corneal topographic changes with excimer laser photorefractive keratectomy. *Arch Ophthalmol* 1992, 110:994–999.

43. Seiler T, Hubscher H-T, Genth U: Corneal curvature change immediately after PRK as detected by Scheimpflug photography [Abstract]. *Association for Research in Vision and Ophthalmology* 1993, 34:703.

44. Lohmann CP, Timberlake GT, Fitzke FW, *et al.*: Corneal light scattering after excimer laser photorefractive keratectomy: the objective measurements of haze. *Refract Corneal Surg* 1992, 8:114–121.

45. Allemann N, Chamon W, Silverman RH, *et al.*: High-frequency ultrasound quantitative analyses of corneal scarring following excimer laser keratectomy. *Arch Ophthalmol* 1993, 111:968–973.

46.•• Belin MW: Intraoperative raster photogrammetry: the PAR Corneal Topography System. *J Cataract Refract Surg* 1993, 19:188–192.

The PAR system does not use Placido disc–reflected images to evaluate corneal curvature, but rather, raster photogrammetry, which does not require a smooth reflective surface. The system is able to evaluate a deepithelialized cornea. By incorporating this system into a laser delivery unit, in the future it may be possible to modify PRK intraoperatively depending on intraoperative corneal topography.

47.• Baer JC, Foster CS: Corneal laser photocoagulation for treatment of neovascularization: efficacy of 577 nm yellow dye laser. *Ophthalmology* 1992, 99:173–179.

The authors found significant reduction in corneal neovascularization after laser treatment in patients with active graft rejection and in patients with lipid or edema threatening the visual axis.

48.• Nirankari VS, Dandona L, Rodrigues MM: Laser photocoagulation of experimental corneal stromal vascularization: efficacy and histopathology. *Ophthalmology* 1993, 100:111–118.

The 577-nm yellow dye laser was found to reduce corneal stromal vascularization effectively in a rabbit model for at least 6 months without damaging deeper stroma or endothelium.

49. Goto S: Q-switched Nd:YAG laser treatment for corneal neovascularization. *Jpn J Ophthalmol* 1992, 36:291–300.

SELECT BIBLIOGRAPHY

Piebenga LW, Matta CS, Deitz MR, *et al.*: Excimer photorefractive keratectomy for myopia. *Ophthalmology* 1993, 100:1335–1345.

Rabinowitz YS: *Color atlas of corneal topography: interpretation of videokeratography*. New York: Igaku-Shoin; 1993.

Seiler T, Fantes FE, Waring GO III: Laser corneal surgery. In *Refractive keratotomy for myopia and astigmatism*. Edited by Waring GO III. Philadelphia: Mosby Yearbook:1992.

Thompson FB, McDonnell PJ: *Color atlas—test of excimer laser surgery: the cornea*. New York: Igaku-Shoin; 1993.

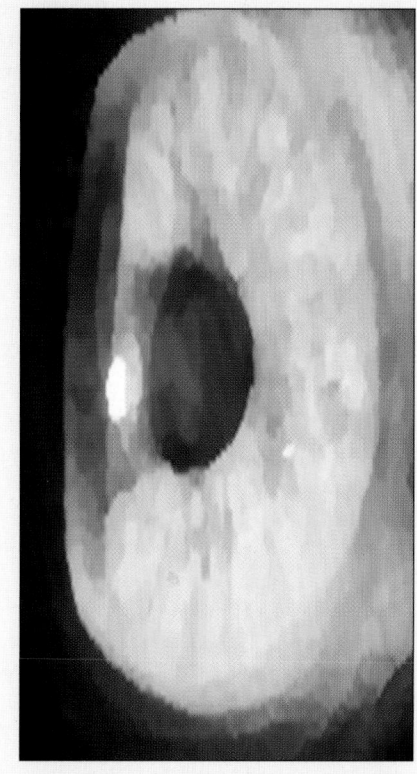

CHAPTER 3

LASERS IN OCULOPLASTIC SURGERY

PATRICK M. FLAHARTY

BHUPENDRA K. PATEL

RICHARD L. ANDERSON

New developments in laser technology and fiberoptic delivery systems have led to an expanded role for lasers in oculoplastic surgery. The potassium titanyl phosphate-yttrium aluminum garnet (KTP:YAG) and holmium-yttrium aluminum garnet (Ho:YAG) lasers continue to show promise in the field of lacrimal surgery. The argon laser has proved a viable alternative to cryotherapy in the treatment of focal trichiasis and the carbon dioxide laser has improved the management of orbital lymphangiomas. Controversy continues to surround the use of the carbon dioxide laser for routine blepharoplasty. New developments include the use of the pulsed dye laser in the treatment of port-wine stains and juvenile hemangiomas, the Q-switched ruby laser in the treatment of nevus of Ota, and the Q-switched neodymium-yttrium aluminum garnet (Nd:YAG) laser for removal of permanent eyeliner. Future advances in laser technology promise to expand the role of lasers in oculoplastic surgery.

The introduction of lasers to the field of oculoplastic surgery has resulted in the development of radical new treatment options for common oculoplastic problems. Surgeons now contemplate no-incision, endoscopic laser–assisted dacryocystorhinostomy (DCR) rather than the external approach to DCR surgery. They can perform selective ablation of individual eyelash follicles with the argon laser rather than administer cryotherapy to the entire eyelid. The new tunable pulsed dye laser (PDL) has shown promising results in the treatment of capillary hemangiomas, which may eliminate the need for local and systemic steroid therapy.

This chapter is an overview of the latest uses of lasers in oculoplastic surgery. Many of the procedures discussed are new techniques at different stages of development. As with all new treatment protocols, results must be duplicated and follow-up extended to verify the success of therapy. With time, the limitations of new procedures become more apparent and the therapeutic role for each more defined. In the field of laser surgery, the rapid pace of new developments renders many relatively new techniques obsolete in a matter of years. It is important to keep this in mind while reading this chapter.

LACRIMAL SURGERY

Conventional external DCR surgery with placement of a silicone stent has achieved a success rate of better than 90% in the treatment of uncomplicated nasolacrimal duct obstruction. In spite of the high success rate, this operation has intimidated both surgeons and patients because of the significant risk for intraoperative and postoperative bleeding, scar formation, and postoperative swelling and ecchymosis.

The initial excitement surrounding the use of lasers for internal DCR surgery has waned somewhat as certain technical limitations of the procedure have become more apparent. Difficulty in creating a large osteotomy has resulted in an unacceptable rate of failure for many surgeons, who have abandoned the procedure. Although the learning curve remains steep, the appeal of no incision, excellent hemostasis, and rapid rehabilitation continues to push the field forward.

Woog and coworkers [1•] describe a technique of endonasal laser–assisted DCR in 40 consecutive patients with the aid of the Ho:YAG laser. The surgical technique was a modification of those previously described by Massaro and coworkers [2] and Gonnering and coworkers [3]. Woog and coworkers used a transnasal approach with the aid of a 0-degree endoscope linked to a videomonitor to visualize the procedure (Fig. 3-1). A 20-gauge fiberoptic light probe was used through the canaliculus to illuminate the lacrimal sac. A 400-μm diameter quartz fiber secured to a suction handpiece was then introduced into the nose. With a laser setting of 0.5 J per pulse at a rate of five pulses per second, an area of nasal mucosa measuring approximately 1 cm in diameter was vaporized. Transillumination from the light pipe was used as a guide for treatment.

Once the mucosa was removed the power was increased to 1.0 J per pulse and the pulse rate to 10 per second to improve efficiency for bone removal. A portion of the anterior ethmoid air cells and lacrimal bone was then vaporized. The laser was then directed toward the thicker anterior lacrimal crest. The authors describe the use of a drill with a 3-mm cutting burr to remove charred tissue, which impedes the efficiency of the laser. This burr was also used to remove additional bone, thus enlarging the osteoto-

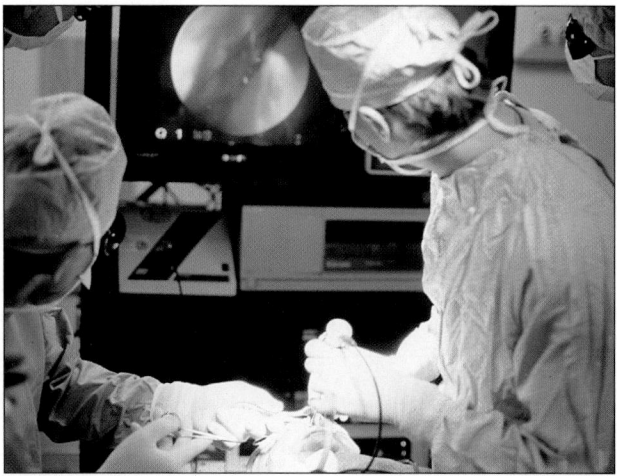

FIGURE 3-1 Surgeons visualize the intranasal anatomy on the video monitor during endoscopic laser–assisted internal dacryocystorhinostomy.

my site to 6 to 10 mm in diameter. The middle turbinate was ablated with the laser when it was located near the osteotomy site.

The medial wall of the lacrimal sac was opened with angled endoscopic forceps, or ablated with the Ho:YAG laser. The angled endoscopic forceps were used to take biopsy specimens from the lacrimal sac when necessary. This opening was expanded to 5 to 10 mm. A 30-degree endoscope was used to identify the lacrimal sac and the common internal punctum. Silicone tubes were passed through the upper and lower canaliculus and retrieved under endoscopic visualization from the middle meatus. During the later part of the study a catheter was used over the silicone stents to aid in maintaining patency of the internal ostium (Fig. 3-2). The silicone tubes and catheter were removed between 2 and 6 months postoperatively.

The authors achieved a success rate of 33 out of 40 (82%) based both on symptomatic improvement and patency of the ostium observed endoscopically. The follow-up period ranged from 6 to 91 weeks, with an average of 55 weeks. Interestingly, the authors noted no failures in the 18 patients who had catheters placed around the silicone tubes, although the follow-up period was not as long for this group. These 18 cases included the 15 cases in which the drill was used to enlarge the osteotomy site.

The authors attribute their success to several modifications from previously published techniques, including 1) use of the intranasal drill to remove char and bone, creating a larger osteotomy site; 2) removing a large amount of mucosa from the medial wall of the lacrimal sac and proximal nasolacrimal duct in an effort to visualize the common internal punctum; and 3) use of a double stent.

Levin and StormoGipson [4] used a transcanalicular approach on six cadavers to investigate the efficacy of the KTP:YAG laser in creating a lacrimal–nasal opening. A 400- to 600-μm blunt-tipped fiberoptic cord was fed through the canaliculus to the medial aspect of the lacrimal sac. Ten to 15 pulses of energy at 10 W and 0.1-second duration were required to create a 2.5 × 1.5–mm fistula. Additional energy was required to create ostia measuring 4 × 6 mm (Fig. 3-3).

The authors report several advantages of the transcanalicular approach when compared with the transnasal approach, including 1) the laser energy is directed toward the nose, reducing the risk for injury to the eye and orbit; 2) the instrumentation and tactile sensation are similar to lacrimal probing; 3) nasal endoscopy and instrumentation may not be required; and 4) conjunctivodacryocystorhinostomy (CDCR) can be performed in a similar fashion.

Silkiss and coworkers [5] reported similar findings with the use of the chromium-sensitized and thulium- and holmium-doped yttrium aluminum garnet laser to create bony ostia measuring 3 to 4 mm in diameter in four human cadavers. They used a 320-μm laser fiber and pulse energies of 250 to 900 mJ with a repetition rate of 5 to 15 pulses per second. Energy levels ranged from 1 to 10 W. The laser creates multiple small perforations in the bone (Fig. 3-4).

These later two reports show that a small osteotomy site can be created internally with the aid of a fiberoptic cord via a transcanalicular approach. The small perforations illustrated in Figure 3-4, however, demon-

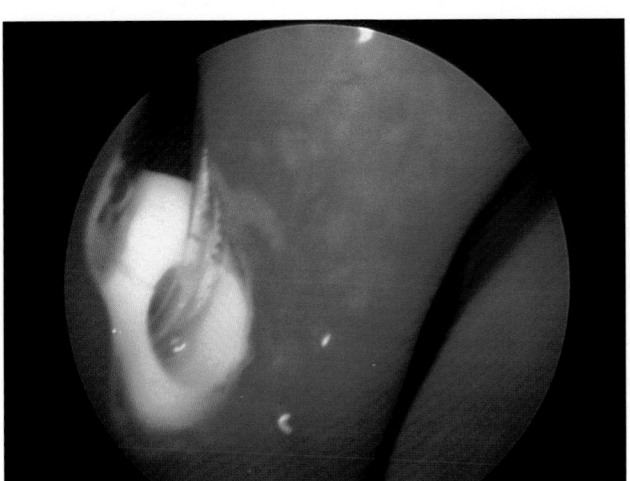

FIGURE 3-2 Endoscopic photograph shows silicone tubing emerging from the central opening of the C-flex catheter. (*From* Woog *et al.* [1•]; with permission.)

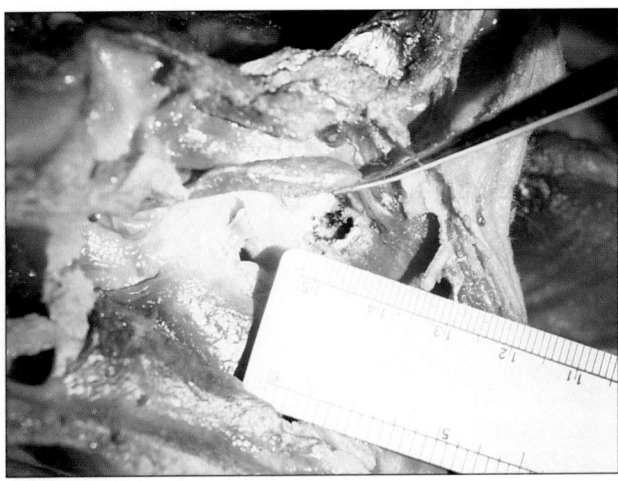

FIGURE 3-3 Middle turbinate is retracted superiorly to reveal the 4- to 6-mm ostium (*arrows*) produced with the potassium titanyl phosphate-yttrium aluminum garnet laser using the endocanalicular fiberoptic. Anterior (A), posterior (P), and superior (S) orientations of the specimen are indicated. (*From* Levin and StormoGipson [4]; with permission.)

strate an important limitation of this technique. In our experience in approximately 16 cases of primary internal laser-assisted DCRs via a transcanalicular approach we found it is relatively easy to create small perforations in the lacrimal bone but exceedingly difficult to create an osteotomy site large enough to ensure long-term patency (10 to 15 mm). Although silicone stents can be passed through small osteotomy sites of 2 to 3 mm, these small openings are unlikely to remain patent once the stents are removed. In our series we had a 50% failure rate after stent removal, with a follow-up of 1 year. For this reason we abandoned the use of primary, internal laser-assisted DCRs.

A second problem encountered with this transcanalicular approach concerns the location of the ethmoid air cells. Linberg [6] has demonstrated that the anterior ethmoid air cells extend past the posterior lacrimal crest in 93% of normal subjects and under the entire lacrimal sac fossa in 40% of normal subjects (Fig. 3-5).

In our early experience with the transcanalicular approach we would often penetrate the lacrimal bone but not visualize the laser tip in the nose, indicating the presence of intervening ethmoid air cells. The small perforations created by the fiberoptic laser tips are ineffective in removing the bulk of bone and mucosa in this area without the aid of additional instrumentation via a transnasal approach.

We agree with the aforementioned authors that the transcanalicular approach provides an added measure of safety by directing the laser energy away from the eye and orbit. This technique reduces the risk for thermal damage to the canaliculi and common internal punctum by directing the energy toward the nose. We use the transcanalicular approach for revision of failed

DCRs when we are confident adequate bone and anterior ethmoid air cells have been removed with the primary DCR procedure. We use the KTP:YAG laser with a blunt-tipped 600-μm fiberoptic cord. Care must be taken when introducing the tip into the canaliculus to avoid false passages. We have also successfully used a transconjunctival approach to CDCR in five patients with this technique.

Familiarity with nasal endoscopy and intranasal instrumentation is essential for surgeons contemplating the use of internal DCR surgery. The intranasal anatomy must be visualized to ensure adequate completion of the procedure. In most cases the transnasal approach is helpful in allowing more freedom of movement of the laser probe and the use of supplemental instrumentation.

The article by Woog and coworkers [1•] emphasizes the many advantages of the intranasal endoscopic approach, including excellent visualization of the intranasal anatomy, ease of removal of the nasal mucosa and middle turbinate, and the ability to use supplemental endoscopic instruments for removal of thick bone, charred tissue, and to perform biopsies on suspicious lesions. The use of additional intranasal instruments, such as a small burring drill and endoscopic forceps as described by Woog, may prove essential in achieving long-term success in laser DCR surgery. Although the laser provides excellent hemostasis, it has limited efficacy in removing large pieces of bone, which is necessary for successful DCR surgery.

There are many potential advantages of the laser-assisted internal DCR procedure, including less intraoperative and postoperative bleeding, avoidance of a cutaneous scar, reduced surgical trauma with less pain and swelling, and a shortened postoperative

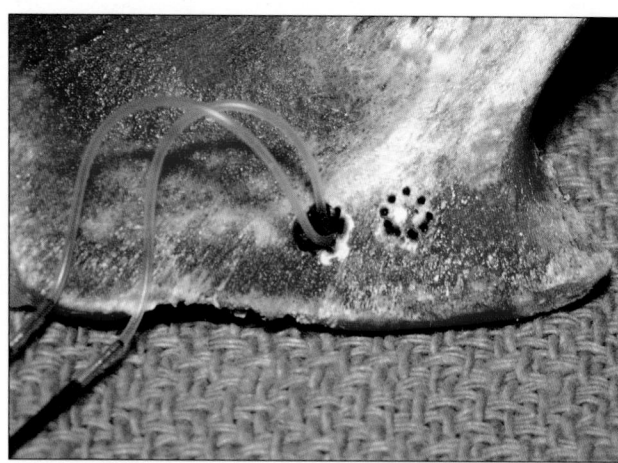

FIGURE 3-4 Multiple small perforations are made in a circular pattern with the fiberoptic tip. The central disc of bone was punched out before passing silicone stents. (*From* Silkiss *et al.* [5]; with permission.)

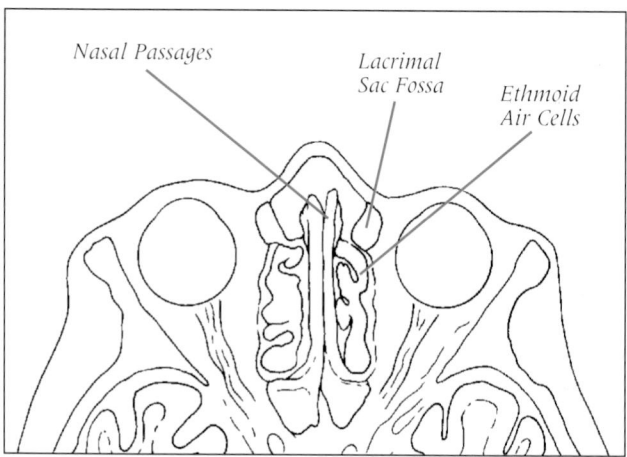

FIGURE 3-5 Computed tomographic scan demonstrates ethmoid air cells extending anteriorly to the posterior lacrimal crest, between the lacrimal sac and the nose. These intervening air cells must be removed during dacryocystorhinostomy. (*From* Linberg *et al.* [6]; with permission.)

recovery. Although the success rate of the laser-assisted internal DCR may not rival the 90% quoted for a well-performed external DCR, important advances such as those discussed by Woog have narrowed the gap. In the future, the laser-assisted internal DCR will likely become an acceptable alternative to external DCR.

ARGON LASER TREATMENT FOR TRICHIASIS

There have been a variety of treatment modalities used over the years for the management of trichiasis, including epilation, electrolysis, cryotherapy, and surgery. Epilation is a temporizing measure because most lashes regrow in 4 to 6 weeks. Electrolysis is a tedious procedure, with recurrence rates as high as 50%. Cryotherapy is currently considered the most effective method of treatment, with cure rates ranging from 70% to 90%. However, this procedure is associated with a significant risk of complication, including eyelid swelling, notching and depigmentation, reactivation of inflammatory conditions such as herpes zoster and pemphigoid, induction of symblepharon, secondary trichiasis, xerosis, corneal ulceration, and visual loss.

In 1979 Berry [7] first published results of the argon laser in the treatment of trichiasis. Seven years later, Arwan [8] reported results in a series of 11 patients in which he used topical tetracaine for anesthesia, a spot size of 50 to 200 µm, exposure time of 0.2 second, and a power setting of 1.0 to 1.2 W. He reported a 45% success rate with one treatment, an 82% success rate with two treatments, and 100% success with three treatments. Regrowth of abnormal lashes was most common in those patients with greater than six abnormal cilia. No complications were reported.

Campbell [9] recently reported an 80% success rate with up to three treatments on 15 eyelids. The author used 15 to 60 shots per cilia with the argon blue-green wavelengths, a spot size of 50 to 100 µm, exposure time of 0.05 to 0.10 second and a power setting of 1.2 to 2.0 W. This procedure was performed with the patients receiving topical anesthesia; no complications were reported. Of the three patients treated who had six or more abnormal lashes per eyelid, one required three treatments to destroy all the abnormal eyelash follicles, and the other two had a recurrence of abnormal lashes even after three treatments. The success rate for patients with fewer than six abnormal lashes was 92% with up to three treatments.

Huneke [10] reported a 62% initial success rate in the treatment of 77 patients with trichiasis. He treated 775 abnormal lashes on 91 eyelids for an average of 8.5 lashes per eyelid. His settings included a 50-µm spot size, 300 mW of power, and a duration of 0.5 second. Treatment was to a depth of 2 to 3 mm with an average of 40 to 50 pulses per eyelash. The author reported no complications and a high degree of patient satisfaction, although 37% of the patients required repeat treatment to the same area.

Bartley and Lowry [11] reported a 59% success rate with one treatment of 44 patients with trichiasis over a 5-year period. They used 1.0 W of power, a 50-µm spot size, 0.2-second duration, and the blue-green wavelength. They did not comment on the number of lashes treated on each eyelid. No complications were reported. The authors concluded that the argon laser is less effective than cryotherapy at destroying abnormal eyelashes. They advocate the use of the argon laser in the treatment of a few scattered eyelashes or in patients with inflammatory disorders such as pemphigoid.

Gossman and coworkers [12•] recently reported results in a prospective study of 60 consecutive eyelids with focal, symptomatic trichiasis. Their laser settings were substantially higher than those of previous authors, with a spot size of 100 µm, an exposure time of 0.5 second, and an energy level of 1.5 W. These higher settings necessitated the use of local infiltrative anesthesia for patient comfort and a white plastic scleral shield to protect the eye. They measured the depth of penetration with a calibrated probe, and at a 2.0-mm depth, the spot size was increased to 200 µm, defocused, and four additional burns were delivered in an attempt to destroy the lash follicle completely. They reported an 88% success rate after one treatment and 100% success rate after two treatments. All recurrences occurred in patients with post-traumatic trichiasis and were attributed to the unpredictable location of the lash follicle. Figure 3-6 illustrates the pre- and post-treatment appearance of the eyelid.

The high degree of success in this series appears to be a result of both patient selection and technique. The authors treated only cases of focal trichiasis. They treated "over 100" lashes on 60 eyelids, suggesting an average of approximately two aberrant lashes per eyelid. Unlike the previous authors, they did not attempt to treat multiple aberrant lashes on a single eyelid. These were the cases found to recur most often as reported in previous publications [8,9]. Secondly, they used higher energy levels than those previously cited, which may account for a more complete destruction of the lash follicles [7–11].

These higher energy levels also account for a higher complication rate. They report an 8% incidence of mild eyelid notching or dimpling, and a 7% incidence of faint hypopigmentation (Fig. 3-7). They also noted more severe eyelid notching when treating lashes involving the marginal tarsus. They therefore do not recommend treating extensive areas of distichiasis for fear of creating subsequent eyelid deformity.

We have used the technique described by Gossman and coworkers [12•] in a small series of patients with focal trichiasis (< six lashes), with excellent early results. Local infiltrative anesthesia allows thorough treatment of the lash follicles while maintaining patient comfort. This is important because the most common mistake made in the early use of this procedure is not treating to the depth necessary to ablate the lash follicle.

In summary, the argon laser appears to be an effective alternative in the treatment of focal areas of trichiasis when compared with the other treatment modalities. It is clearly more effective than epilation or electrolysis, with a success rate similar to that of cryotherapy. Unlike cryotherapy, however, this technique uses a selective ablation of the abnormal lash follicle, which spares most of the normal adjacent eyelid tissue and reduces the risk for swelling, notching, depigmentation, atrophy, symblepharon formation, and reactivation of inflammatory conditions. If lashes recur, repeat treatment can be administered with relative ease.

The argon laser treatment of trichiasis does have certain limitations. It is clearly less effective than cryotherapy in treating extensive areas of trichiasis (< six lashes) and may be less effective in the treatment of traumatic trichiasis where the location of the follicle is unpredictable. This technique may be inappropriate in the treatment of distichiasis where notching of the tarsus may occur. It is more technically demanding than cryotherapy but is relatively easy to learn. It requires the patient to remain still at the slit lamp during the procedure and may be difficult to perform in children, bedridden individuals, and patients with tremors or movement disorders.

LASERS IN CUTANEOUS AND ORBITAL SURGERY

Pulsed dye laser

The PDL is the most exciting new advance in the treatment of cutaneous vascular lesions. This tunable laser can be set at a wavelength of 580 nm, thereby allowing selective absorption by oxyhemoglobin and limiting the absorption by melanin. This setting increases penetration of the skin and decreases the risk of pigment loss. The flashlamp-pumped PDL gives out short pulses

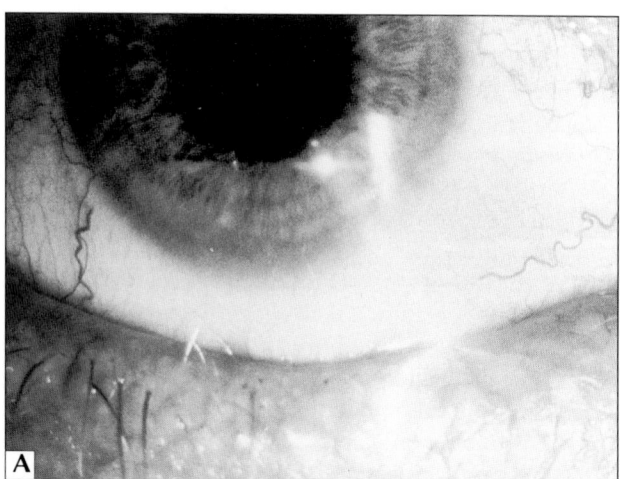

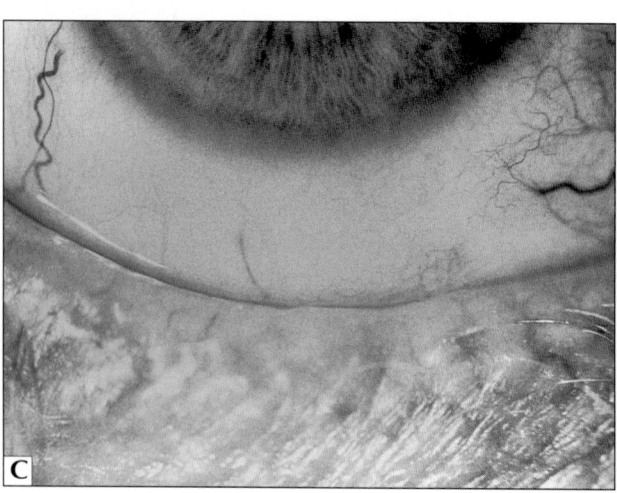

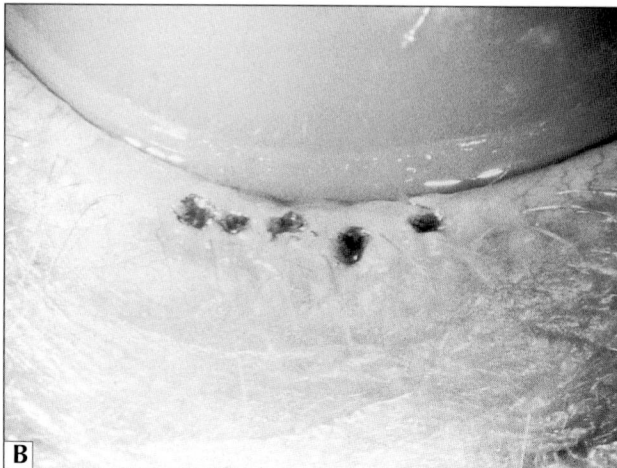

FIGURE 3-6 A, Focal trichiasis contacting the conjunctiva before treatment. **B**, Eyelid immediately after treatment. **C**, Eyelid 2 months after treatment. Healing occurred by secondary intention, preserving eyelid color and contour. (*From* Gossman *et al.* [12•]; with permission.)

of energy that are selectively absorbed by blood vessels, thus producing intravascular coagulation. Most of the energy from each pulse is absorbed by blood vessels, limiting nonspecific thermal damage to adjacent structures. This selective photothermolysis has greatly reduced the incidence of scarring and pigmentary change when compared with the argon laser.

Holy and Geronemus [13••] reported their results with the use of flashlamp-pumped PDL in the treatment of 67 patients with periorbital port-wine stains. Their most effective setting was at a wavelength of 585 nm, a pulse duration of 450 μs, and a 5-mm spot size. They treated 36 children and 31 adults and noted good to excellent results in 93% of all patients, with no incidence of scarring or permanent pigmentary change. They strongly advocate the use of the flashlamp-pumped PDL in the treatment of flat and mildly hypertrophic port-wine stains in persons of all ages.

Goldman and coworkers [14••] reported on the treatment of 43 children with 49 separate port-wine–stain vascular malformations with the flashlamp-pumped PDL. Patients ranged in age from 2 weeks to 14 years. They treated at a wavelength of 585 nm, pulse duration of 450 μs, and a spot size of 5 mm. Patients received one to 11 treatments, with an average of 3.6 treatments per lesion. The authors noted an average improvement of 50% with the initial treatment and a 10% improvement with each successive treatment. After six treatments 40% of the lesions had completely cleared, and the remainder had an average improvement of 80%. Lesions treated in children under the age of 4 years had a greater overall improvement with fewer treatment sessions. Treated areas became purpuric within a few hours, but the swelling and erythema faded in 24 to 48 hours. Transient hyperpigmentation occurred in 25% to 30% of patients but resolved within 2 to 3 months. Transient hypopigmentation was rare and resolved within 3 to 6 months in all cases. There were no cases of scarring or persistent pigmentary change. Figure 3-8 demonstrates the pre- and post-treatment appearance of port-wine stains.

Gonzalez and coworkers [15] used the PDL in the treatment of 92 adults with telangiectases of the face. They used the flashlamp-pumped PDL at a wavelength of 577 nm, a pulse duration of 300 μs, and a 5-mm spot size to treat linear, spider, and matted vascular ectases. A single pulse was used for most small lesions (< 5 mm), whereas multiple, contiguous pulses were necessary for larger or deeper lesions. Ninety-one percent of the subjects treated showed good to excellent results with only one treatment. Adverse reactions included hyperpigmentation in five patients and hypopigmentation in three patients, all of which resolved in 4 to 6 months. Four patients demonstrated some degree of depression over the treated area as a result of dermal and epidermal atrophy. The authors conclude that the PDL is superior to the argon laser in the treatment of vascular lesions of the face, with improved cosmetic results and a much lower incidence of serious complications.

The above-mentioned studies demonstrated the efficacy of the flashlamp-pumped PDL in the treatment of flat, superficial vascular lesions such as the nevus flammeus of the Stürge-Weber syndrome. The flashlamp-pumped PDL appears superior to the argon laser in achieving better resolution of these vascular malformations with a much lower incidence of serious complication, especially scarring. These studies support the early treatment of these lesions prior to the onset of thickening and hypertrophy.

Garden and coworkers [16•] used the flashlamp-pumped PDL in the treatment of 33 cutaneous capillary and mixed hemangiomas in 24 patients. Patients ranged in age from 2 weeks to 7 months. The treatment protocol included a wavelength of 585 nm, a pulse duration of 360 to 400 μs, and a 5-mm spot size. Eighteen patients with 25 lesions were given maximum therapy, which entailed treating until the lesion completely resolved, or until no further improvement was noted with successive sessions. This group showed an overall lightening of 93%, with an average of five treatment sessions per lesion. The thickness of these lesions decreased from an average of 3.4 mm to an average of 1.3 mm. Thin lesions (< 3 mm) responded better than did thick lesions and the cavernous component of mixed hemangiomas responded poorly to treatment. Six patients received therapy only until capillary proliferation halted, which required an average of 2.2 treatments.

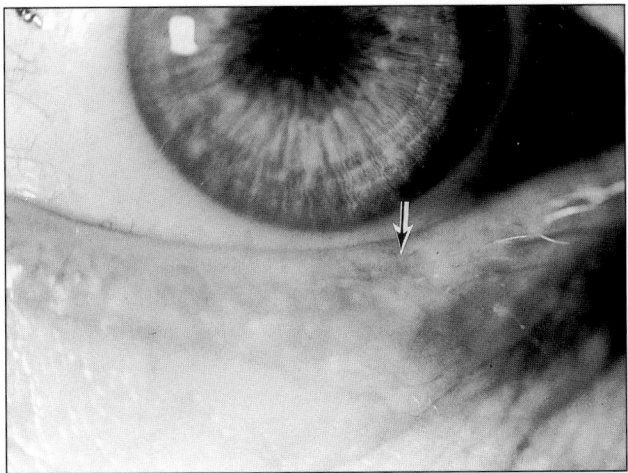

FIGURE 3-7 Dimpling at the treatment site 3 months after treatment (*arrow*). (*From* Gossman *et al.* [12•]; with permission.)

Complications included atrophy in four of the 25 lesions that were treated with maximum therapy. There was transient hyperpigmentation in 21% of lesions and transient hypopigmentation in 10% of lesions. There were no cases of fibrosis or hypertrophic scar formation.

The authors conclude that the flashlamp-pumped PDL yields satisfactory lightening and thinning of capillary and mixed hemangiomas. It is most effective when treating thinner lesions. The authors note, however, that 50% of juvenile hemangiomas will completely involute by 5 years of age and 90% by 9 years, with less than 20% resulting in permanent skin changes. Although the complications reported in this study were minimal, the longest follow-up was only 22 months. Longer follow-up is needed before an accurate comparison can be made between this and other treatment modalities in the management of juvenile capillary hemangiomas.

Tappero and coworkers [17] reported on the use of the PDL in the treatment of 15 patients with AIDS and Kaposi's sarcoma. A complete or partial clinical response was seen in 44% of the treated lesions; however, all treated lesions recurred at 12 weeks. Based on these results, the authors concluded that the PDL is ineffective in the management of Kaposi's sarcoma of AIDS.

Goldberg and Nychay [18] reported their results in the treatment of two patients with the nevus of Ota with the Q-switched ruby laser. At a wavelength of 694 nm and a pulse duration of 40 ns, the two patients were treated with slightly overlapping pulses. One patient was lost to follow-up, but the second showed good results at a follow-up of 1 year. There was no evidence of scarring or recurrent pigmentation (Fig. 3-9).

Watts and coworkers [19] reported their results with the use of the Q-switched Nd:YAG laser for removal of permanent eyeliner. They treated 14 eyelids in six patients who desired a generalized reduction in pigment thickness and intensity, or removal of a small area of pigment migration or imperfection. Patients had two to 10 treatment sessions. Treatment consisted of triple pulses of energies not exceeding 11.5 mJ, with a pulse duration of 3 ns set at a wavelength of 1064 nm. They noted an initial blanching lasting several hours followed by a more gradual but permanent fading of the pigment over a period of weeks, although complete removal was not achieved. The response was varied, with three patients achieving greater than 60% fading of pigment and three patients, less than 60%. Complications were limited to transient periocular bruising, with no evidence of scar formation. The authors conclude that this is a precise and safe method of reducing blepharopigmentation and is best suited to treating localized areas of imperfection. It is important to recognize the limitations of this technique as reported by the authors, including 1) the individual response to treatment was highly variable, ranging from minimal fading to nearly complete removal of the pigment, and 2) in no cases was there complete removal of the pigmentation.

Carbon dioxide laser

The major advantage of the carbon dioxide (CO_2) laser is its hemostatic properties. In the field of oculoplastic surgery, the CO_2 laser has been most noted for its use in the management of orbital lymphangiomas [20,21].

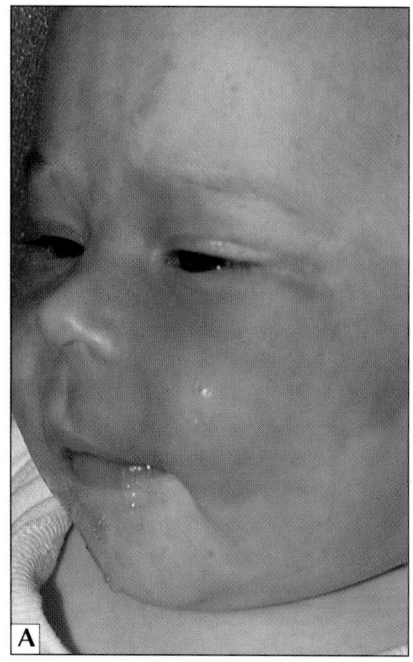
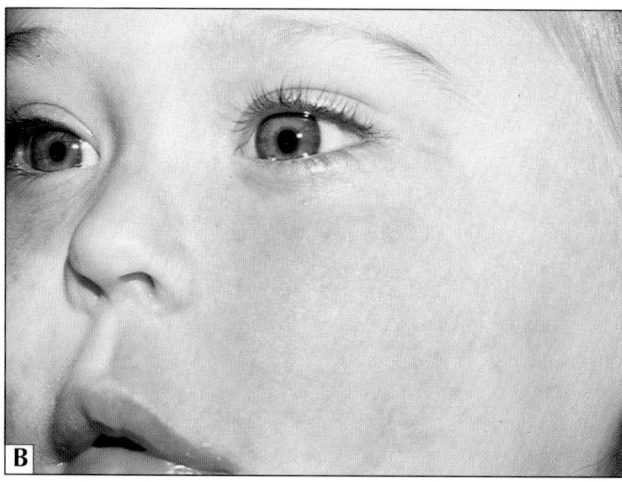

FIGURE 3-8 A, Initial appearance of extensive port-wine hemangioma on a 10-week-old girl. **B**, The patient 4 months after her fourth treatment with the pulsed dye laser. The parents and the physician noted nearly 90% resolution of the port-wine hemangioma. (*From* Goldman *et al.* [14••]; with permission.)

These unencapsulated infiltrative tumors are extremely difficult to excise with traditional surgical techniques because of their extreme friability and intimate relationship to vital orbital structures. These lesions can be debulked with excellent hemostasis and minimal risk of damage to adjacent orbital structures through the use of the CO_2 laser. The CO_2 laser has also been used in the excision of multiple facial syringomas and xanthelasma palpebrarum [22–24]. With the advent of PDL, its use in the treatment of vascular tumors such as capillary hemangiomas will likely become less popular. Morrow and Morrow [25] compared the CO_2 laser with the conventional scalpel in 10 patients who underwent cosmetic upper and lower eyelid blepharoplasty. They used the CO_2 laser on one side as the exclusive cutting and cauterizing instrument and the scalpel and electrocautery on the other side. They noted less discomfort and swelling, and a shorter operative time on the side treated with the CO_2 laser. There were no complications on either side. Disadvantages reported with the use of the CO_2 laser included the cost of purchasing and maintaining the equipment, the time and effort required to become proficient with the use of this laser in blepharoplastic surgery, and the need for an additional surgical assistant.

CONCLUSIONS

The appeal of the rapidly evolving field of laser surgery has fostered continued experimentation on all fronts of oculoplastic and orbital surgery. Many new laser systems have given the surgeon a real advantage when compared with existing techniques. These newer techniques may revolutionize the way physicians approach such common oculoplastic problems as nasolacrimal duct obstruction and capillary hemangiomas. Some laser applications, however, have proved to be no more than an expensive alternative to existing techniques and one must consider the cost-benefit ratio when contemplating new laser applications. In years to come, the development of new lasers and refinement in the fiberoptic delivery systems will certainly result in an expanded role for lasers in the field of oculoplastic surgery.

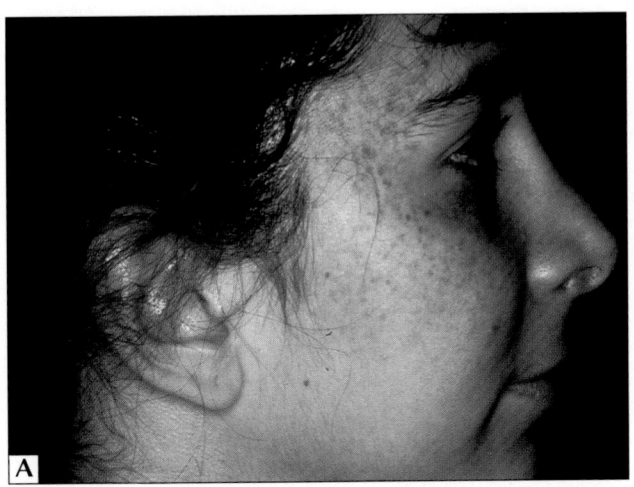 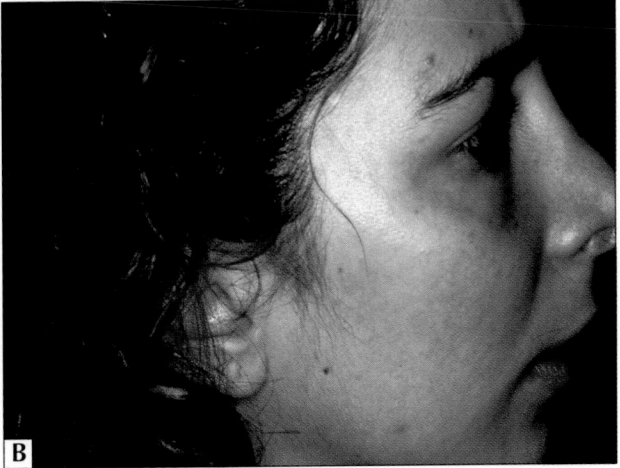

FIGURE 3-9 A, Nevus of Ota after test spots with Q-switched ruby laser to right cheek (note small lightened area). **B**, Nevus of Ota 1 year after treatment of right temple and right cheek. Note right infraorbital region requires further treatment. (*From* Goldberg and Nychay [18]; with permission.)

REFERENCES AND RECOMMENDED READING

Recently published papers of particular interest have been highlighted as:
• Of interest
•• Of outstanding interest

•1.   Woog JJ, Metson R, Puliafito CA: Holmium:YAG endonasal laser dacryocystorhinostomy. *Am J Ophthalmol* 1993, 116:1–10.
Describes a new technique of laser-assisted endonasal DCR used with good success in 40 consecutive patients. Important modifications from previously described techniques include the use of an intranasal drill, endoscopic instrumentation, and a double stent.

2.   Massaro BM, Gonnering RS, Harris GJ: Endonasal laser dacryocystorhinostomy. *Arch Ophthalmol* 1990, 108:1172–1176.

3.   Gonnering RS, Lyon DB, Fisher JC: Endoscopic laser-assisted lacrimal surgery. *Am J Ophthalmol* 1991, 111:152–157.

4. Levin PS, StormoGipson J: Endocanalicular laser-assisted dacryocystorhinostomy. *Arch Ophthalmol* 1992, 110:1488–1490.

5. Silkiss RZ, Axelrod RN, Iwach AG, *et al.*: Transcanalicular THC:YAG dacryocystorhinostomy. *Ophthalmic Surg* 1992, 23:351–353.

6. Blaylock WK, Moore CA, Linberg JV: Anterior ethmoid anatomy facilitates dacryocystorhinostomy. *Arch Ophthalmol* 1990, 108(suppl 12):1774–1777.

7. Berry J: Recurrent trichiasis: treatment with laser photo-coagulation. *J Ophthalmic Surg* 1979, 10:36–38.

8. Arwan KJ: Argon laser treatment of trichiasis. *J Ophthalmic Surg* 1986, 17:658–660.

9. Campbell DC: Thermoablation treatment for trichiasis using the argon laser. *Aust NZ J Ophthalmol* 1990, 18:427–430.

10. Huneke JW: Argon laser treatment for trichiasis. *Ophthalmic Plast Reconstr Surg* 1992, 8:50–55.

11. Bartley GB, Lowry JC: Argon laser treatment of trichiasis. *Am J Ophthalmol* 1992, 113:71–74.

•12. Gossman D, Yung R, Berlin J, *et al.*: Prospective evaluation of the argon laser in the treatment of trichiasis. *Ophthalmic Surg* 1992, 23:183–187.

Describes use of the argon laser in the treatment of 60 consecutive cases of focal trichiasis with excellent results. Discussion includes details of the technique and complications.

••13. Holy A, Geronemus RG: Treatment of periorbital port-wine stains with the flashlamp-pumped pulsed dye laser. *Arch Ophthalmol* 1992, 110:793–797.

A series of 67 patients with periorbital port-wine stains treated with the flashlamp-pumped pulsed dye laser. The authors report good-to-excellent results in 93% of patients, with no incidence of scarring or permanent pigment change.

••14. Goldman MP, Fitzpatrick RE, Ruiz-Esparza J: Treatment of port-wine stains (capillary malformation) with the flashlamp-pumped pulsed dye laser. *J Pediatr* 1993, 122:71–77.

Report of impressive results in the treatment of 49 separate port-wine stains in children with the flashlamp-pumped pulsed dye laser. Children under the age of 4 years had the best response to treatment and there were no cases of scarring or permanent pigmentary change.

15. Gonzalez E, Gange RW, Momtaz KT: Treatment of telangiectases and other benign vascular lesions with the 577 nm pulsed dye laser: *J Am Acad Dermatol* 1992, 27:220–226.

•16. Garden JM, Bakus AD, Paller AS: Treatment of cutaneous hemangiomas by the flashlamp-pumped pulsed dye laser: prospective analysis. *J Pediatr* 1992, 120:555–560.

Describes the use of the flashlamp-pumped pulsed dye laser in the treatment of 33 cutaneous capillary and mixed hemangiomas. Thin capillary lesions responded better than did thick cavernous lesions. Some atrophy of the skin was noted in treated areas.

17. Tappero JW, Grekin RC, Zanelli GA, *et al.*: Pulsed-dye laser therapy for cutaneous Kaposi's sarcoma associated with acquired immunodeficiency syndrome. *J Am Acad Dermatol* 1992, 27:526–530.

18. Goldberg DJ, Nychay SG: Q-switched ruby laser treatment of nevus of ota. *J Dermatol Surg Oncol* 1992, 18:817–821.

19. Watts MT, Downes RN, Collin JRO, *et al.*: The use of q-switched Nd:Yag laser for removal of permanent eyeliner tattoo. *Ophthalmic Plast Reconstr Surg* 1992, 8:292–294.

20. Kennerdell JS, Maroon JC, Garrity JA, *et al.*: Surgical management of orbital lymphangioma with the carbon dioxide laser. *Am J Ophthalmol* 1986, 102:308–314.

21. Jordan DR, Anderson RL: Carbon dioxide laser therapy for conjunctival lymphangioma. *Ophthalmic Surg* 1981, 18:728–730.

22. Wheeland RG, Bailin PL, Reynolds OD, *et al.*: Carbon dioxide laser vaporization of multiple facial syringomas. *J Dermatol Surg Oncol* 1987, 13:149–151.

23. Gladstone GJ, Beckman H, Elson LM: CO_2 laser excision of xanthelasma lesions. *Arch Ophthalmol* 1985, 103:440–442.

24. Apfelberg DB, Maser MR, Lash H, *et al.*: Treatment of xanthelasma palpebrarum with the carbon dioxide laser. *J Dermatol Surg Oncol* 1987, 13:149–151.

25. Morrow DM, Morrow LB: CO_2 laser blepharoplasty: a comparison with cold-steel surgery. *J Dermatol Surg Oncol* 1992, 18:307–313.

SELECT BIBLIOGRAPHY

Anderson RR, Parrish JA: Selective photothermolysis: precise microsurgery by selective absorption of pulsed radiation. *Science* 1983, 220:524–527.

Dover JS, Arndt KA, Geronemus RG, *et al.*: *Illustrated cutaneous laser surgery, a practitioner's guide*. Norwalk, CT: Appleton & Lange; 1990:73–106.

Hornblass A, Coden DJ: Lasers in oculoplastic and orbital surgery. *Int Ophthalmol Clin* 1989, 29:265–274.

Tan OT, Sherwood K, Glichrest BA: Treatment of children with port-wine stains using the flashlamp-pulsed tunable dye laser. *N Engl J Med* 1989, 320:416–421.

Wesley RE, Bond JB: Carbon dioxide laser in ophthalmic plastic and orbital surgery. *Ophthalmic Surg* 1985, 16:631–633.

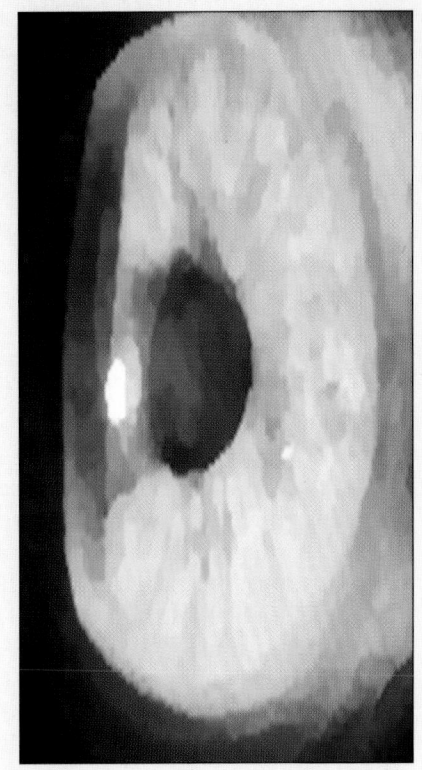

CHAPTER 4

LASER TREATMENT OF CYSTOID MACULAR EDEMA

STEPHEN S. PAPPAS, JR.
DARMAKUSUMA IE
ROBERT P. MURPHY

Laser surgery has been used in the practice of ophthalmology for the past three decades. Since the late 1970s, a number of randomized controlled clinical trials have established the use and expanded the indications of laser photocoagulation in a variety of retinal disorders such as diabetic retinopathy and vascular occlusive disease. Cystoid macular edema (CME), the accumulation of fluid and exudates in the extracellular space of the retina, represents a common cause of significant central visual loss associated with retinal vascular disease, ocular inflammation, and cataract surgery. This chapter will address the current indications, methods, and results of laser therapy for CME from various etiologies.

PATHOPHYSIOLOGY OF CYSTOID MACULAR EDEMA

The passage of molecules and fluid from the vasculature into the retina normally is restricted by the blood-retinal barriers. These blood-retinal barriers occur in two locations: the tight junctions between retinal vascular endothelial cells (inner blood-retinal barrier) and the tight junctions between adjacent retinal pigment epithelial cells (outer blood-retinal barrier). In addition, active transport mechanisms move fluid from the eye across the retinal pigment epithelium (RPE) into the bloodstream.

Disruption of the blood-retinal barriers results in the accumulation of plasma components within the extracellular space of the retina. Histologically, macular edema is defined as an abnormal collection of fluid in the extracellular compartment of the retina in the macula. The exact mechanism of leakage as it relates to histologic changes seen is not well understood. The accumulation of fluid within the macular area may be related to leakage of perifoveal capillaries or from more distant retinal vascular leakage. Distinct retinal microaneurysms or larger areas of abnormal telangiectatic retinal capillaries may leak and produce macular edema. The leakage also may be secondary to abnormalities in the RPE, but mechanisms at this level are even less well understood. Breakdown of the inner and outer blood-retinal barriers permit extravasation of ions, along with both low and high molecular weight molecules. The presence of these osmotically powerful substances in the retina creates an oncotic gradient that permits further extravasation of fluid into the retina.

Macular edema is evaluated clinically by slit-lamp biomicroscopy, which demonstrates retinal thickening. In chronic cases, one may see cyst-like spaces within the retina. The distribution of retinal thickening may be described as focal or diffuse, depending on its extent.

Examining the macula with stereoscopic technique is essential to making the diagnosis of macular edema. It is important to determine whether the center of the macula is thickened, because the prognosis and management is different with central involvement. Most observers agree the best way to determine macular thickening is with the stereoscopic view provided by a macular contact lens at the biomicroscope. Indirect lenses, such as a 78- or 90-diopter lens, at the biomicroscope are helpful in screening patients. If macular thickening is detected using these lenses, it is undoubtedly present, but subtle thickening can be missed. Examination with the indirect ophthalmoscope is not an effective method of detecting thickening.

Fluorescein angiography should be obtained only when the clinical diagnosis of macular edema has been made and treatment is being planned. Fluorescein angiography can be very helpful in identifying the areas of leakage. With an intact inner blood-retinal barrier, fluorescein dye remains within the retinal vasculature. Disruption of endothelial cell tight junctions, however, permits extravasation of dye into the retina.

Angiographically, this pattern of dye leakage around the macula assumes a characteristic petaloid pattern produced by the obliquely arranged middle retinal layers, namely the outer plexiform layer of Henle. Although this characteristic fluorescein pattern is most often seen after cataract surgery, more diffuse, irregular patterns of dye leakage are seen in other forms of retinal vascular disease, such as diabetic retinopathy.

LASERS

Photocoagulation exerts its therapeutic effect on the macula by heating the retina and underlying choroid to produce coagulation necrosis, which results in a chorioretinal scar. The exact biochemical and pathophysiologic processes that determine therapeutic response are poorly understood. The conversion of light to heat energy at a particular tissue site is a function of effective light absorption at that site [1]. The pigments involved with light absorption during macular photocoagulation are xanthophyll (inner and outer plexiform layers of the retina), melanin (RPE and choroidal melanocytes), and hemoglobin (in retinal and choroidal blood vessels).

Wavelength selection helps determine where light will be absorbed to produce its desired effect. Blue wavelengths are absorbed by xanthophyll in the inner retinal layers, while the other visible wavelengths—red, yellow, and green—are absorbed by the RPE (mostly by melanin) [1]. Although melanin may absorb light most effectively, its ability to do so varies little with change in wavelength [1]. Because xanthophyll, located primarily around the macula, absorbs blue light better than green light, the latter wavelength is preferred for macular laser treatments to avoid damage to the inner retinal layers. Hemoglobin has poor red light absorption, whereas blue, yellow, and green wavelengths are easily absorbed. With vitreous, intraretinal, or subretinal hemorrhages, krypton red laser may provide a selective advantage, because it theoretically can penetrate hemorrhagic tissues with less damage.

The argon green (514 nm) and krypton red (647 nm) wavelength lasers are currently the most commonly used lasers in the treatment of retinal disorders. Most of the collaborative randomized retinal studies were done with the argon laser, but the advantages of the krypton red laser in penetrating cataracts and hemorrhages, while sparing the inner retinal layers, have established the utility of this wavelength in the management of neovascular retinal disease. The more recently developed tunable dye lasers provide a wider selection of red (630 nm), orange (600 nm), and yellow (577 nm) wavelengths, which may potentially provide the ability to exert more selectively a therapeutic effect on tissues. There are a number of longer wavelength lasers, but these, in general, create a deeper retinal or choroidal burn. The treatment benefit demonstrated in most of the collaborative studies resulted from treatment with green or blue-green wavelength lasers.

DIABETIC MACULAR EDEMA

Diabetic macular edema is the leading cause of visual impairment in individuals with diabetic retinopathy [2–4]. It is estimated that 10% of people with diabetes have macular edema [5]. Although uncommon in the first 7 years of diabetes, macular edema is increasingly frequent after 10 years. For individuals with disease duration of 15 years, the prevalence of edema (defined as thickening within one disc diameter of the center of the macula) rises to approximately 30%. Older onset diabetics who are not taking insulin are less likely to have macular edema [5]. The risk of having macular edema increases with time and with increasing severity of retinopathy [5].

The usefulness of laser treatment for diabetic macular edema began to be apparent when three prospective randomized clinical trials demonstrated a treatment benefit [6–9]. Studies by Patz and coworkers [6], Blankenship [7], and the multicentered British Diabetes trial [8] all demonstrated reduction of visual loss with photocoagulation for diabetic macular edema compared to no treatment. All studies were relatively small, but the conclusions were similar. The study authors agreed that a larger, more rigorous study was warranted, and all supported a prospective randomized clinical trial with longer follow-up. One such study was the Early Treatment Diabetic Retinopathy Study. With 3711 persons followed for over 7 years, the Early Treatment Diabetic Retinopathy Study was designed to evaluate multiple laser treatment strategies for diabetic macular edema. Information from Early Treatment Diabetic Retinopathy Study reports on macular edema remains the best source of natural history data for this condition and offers the clearest guidelines for the management and laser treatment of macular edema [10–14].

Clinically, diabetic macular edema is defined as abnormal thickening of the macula with fluid. The diagnosis is made on the basis of a stereoscopic evaluation of the macula at the biomicroscope. Fluorescein angiography is not required to make the diagnosis; in some cases angiographic leakage in the macula is not associated with clinical edema. Thickening of the macula must be determined from clinical experience. Hard exudates are often, but not always, associated with macular edema and are often a useful clinical clue. Chronic edema can cause microcystic changes in the retina, especially in the central macula.

Fluorescein angiography is usually needed to determine patterns of leakage. Discrete leakage from individual microaneurysms or localized microvascular abnormalities is called "focal" leakage. Less well-localized leakage from larger areas of abnormal retinal capillaries is termed "diffuse" leakage. Diffuse leakage can come from localized areas of the macula or from the entire macular areas in severe cases. Macular edema can also be associated with distinct microaneurysms or larger areas of abnormal capillaries.

Macular edema can range widely in severity. To identify the more severe and visually threatening forms of macular edema, the Early Treatment Diabetic Retinopathy Study developed the term *clinically significant macular edema* to define retinal thickening that involves or threatens the center of the macula. Visual acuity is not part of the definition. Macular edema is assessed by stereo contact lens biomicroscopy or stereo photography. The Early Treatment Diabetic Retinopathy Study definition of "clinically significant" macular edema includes one or more of the following three criteria: 1) thickening of the retina at or within 500 μm of the center of the macula; 2) hard exudates at or within 500 μm of the center of the macula, if associated with thickening of adjacent retina (but not residual hard exudates remaining after disappearance of retinal thickening); 3) a zone or zones of retinal thickening one disc area or larger in size, any part of which is within 1 disc diameter of the center of the macula (Table 4-1).

However, in more recent analyses of Early Treatment Diabetic Retinopathy Study data, eyes with macular edema involving the center of the macula have been evaluated separately. These eyes may be designated as having "central macular involvement" with edema and appear to be at highest risk of visual loss without treatment [4]. Investigators in the Early Treatment Diabetic Retinopathy Study used argon blue-green and argon green wavelengths for macular treatment. Tunable dye lasers have been developed, allowing for a selection of a variety of wavelengths. Some investigators prefer dye yellow to treat individual microaneurysms. In general, the longer wavelength lasers appear to be less suitable for treatment of diabetic macular edema unless opacities in the optical media prevent adequate treatment with the shorter laser wavelengths.

The Early Treatment Diabetic Retinopathy Study was designed to answer three clinical questions regarding diabetic retinopathy:

1) When in the course of diabetic retinopathy is it most effective to initiate photocoagulation therapy?
2) Is photocoagulation effective in the treatment of macular edema?
3) Is aspirin effective in altering the course of diabetic retinopathy?

The first two questions address the issue of macular edema. Between April 1980 and July 1984, the Early Treatment Diabetic Retinopathy Study enrolled 3711 patients with diabetes mellitus and diabetic retinopathy in both eyes. This review concentrates on the patients who entered the Early Treatment

Diabetic Retinopathy Study with macular edema who had a visual acuity of 20/200 or better and mild to severe nonproliferative diabetic retinopathy or early proliferative diabetic retinopathy. One eye was randomly assigned to early photocoagulation with one of three possible treatments: 1) initial mild scatter, 2) initial full scatter, or 3) initial focal laser. The initial type of laser treatment could subsequently be followed by another type of laser treatment. For example, eyes treated initially with focal treatment could have full scatter treatment later, or eyes initially treated with scatter treatment could have focal treatment later. The other eye was assigned to deferral of photocoagulation.

The primary endpoint for comparing the effects of laser treatment on macular edema was the development of "moderate visual loss", which was defined as a loss of 15 or more letters on the Early Treatment Diabetic Retinopathy Study chart between baseline and follow-up visit (Fig. 4-1, and Table 4-1) [10,13]. This loss is equivalent to a doubling of the visual angle. Scatter laser treatment used in the Early Treatment Diabetic Retinopathy Study could be mild or full, depending on the number of burns placed. Mild scatter treatment consisted of 400 to 650 burns spaced more than one burn width apart, whereas full scatter consisted of 1200 to 1600 burns spaced a half burn width apart. The spot-size diameter used was 500 µm, creating burns of moderate intensity. The treatment technique described by the Early Treatment Diabetic Retinopathy Study for macular edema specified argon blue-green or argon green laser applications (Table 4-2). Treatable lesions consisted of microaneurysms, focal leaks, or diffuse leakage, all of which cause thickening of the retina and are identified by slit-lamp biomicroscopy or fluorescein angio-

---

TABLE 4-1   EARLY TREATMENT DIABETIC RETINOPATHY STUDY DEFINITIONS

Macular edema
    Thickening of retina within 1 disc diameter of the center of the macula; or hard exudates ≥ standard photograph 3 in a standard 30° photographic field centered on the macula (field 2), with some hard exudates within 1 disc diameter of the center of the macula
Clinically significant macular edema
    Retinal thickening at or within 500 µm of the center of the macula; or hard exudates within 500 µm of the center of the macula, if associated with thickening of the adjacent retina; or a zone or zones of retinal thickening 1 disc area in size, at least part of which was within 1 disc diameter of the center
Severe visual loss
    Visual acuity < 5/200 at two consecutive follow-up visits (scheduled at 4-month intervals)
Moderate visual loss
    Loss of 15 or more letters between baseline and follow-up visit, equivalent to doubling the initial visual angle (ie, 20/20 to 20/40 or 20/50 to 20/100)

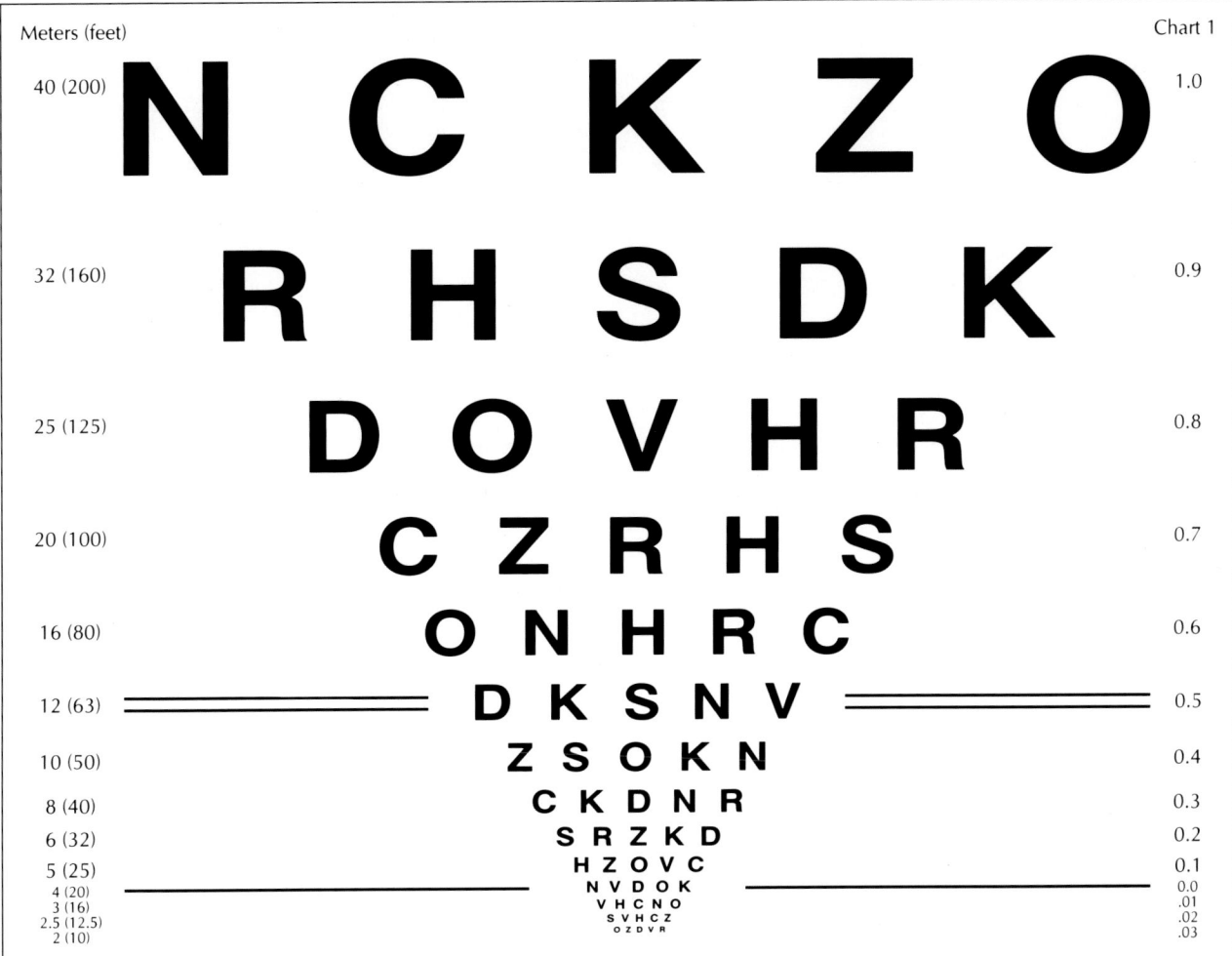

FIGURE 4-1 One of three Early Treatment Diabetic Retinopathy Study visual acuity charts used in the Early Treatment Diabetic Retinopathy Study. Moderate visual loss, defined as a loss of 15 or more letters (three lines) on the Early Treatment Diabetic Retinopathy Study chart, is equivalent to a doubling of the visual angle. Moderate visual gain, defined as a gain of 15 or more letters (three lines) is equivalent to a halving of the visual angle.

TABLE 4-2 EARLY TREATMENT DIABETIC RETINOPATHY STUDY TECHNIQUES—BURN CHARACTERISTICS

Focal	Direct	Grid
Size	50–100μm	< 200 μm (at retina)
Exposure	0.05–0.1 s	0.05–0.1 s
Intensity	Sufficient to whiten or darken large microaneurysms	Mild
Number	Sufficient to satisfactorily treat all focal leaks	Sufficient to cover areas of diffuse leakage and nonperfusion
Placement	500–3000 μm from center of fovea	Spaced greater than one burn wodth apart 500–3000 μm from center of fovea
Number of episodes	1	1
Indications for follow-up treatment	Presence of CSME and treatable lesions at ≥ 4 months	Presence of CSME and treatable lesions at ≥ 4 months

CSME—clinically significant macular edema.

graphy. Focal leakage and microaneurysms were treated directly using 50- to 100-µm–size burns of 0.1 second duration or less. The treatment goal was to achieve whitening around larger microaneurysms. Achieving a color change in smaller microaneurysms was not required. Milder, not more intense, laser burns were recommended. Initial laser treatment avoided areas within 500 µm of the center of the macula, but treatment could be extended to within 300 µm of the center of the fovea at later treatment sessions if edema persisted. Areas of diffuse leakage received a grid pattern, using 50- to 200-µm spot size and spacing them at least one burn width apart. Grid treatments were not placed within 500 µm of the center of the macula or within 500 µm of the disc margin, but could be placed in the papillomacular bundle.

In summary, the Early Treatment Diabetic Retinopathy Study treatment recommendations for macular edema followed these guidelines:

• Treat leaking microaneurysms with focal photocoagulation using small, mild burns. More diffuse

areas of leakage are treated with scatter or grid patterns of photocoagulation.
• Reevaluate each patient every 2 to 4 months.
• Re-treat at intervals of 3 to 4 months if clinically significant macular edema persists. The need to treat again is common; for additional treatment, the same treatment protocol is used.

The Early Treatment Diabetic Retinopathy Study showed that focal photocoagulation of clinically significant diabetic macular edema substantially reduces the risk of visual loss. After 3 years of follow-up, 29% of untreated eyes with less severe retinopathy and macular edema with central thickening developed moderate visual loss ($\geq$ a doubling of the visual angle). In contrast, only 13% of similar eyes treated with focal laser treatment as the initial treatment strategy developed such a degree of visual loss. This difference was evident from the 1st year of follow-up and continued throughout the 7-year follow-up period. The benefit of treatment was statistically significant at each follow-up visit. Focal treatment also increases the chance of visual improvement, decreases the frequency of persistent

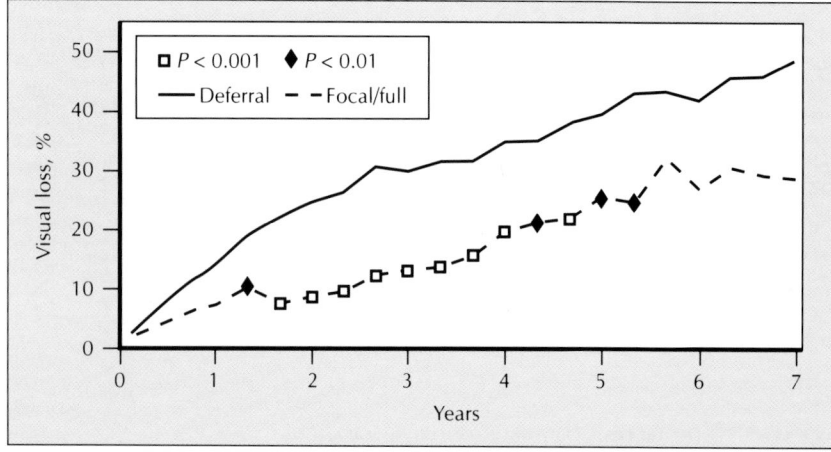

FIGURE 4-2 Occurrence of moderate visual loss in eyes with less severe retinopathy and central macular edema assigned to immediate focal photocoagulation and delayed full scatter treatment (*dotted line*) versus deferral of photocoagulation (*solid line*). The beneficial effect of focal photocoagulation as the initial laser treatment strategy is clearly demonstrated; this treatment strategy is associated with the best visual outcome. Focal treatment decreases the risk of moderate visual loss by over 50%. The beneficial treatment effect is sustained for the 7-year study period.

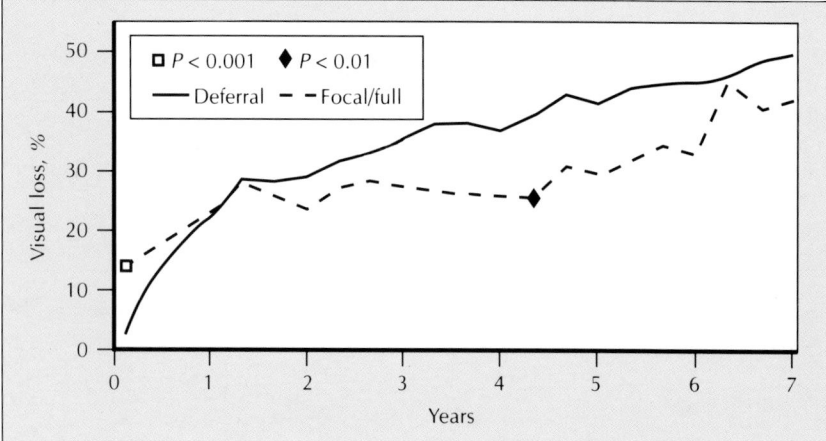

FIGURE 4-3 Occurrence of moderate visual loss in eyes with more severe retinopathy and central macular edema assigned to immediate focal photocoagulation and delayed mild scatter treatment (*dotted line*) versus deferral of photocoagulation (*solid line*). The beneficial effect of focal photocoagulation becomes evident only after the 1st year following treatment, but treated eyes develop less moderate visual loss than untreated eyes do.

macular edema, lessens loss of color vision, and causes only minor visual field losses.

For eyes with macular edema that was **not** clinically significant, there was little difference in development of moderate visual loss between treated and untreated eyes in the first 2 years of follow-up. After 2 years, treated eyes developed moderate visual loss at approximately one half the rate as untreated eyes. Any difference between the two groups after 2 years probably results from the development of central macular edema. It seems reasonable, therefore, to defer laser treatment in eyes that do not have clinically significant macular edema, but to follow them carefully at intervals of 4 months (Fig. 4-2). Eyes that subsequently develop clinically significant macular edema should be considered for laser treatment [10]. There was a similar but somewhat less pronounced treatment effect in eyes with macular edema and more severe retinopathy (Fig. 4-3).

Full scatter photocoagulation as an initial treatment for eyes with macular edema and less severe retinopathy was not a good treatment strategy. For these eyes there was an initial adverse effect on the risk of moderate visual loss in the first 2 years when full scatter photocoagulation was initiated before focal treatment (Fig. 4-4). The visual outcome in these eyes was never better than the outcome for the deferred treatment group. In eyes with less severe retinopathy and macular edema with central involvement receiving mild scatter treatment initially followed by focal treatment, a beneficial effect on the risk of moderate visual loss was seen, but only after about 4 years following treatment (Fig. 4-5).

Eyes receiving focal laser treatment were also more likely to have improved vision. Only 5% of untreated eyes gained 3 or more lines of vision, whereas 17% of treated eyes experienced this degree of improvement. These data suggest that the main benefit of focal laser treatment for diabetic edema is prevention of further visual loss, with only a small chance of visual improvement. For this reason, treatment is recommended for eyes that have developed clinically significant macular edema or macular edema with central involvement before there has been a decrease in visual acuity.

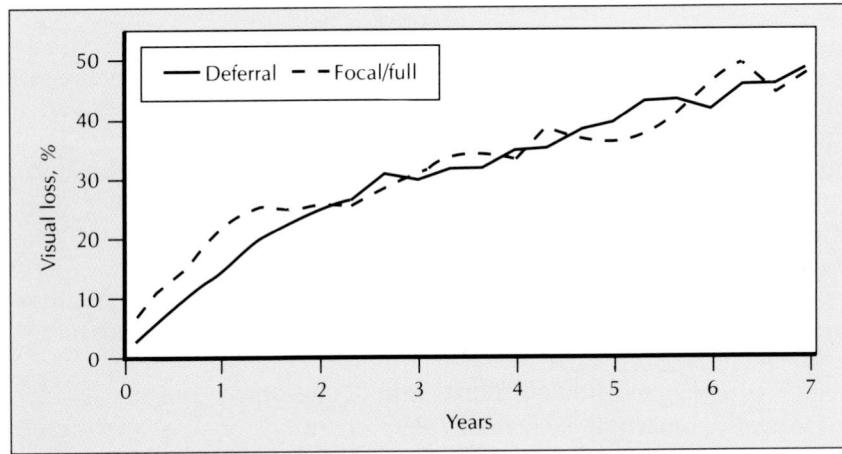

FIGURE 4-4 Occurrence of moderate visual loss in eyes with less severe retinopathy and central macular edema assigned to immediate full scatter treatment followed by focal photocoagulation (*dotted line*) versus deferral of photocoagulation (*solid line*). The adverse effect of full scatter photocoagulation as an initial treatment strategy on moderate visual loss is seen. Eyes with central macular edema treated with full scatter treatment develop more moderate visual loss initially than do deferral eyes; after the 1st year, the rates of moderate visual loss are similar in treated and untreated eyes. Visual acuity in eyes treated with this strategy is considerably worse than similar eyes receiving focal treatment as the initial strategy. (See Fig. 4-2.)

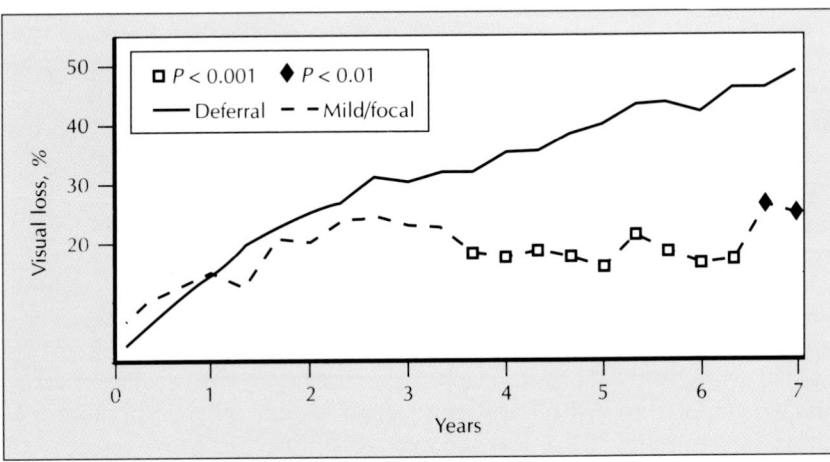

FIGURE 4-5 Occurrence of moderate visual loss in eyes with less severe retinopathy and central macular edema assigned to immediate mild scatter treatment followed by focal photocoagulation (*dotted line*) versus deferral of photocoagulation (*solid line*). Here, the beneficial effect of photocoagulation can also be seen, but not until 4 years following initial treatment. (See Fig. 4-2.)

The beneficial effects of treatment demonstrated in this Early Treatment Diabetic Retinopathy Study support the following:

1) Focal photocoagulation treatment as an initial treatment strategy should be considered for all eyes with clinically significant macular edema and mild or moderate nonproliferative diabetic retinopathy.
2) Scatter treatment, or panretinal photocoagulation, was not shown to be effective for macular edema in the Early Treatment Diabetic Retinopathy Study. It may worsen the visual acuity in untreated eyes. Some patients also had side effects such as mild decreases in central or peripheral vision following scatter treatment.
3) In cases of macular edema with more severe nonproliferative or proliferative retinopathy requiring immediate scatter treatment, the strategy associated with the least visual loss was a combination of mild scatter and focal treatment at the same sitting.

The Early Treatment Diabetic Retinopathy Study has shown the beneficial effects of focal laser treatment with delayed scatter photocoagulation in the management of diabetic macular edema (Fig. 4-6). Focal laser photocoagulation should be considered for all eyes with clinically significant macular edema and mild or moderate nonproliferative diabetic retinopathy or with more severe nonproliferative or proliferative retinopathy.

Complications of the treatment of diabetic macular edema were evaluated in the Early Treatment Diabetic Retinopathy Study, but, in general, were few and difficult to measure. However, in individual cases this treatment is not without complications. Development of scotomata after focal laser therapy close to the center of the macula is a well-recognized problem. Recently, other complications have been reported. Fortunately, these other complications are uncommon and, for the most part, are avoidable. Choroidal neovascularization has been reported following treatment of diabetic macular edema by Varley and coworkers [15]. Lewis and coworkers [16] presented a series of eight patients with choroidal neovascularization developing from a previous laser scar. The patients were diagnosed 2 weeks to 5 months after treatment, and despite further laser treatment to the choroidal neovascularization, visual acuity remained poor. Schatz and coworkers [17] describe enlargement of laser scars following grid laser treatments for diffuse diabetic macular edema. They reported 11 patients with progressive enlargement of focal photocoagulation scars and decreased visual acuity over months to years after treatment. Enlargement of the scars into the central macula as well as hyperplastic changes in the RPE were seen in these eyes. This type of scar can be formed only from relatively intense laser applications. Excessively intense laser burns are to be avoided in the macula to avoid this potential complication. Both complications of choroidal neovascularization and of enlargement of laser scars can be avoided with avoidance of intense laser applications in the macula.

Another potentially vision-limiting complication following laser photocoagulation of diabetic macular edema is the development of submacular fibrosis. Han and coworkers [18] reported on 10 eyes and Guyer and coworkers [19] reported on seven eyes with subretinal fibrous strands emanating from the treated areas. In some eyes, these strands extended from laser scars, suggesting a role of the laser treatment in this process. This complication is associated with a decline in visual acuity. Again, avoidance of excessively intense laser applications will avoid this complication.

VENOUS OCCLUSIVE DISEASE

Overview

Retinal venous occlusive disease, including central and branch retinal vein occlusion (BRVO), represents a common cause of visual loss in older age groups, ranking second behind diabetic retinopathy. This condition has no sex predilection and usually affects patients between age 60 to 70 years. Retinal neovascularization (with secondary vitreous hemorrhage), macular ischemia, and persistent macular edema can all cause significant visual deterioration as a result of venous occlusive disease. Although the exact mechanism of macular edema is unknown, leakage from dysfunctional capillaries or macular capillary nonperfusion are thought to contribute to extracelluar fluid accumulation around the macula.

Branch retinal vein occlusion

Branch retinal vein occlusions occur at the site of an arteriovenous crossing. The location of the venous blockage determines the distribution of intraretinal hemorrhage. When tributary veins involving the macula are involved, macular edema may result, causing a decrease in visual acuity. Recent data from the Eye Disease Case Control Study Group demonstrate that risk factors for BRVO include systemic hypertension, history of cardiovascular disease, age, and glaucoma [20]. Fluorescein angiography will show the extent of capillary leakage or nonperfusion, as well as the extent of the macular edema. These factors, as well as the duration of the disease, are important considerations in determining the cause of decreased visual acuity. Conventional thinking holds that macular capillary nonperfusion appears to cause an irreversible vision loss with transient macular edema, whereas perifoveal capillary leakage may produce a persistent but reversible form of macular edema that seems to be more amenable to laser photocoagulation. The mechanism of therapeutic response remains unclear.

Finkelstein [21] compared potential mechanisms of macular edema in BRVOs by examining the integrity of the perifoveal capillary ring during fluorescein angiography. Breaks in the ring attributable to capillary nonperfusion produced macular edema from the cytotoxic effects of ischemia. Such "ischemic macular edema" was detectable clinically but not angiographically, because the extracellular fluid did not originate from damaged capillaries containing fluorescein. In over 3 years of follow-up, 91% of patients with ischemic macular edema demonstrated spontaneous improvement in visual acuity, whereas only 29% of patients with vasogenic macular edema, produced from vascular hyperpermeability, spontaneously improved. These results suggested that the latter subset of patients may fare better with laser treatment under Branch Vein Occlusion Study criteria as opposed to observation.

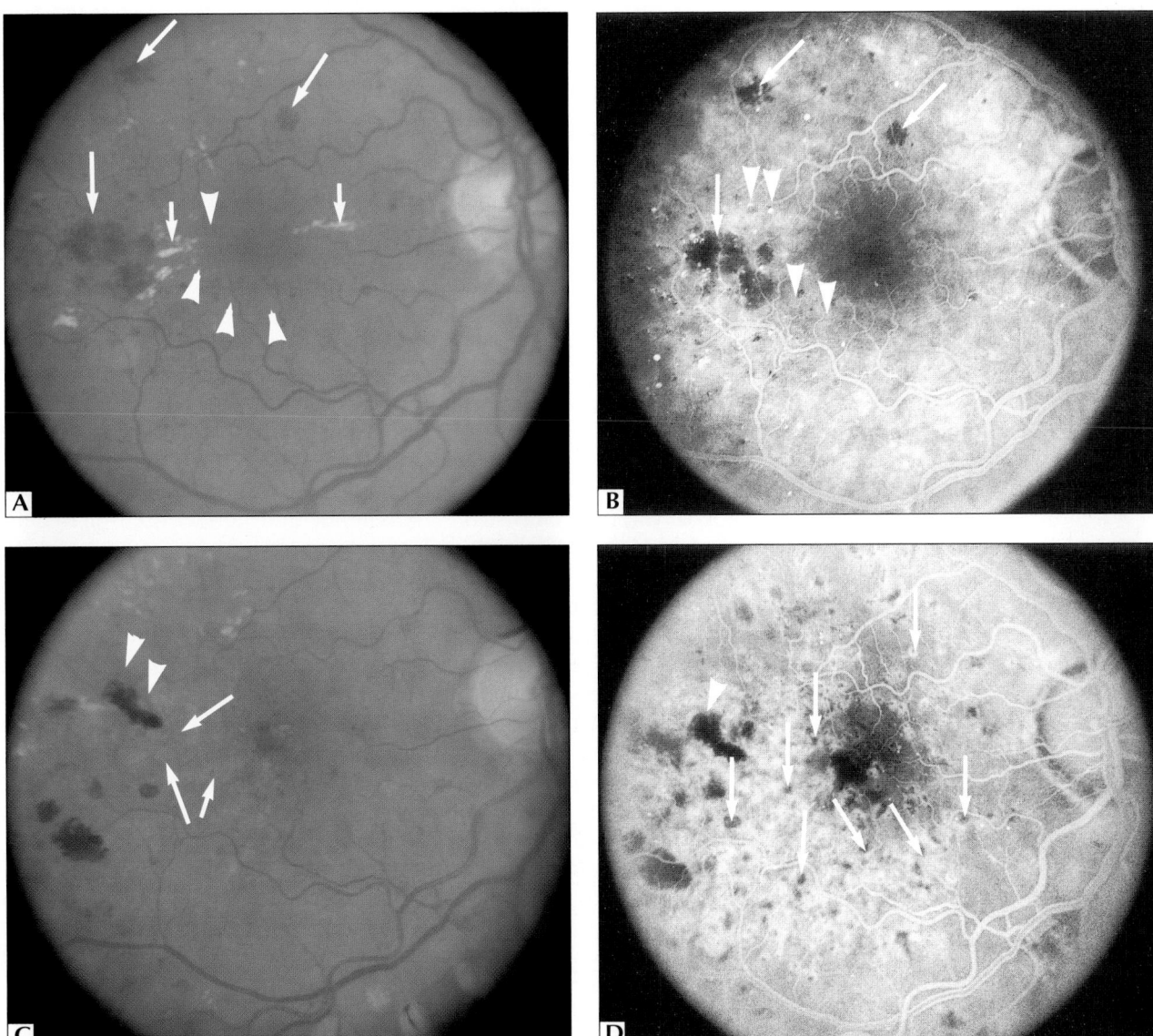

FIGURE 4-6 **A**, Pretreatment red-free photograph of an eye with multiple retinal hemorrhages (*long arrows*), microaneurysms (*arrowheads*), and lipid exudates (*shorter arrows*) in the posterior pole. Stereo photography is required to recognize retinal thickening. **B**, Pretreatment fluorescein angiogram of the same eye shows blockage of fluorescence (*long arrows*) in the areas of retinal hemorrhage. Multiple microaneurysms (*small arrowheads*) can be seen temporal to the fovea. **C**, Red-free photograph of the same eye 3 years following focal laser photocoagulation to areas of leakage. Note reabsorption of intraretinal hemorrhages (*area between long arrows*) and reabsorption of lipid exudates (*area superior to short arrow*) temporal to fovea. Only small residual foci of intraretinal hemorrhage (*arrowheads*) remain around the fovea. **D**, Post-treatment fluorescein angiogram clearly shows areas of laser treatment (*arrows*). Focal laser burns corresponding to treated microaneurysms are seen temporal and superior to the fovea. A grid pattern of laser burns has also been applied inferiorly. In comparison to Figure 4-6*B*, note disappearance of microaneurysms temporal to the fovea. A small focus of intraretinal hemorrhage remains temporal to fovea (*small arrowheads*).

Branch vein occlusion study

Design

The Branch Vein Occlusion Study was a multicenter, randomized, controlled clinical trial sponsored by the National Eye Institute that evaluated the effects of laser photocoagulation for the potential complications of BRVO, retinal neovascularization, and macular edema [22–24]. One arm of the study randomly assigned 139 eyes with macular edema and reduced vision to either laser treatment or no laser treatment. Eligibility criteria included the following:

- Duration of 3 to 18 months
- Visual acuity of 20/40 or worse
- Fluorescein angiographic evidence of foveal involvement
- Absence of retinal hemorrhage involving the fovea
- Absence of other ocular disease threatening visual acuity
- No anticoagulant therapy

No patients were eligible before 3 months after onset of the BRVO, because spontaneous resolution of the macular edema and concurrent visual improvement occur most often within this time period.

Technique

A fluorescein angiogram less than 1 month old was used for diagnostic and treatment purposes. Argon blue-green laser treatment was applied in a grid pattern, with photocoagulation extending no closer to the fovea than the edge of the capillary-free zone and no further peripherally than the major vascular arcades. The grid was applied to areas demonstrating leakage on fluorescein angiography. Treatment parameters included a duration of 0.1 second, a 100-μm-diameter spot size, and a power setting sufficient to produce a medium white burn. Eyes were reevaluated at 4-month intervals, and additional photocoagulation was applied if macular edema persisted with continued visual deterioration. In most cases, only one treatment was sufficient.

Results

The study demonstrated a beneficial treatment effect for eyes with macular edema. Of eyes receiving photocoagulation, 63% gained two or more lines of visual acuity, whereas only 36% of untreated eyes showed similar improvement. Almost twice as many treated eyes had a visual acuity of 20/40 or better compared with those in the nontreatment group after 3 years of follow-up. Because more eyes improved within 1 year after diagnosis than afterward, it appeared that longer duration of BRVO adversely affected the likelihood of regaining visual acuity. The benefit of laser photocoagulation, however, persisted independent of the duration of the occlusion. In addition, hypertension (defined as taking antihypertensive medication) appeared to have an adverse effect on visual acuity. Complications from grid laser photocoagulation were rare. The most common side effect was the production of paracentral scotomas. These symptoms were transient and usually resolved several weeks to months after treatment. The study emphasized careful study of the fluorescein angiogram to identify the capillary-free zone that surrounds the center of the macula and intraretinal hemorrhage to avoid direct laser treatment to such areas.

Central retinal vein occlusion

In central retinal vein occlusion (CRVO), the obstruction is secondary to thrombosis of the central retinal vein at the level of the lamina cribrosa. Clinically, the diagnosis is based on the presence of dilated retinal veins and retinal hemorrhages in all four quadrants of the retina. Macular edema can result from retinal capillary leakage or nonperfusion identified by fluorescein angiography. Risk factors associated with CRVO include hypertension, cardiovascular disease, and diabetes mellitus.

Central retinal vein occlusions are classified as perfused or nonischemic and nonperfused or ischemic, based on fluorescein angiographic perfusion characteristics. Retinal capillary nonperfusion of 10 disc areas or greater is associated with development of iris or retinal neovascularization. Iris neovascularization represents an ominous precursor of neovascular glaucoma, because fibrovascular contraction of new abnormal iris vessels closes the anterior chamber angle, causing an acute rise of intraocular pressure. Identifying patients with nonperfused CRVO is partially important, because laser treatment can promote regression of new iris vessels.

The natural history of macular edema in CRVO is poorly understood [25]. In perfused CRVO, macular edema is presumably the primary cause of significant visual loss [26]. Other investigators have found that edematous (nonperfused) CRVO carries a guarded to unfavorable visual prognosis [27]. For these reasons, a study is currently underway to investiate the potential benefit of laser photocoagulation for this vascular disorder.

Central vein occlusion study

Design

The Central Vein Occlusion Study was a collaborative multicenter, randomized, clinical trial initiated to study the effect of laser photocoagulation on the management of ocular complications associated with CRVOs. This large trial is based on a small pilot study that noted improvement in macular edema following grid pattern photocoagulation [28]. As part of this study, grid pattern photocoagulation therapy is being evaluated for efficacy in the treatment of macular edema associated with CRVOs and capillary leakage. Eligibility criteria for this group of patients includes the following:

- Macular edema involving the fovea
- Visual acuity between 5/200 and 20/50 with no other apparent explanation for decreased acuity
- Ocular media compatible with 20/20 Snellen acuity

The study is scheduled for completion in February 1994, with the results to be published shortly thereafter. Until that time, by extrapolating Branch Vein Occlusion Study data, grid laser treatment of macular edema secondary to capillary leakage in CRVO appears to be a reasonable option in cases where visual acuity is diminished.

Technique

The technique described for treating macular edema associated with CRVOs is similar to the technique used in the Branch Vein Occlusion Study. Argon laser is being used in the Central Vein Occlusion Study. Recommended treatment parameters are as follows:

1. 100-µm spot size
2. 0.1-second duration
3. Laser spots one burn width apart
4. Light to medium white burn
5. Application to areas of leaking capillaries

OTHER CONDITIONS

Aphakic cystoid macular edema

Aphakic and pseudophakic CME, commonly referred to as the Irvine-Gass syndrome, remains a frustrating complication responsible for visual loss following uneventful cataract surgery. The pathogenesis remains unclear but has been attributed to a variety of causes, ranging from operative technique to prostaglandin-mediated postoperative inflammation. Many cases resolve spontaneously, but a small percentage develop significant and sometimes permanent visual disability. Various modalities have been tried to treat this disorder, with varying degrees of success [29–31].

Pharmacologic therapy is the mainstay of treatment in aphakic CME. Anti-inflammatory prostaglandin

inhibitors and corticosteroid drugs, both topically and systemically, have been advocated. However, no large trials to document their efficacy have been performed.

In cases where vitreous incarceration to the wound is associated with aphakic CME, a prospective randomized trial has shown that the use of vitrectomy in removing the vitreous strands will improve the macular edema [32].

With the development of the neodymium-yttrium aluminum garnet (Nd:YAG) laser, vitreous strands can now be treated without surgery [33,34]. Katzen and coworkers [33] reported visual improvement greater than or equal to 2 lines of Snellen acuity in 12 of 14 eyes that underwent Nd:YAG laser vitreolysis. Levy and coworkers [34] had visual improvement of at least 2 Snellen lines in eight of 20 eyes that underwent Nd:YAG laser vitreolysis.

Macroaneurysms

Arterial macroaneurysms are acquired round or fusiform dilatations of retinal arterioles associated with lipid exudation and retinal fluid accumulation. Such vascular changes are seen often in hypertension and arteriosclerotic cardiovascular disease [35]. Extension of fluid and exudate into the macula can result in visual loss. Although retinal macroaneurysms usually thrombose and spontaneously involute with reabsorption of vascular leakage, laser photocoagulation can minimize the possibility of foveal involvement. No formal treatment guidelines have been established by controlled clinical trials. Laser treatment of light intensity applied over the lesion can cause attenuation of the macroaneurysm over a period of weeks to months, with subsequent clearing of the macular edema and accompanying lipid exudation.

Other exudative retinal vasculopathies

Macular edema associated with lipid exudation is also seen with other less commonly diagnosed conditions, such as Coats' disease, Hippel's disease, parafoveal telangiectasis, and radiation retinopathy.

Coats' disease is an idiopathic exudative retinopathy characterized by abnormal telangiectatic, dilated vessels, with massive subretinal and intraretinal fluid accumulation. This unilateral condition affects males primarily without evidence of genetic transmission or racial predilection [36]. Two forms have been recognized clinically: 1) a juvenile form diagnosed before age 16 and associated with strabismus or leukocoria and 2) a less common adult form associated with hypercholesterolemia [37]. Fluorescein angiography can identify areas of capillary nonperfusion and loss of blood-retinal barrier integrity not otherwise detectable clinically.

Although many cases may be followed conservatively, macular involvement usually requires intervention with angiographically guided laser photocoagulation [36]. Not infrequently, lesions in the peripheral retina may produce pathology in the posterior pole. Cryotherapy and diathermy have also been used to treat this condition with some success [37].

Retinal capillary hemangioma is a retinal vascular tumor associated with exudative maculopathy. The presence of multiple or bilateral lesions suggest a diagnosis of the autosomal dominant Hippel-Lindau disease [38]. Ophthalmoscopically, a dilated, tortuous afferent arteriole feeds a distinct, red nodule that is drained by an efferent venule [38]. These lesions will leak subretinal fluid and a lipid exudate that will cause visual loss with macular involvement. Like Coats' disease, peripheral lesions can produce macular changes. Fluorescein angiography demonstrates rapid filling of the afferent arteriole and a lacy capillary network in the early phase with leakage into the retina and overlying vitreous in the late phases. Photocoagulation with argon laser is suggested for smaller lesions (2 mm) posterior to the equator of the globe [39]. Additional treatment of feeder vessels may be necessary for larger lesions (3 to 5 mm). Peripheral lesions should be treated with cryotherapy.

Parafoveal telangiectasis can also be associated with macular edema. Small leaking telangiectatic vessels are often found temporal to the fovea and can easily be seen on fluorescein angiography. An association with diabetes mellitus has been reported [40]. Laser treatment has been attempted in selected subtypes of this disorder, with varying degrees of success [40].

Radiation retinopathy represents a slowly progressive microangiopathy produced from toxic levels of radiation exposure. Visual loss may result from capillary nonperfusion, macular edema, or vitreous hemorrhage from proliferation of abnormal retinal vessels. Although scatter photocoagulation for optic disc and retinal neovascularization may prevent complications of vitreous hemorrhage and neovascular glaucoma, grid laser treatment for macular edema provides only transient visual improvement [41]. This condition usually progresses from an exudative to nonperfused phase not amenable to laser treatment.

Retinitis pigmentosa

Retinitis pigmentosa is a hereditary dystrophy characterized by the onset of night blindness in childhood or young adulthood with progressive contraction of the peripheral visual field. Macular edema has been reported with this condition [42,43]. Cystic changes, evident as leakage on fluorescein angiography, can cause a decrease in vision. Occasionally, no staining or leakage is found on angiography, even though it is appreciated biomicroscopically. Such findings may be compatible with a form of macular edema recently described with BRVO, namely the hypertonic extracellular accumulation of fluid produced from cell death [21]. The mechanism for the macular edema in retinitis pigmentosa is unknown. Newsome and Blacharski [44] treated macular edema associated with retinitis pigmentosa in 16 patients. The fellow eye served as the control. Following laser treatment, 13 of 16 eyes showed resolution of fluorescein leakage, but only three eyes had improved Snellen visual acuity more than 2 lines. Heckenlively [45] cautions against the use of such grid treatment in these patients because it may impair the minimal central visual field that remains. Treatment of the edema with oral carbonic anhydrase inhibitors has been demonstrated to be beneficial in some cases [46].

CONCLUSIONS

Macular edema remains a cause of significant visual loss in many retinal diseases. Laser surgery has allowed the ophthalmologist to treat this condition with increasing success. Large, prospective, randomized clinical trials have added invaluable information to our knowledge of these disease processes. The Early Treatment Diabetic Retinopathy Study has shown that focal treatment of diabetic macular edema is beneficial in the prevention of visual loss. The Branch Vein Occlusion Study has also shown a benefit of focal laser treatment for macular edema secondary to venous occlusive disease. The results of the Central Vein Occlusion Study will be available shortly to provide appropriate treatment parameters for macular edema in this form of vascular occlusive disease. Other less common etiologies of exudative retinopathies, such as intraocular tumors, are also treatable by laser photocoagulation in the appropriate clinical setting. Future observations, clinical studies, and advances in laser technology will more clearly define and possibly expand the role of laser treatment for the various causes of macular edema.

REFERENCES AND RECOMMENDED READING

Recently published papers of particular interest
have been highlighted as:

• Of interest

•• Of outstanding interest

1. Mainster MA: Wavelength selection in macular photoco-agulation: tissue optics, thermal effects, and laser systems. *Ophthalmology* 1986, 93:952–958.

2. Ferris FL III, Patz A: Macular edema. A complication of diabetic retinopathy. *Surv of Ophthalmol* 1984, 28:452–461.

3. Bresnick GH: Diabetic maculopathy. A critical review highlighting diffuse macular edema. *Ophthalmology* 1984, 90:1301–1317.

4. Bresnick GH: Diabetic macular edema. A review. *Ophthalmology* 1986, 93:989–997.

5. Klein R, Klein BEK, Moss SE, *et al.*: The Wisconsin Epidemiologic Study of Diabetic Retinopathy. IV. Diabetic macular edema. *Ophthalmology* 1984, 91:1464–1474.

6. Patz A, Schatz H, Berkow JW, *et al.*: Macular edema—an overlooked complication of diabetic retinopathy. *Trans Am Acad Ophthalmol Otolaryngol* 1973, 77:34–42.

7. Blankenship GW: Diabetic macular edema and argon laser photocoagulation: a prospective randomized study. *Ophthalmology* 1979, 86:69–78.

8. Multicentered Controlled Study: Photocoagulation in treat-ment of diabetic maculopathy. *Lancet* 1975, ii:1110–1113.

9. Townsend C, Bailey J, Kohner E: Xenon arc photocoagu-lation for the treatment of diabetic maculopathy: interim report of a multicentre controlled clinical study. *Br J Ophthalmol* 1980, 64:285–291.

10. Early Treatment Diabetic Retinopathy Study Research Group: Photocoagulation for diabetic macular edema. Early Treatment Diabetic Retinopathy Study Report Number 1. *Arch Ophthalmol* 1985, 103:1796–1806.

11. Early Treatment Diabetic Retinopathy Study Research Group: Treatment techniques and clinical guidelines for photocoagulation of diabetic macular edema. Early Treatment Diabetic Retinopathy Study Report Number 2. *Ophthalmology* 1987, 94:761–774.

12. Early Treatment Diabetic Retinopathy Study Research Group: Photocoagulation for diabetic macular edema. Early Treatment Diabetic Retinopathy Report Number 4. *Int Ophthalmol Clin* 1987, 27:265–272.

13. Early Treatment Diabetic Retinopathy Study Research Group: Early Treatment Diabetic Retinopathy Report Number 7. *Ophthalmology* 1991, 98(suppl):741–756.

14. Early Treatment Diabetic Retinopathy Study Research Group: Early photocoagulation for diabetic retinopathy. Early Treatment Diabetic Retinopathy Report Number 9. *Ophthalmology* 1991, 98(suppl):766–785.

15. Varley MP, Frank E, Purnell EW: Subretinal neovascular-ization after focal argon laser for diabetic macular edema. *Ophthalmology* 1988, 95:567–573.

16. Lewis H, Schachat AP, Haimann MH, *et al.*: Choroidal neovascularization after laser photocoagulation for diabet-ic macular edema. *Ophthalmology* 1990, 97:503–511.

17. Schatz H, Madeira D, McDonald R, *et al.*: Progressive enlargement of laser scars following grid laser photocoag-ulation for diffuse diabetic macular edema. *Arch Ophthalmol* 1991, 109:1549–1551.

18. Han DP, Mieler WF, Burton TC: Submacular fibrosis after photocoagulation for diabetic macular edema. *Am J Ophthalmol* 1992, 113:513–521.

19. Guyer DR, D'Amico DJ, Smith CW: Subretinal fibrosis after laser photocoagulation for diabetic macular edema. *Am J Ophthalmol* 1992, 113:652–656.

20. The Eye Disease Case-Control Study Group: Risk factors for branch retinal vein occlusion. *Am J Ophthalmol* 1993, 116:286–296.

21. Finkelstein D: Ischemic macular edema: recognition and favorable natural history in branch vein occlusion. *Arch Ophthalmol* 1992, 110:1427–1434.

22. The Branch Vein Occlusion Study Group: Argon laser photocoagulation for macular edema in branch vein occlusion. *Am J Ophthalmol* 1984, 98:271–282.

23. Finkelstein D: Argon laser photocoagulation for macular edema in branch vein occlusion. *Ophthalmology* 1986, 93:975–977.

24. Finklestein D: Laser treatment of branch and central reti-nal vein occlusion. *Int Ophthalmol Clin* 1990, 30:84–88.

25. Central Vein Occlusion Study Group: Baseline and early natural history report: the central vein occlusion study. *Arch Ophthalmol* 1993, 111:1087–1095.

26. Hayreh SS: Classification of central retinal vein occlusion. *Ophthalmology* 1983, 90:458–474.

27. Coscas G, Dhermy P: *Occlusions Veineuses Retiniennes* Paris: Masson; 1978:284–314.

28. Klein ML, Finkelstein D: Macular grid photocoagulation for macular edema in central retinal vein occlusion. *Arch Ophthalmol* 1989, 107:1297–1302.

29. Yannuzzi LA: A perspective on the treatment of aphakic cystoid macular edema. *Surv Ophthalmol* 1984, 8(suppl):540–553.

30. Jampol LM, Sanders DR, Kraff MC: Prophylaxis and ther-apy of aphakic cystoid macular edema. *Surv Ophthalmol* 1984, 28(suppl):535–539.

31. Milch FA, Yannuzzi LA: Medical and surgical treatment of aphakic cystoid macular edema. *Int Ophthalmol Clin* 1987, 27:205–217.

32. Fung WE: Vitrectomy for chronic aphakic cystoid macular edema: results of a national, collaborative, prospective, randomized investigation. *Ophthalmology* 1985, 92:1102–1111.

33. Katzen LE, Fleischman JA: YAG laser treatment of cystoid macular edema. *Am J Ophthalmol* 1983, 95:589–592.

34. Levy JH, Pisacano AM: Clinical experience with Nd:YAG laser vitreolysis in the anterior segment. *J Cataract Refract Surg* 1987, 13:548–550.

35. Robertson DM: Macroaneurysms of the retinal arteries. *Trans Am Acad Ophthalmol Otolaryngol* 1973, 77:55–67.

36. Haller JA: Coats' disease. In *Retina*, vol 2. Edited by Ryan SJ, Schachat AP, Murphy RP, *et al*. St. Louis: CV Mosby; 1989:491–495.

37. Pauleikoff D, Kruger K, Heinrich T, *et al*.: Epidemiologic features and therapeutic results in Coats' disease. *Invest Ophthalmol* 1988, 29(suppl):335.

38. Shields JA, Shields CL: Vascular tumors of the retina and optic disc. In *Intraocular Tumors: A Text and Atlas*. Edited by Shields JA, Shields CL. Philadelphia: WB Saunders; 1992:393–419.

39. Shields JA: Therapeutic approaches to intraocular tumors. In *Ophthalmic Surgery: Principles and Practice*, edn 2. Edited by Spaeth GL. Philadelphia: WB Saunders; 1990:702–722.

40. Chew EY, Murphy RP, Newsome DA, *et al*.: Parafoveal telangiectasis and diabetic retinopathy. *Arch Ophthalmol* 1986, 104:71–75.

41. Schachat AP: Radiation retinopathy. In *In Retina*, vol 2. Edited by Ryan SJ, Schachat AP, Murphy RP, *et al*. St. Louis: CV Mosby; 1989:541–545.

42. Spalton DJ, Bird AC, Cleary PE: Retinitis pigmentosa and retinal edema. *Br J Ophthalmol* 1978, 62:174.

43. Gass JDM: *Stereoscopic Atlas of Macular Diseases* St. Louis: CV Mosby; 1987:274–284.

44. Newsome DA, Blacharski PA: Grid photocoagulation for macular edema in patients with retinitis pigmentosa. *Am J Ophthalmol* 1987, 103:161–166.

45. Heckenlively JR: Grid photocoagulation for macular edema in patients with retinitis pigmentosa. *Am J Ophthalmol* 1987, 104:94–95.

46. Cox SN, Hay E, Bird AC: Treatment of chronic macular edema with acetazolamide. *Arch Ophthalmol* 1988, 106:1190–1195.

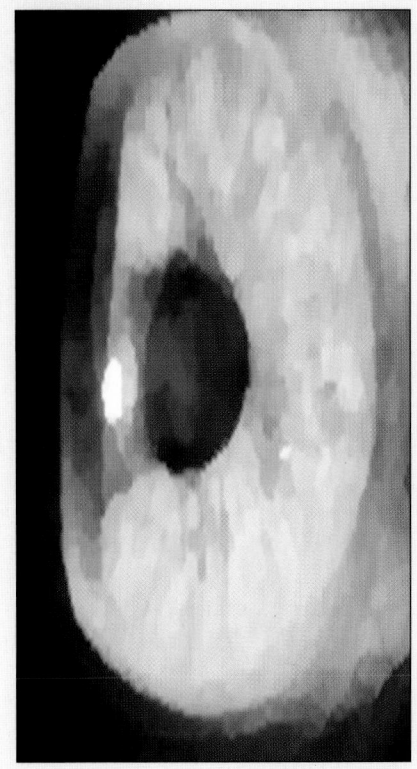

CHAPTER 5

LASERS IN THE TREATMENT OF PROLIFERATIVE RETINOPATHIES

DOMINIC MCHUGH

LUKE HERBERT

EVA M. KOHNER

Proliferative retinopathies are characterized by the presence of abnormal neovascularization that may arise from the optic disc or from vessels in the retinal periphery—most commonly from veins. Whatever the cause of the new vessels, they always represent a sight-threatening condition, which is the worse for not being associated with any visual symptoms. Patients are thus not aware of the presence of abnormal vessels until complications arise. These complications include vitreous hemorrhage and tractional abnormalities, including peripheral retinal and macular detachment. Until the advent of photocoagulation, no effective treatment was available for most of the proliferative retinopathies. These retinopathies have been a common cause of blindness, much of which can be avoided today by early recognition and treatment with lasers.

In the first part of this review we concentrate on the background, technology, and rationale of using lasers to treat proliferative retinopathy. In the second part, the treatment of the different conditions characterized by neovascularization, diabetic retinopathy in particular, is considered, and complications of treatment are addressed. Although important previous work is considered, emphasis is on more recent work, between 1990 and the present.

BACKGROUND

Photocoagulation for the treatment of retinal conditions has been used for more than 40 years. Meyer-Schwickerath [1] initially used focused sunlight to produce retinal lesions, but this use was superseded by the use of a modified Beck arc. The development of the xenon arc photocoagulator provided a source of broadband optical radiation, which was effective in producing full-thickness chorioretinal lesions. Xenon arc devices are of proven effectiveness in the treatment of proliferative diabetic retinopathy and are still commonly used for retinal therapeutic procedures [2].

Lasers

The first laser to be used in the treatment of proliferative retinopathies was the Ruby laser (emitting 694.3 nm). Aiello and coworkers [3] were the first to describe scatter treatment for the management of diabetic retinopathy with the use of this laser. The most widely used laser currently is the argon laser (emitting at 488 and 514.5 nm). Its clinical potential was first investigated by L'Esperance [4], and it became commercially available in 1971. The effectiveness of the argon laser in the treatment of proliferative retinopathies, including subretinal neovascular membranes, was quickly established [5–7].

Other lasers, such as the krypton laser (647 nm) and dye lasers (575 to 630 nm), came into use in the late 1970s and early 1980s, but do not offer any special advantage over the argon laser in the treatment of retinal neovascularization [8–10]. The most recent commercially available lasers for the treatment of proliferative retinopathies are the neodymium-yttrium aluminum garnet (Nd:YAG) and diode lasers.

Neodymium-yttrium aluminum garnet laser

The advent of the Q-switched Nd:YAG laser, emitting at 1064 nm, introduced the phenomenon of nonlinear damage processes, or tissue "photodisruption" [11]. The production of high energy pulses of laser energy concentrated in both time and space allowed transparent tissues to be cut within the eye. The Q-switched Nd:YAG laser has been successfully used in the incision of vitreous membranes in patients with severe proliferative retinal disease [12]. Nd:YAG lasers that emit laser energy in a continuous-wave mode and therefore have a thermal, photocoagulative mode

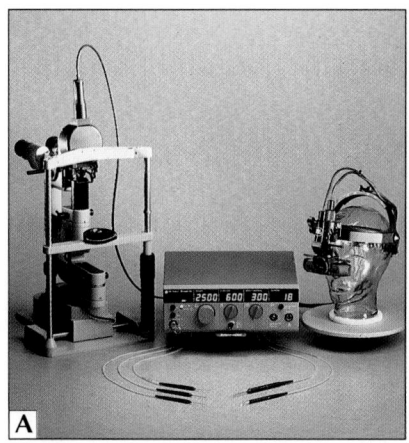 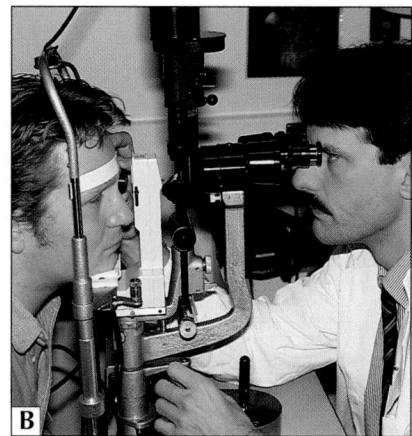 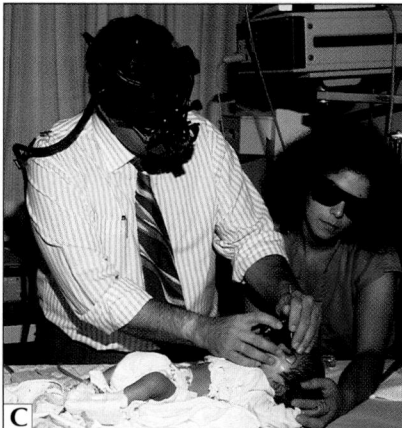

FIGURE 5-1 Ophthalmic diode lasers. **A,** Slit-lamp mounted version. **B,** Indirect diode laser. **C,** Transscleral endolaser.

of action have been recently introduced. Successful treatment of proliferative retinopathy has been reported with the use of infrared (1064 nm) and frequency-doubled (532 nm, green) continuous-wave Nd:YAG lasers [13,14•].

Diode lasers

Advances in semiconductor technology have allowed the development of infrared diode lasers (750 to 950 nm) measuring a few millimeters. These lasers are used in compact disc players and have important applications in the field of optical printing and communication.

The recent availability of laser diodes with an output power of 1 to 3 W has stimulated interest in their potential applications in ophthalmic surgery. These diodes are compact (being less than 1 mm), and the laser system is portable (typically weighing 10 kg). The diodes may be powered by either a standard 13-A power supply or a 6-V battery, and no ancillary cooling facilities are needed.

Currently, most high-powered diodes emit in the infrared region of the spectrum (810 nm), which confers a number of biophysical advantages to their use. The laser emission is invisible to the patient, and therefore there is an absence of bright flashes during each exposure. There is high transmission of this wavelength through blood, allowing more effective delivery of the incident energy to the retina through preretinal and vitreous blood [15]. Because there is low absorption by macular luteal pigment, the risk for inner retinal damage after photocoagulation in the macular region is reduced [16]. There is low scleral absorption and scattering, thus allowing transscleral photocoagulation to be performed [17]. Finally, the use of near-infrared radiation eliminates the adverse photochemical effects on macular cones that may occur secondary to short wavelength exposure. This phenomenon has been dubbed the "blue light hazard," and use of the argon blue-green laser can produce tritanopic defects in both the patient and the surgeon [18].

Ophthalmic diode lasers are available that can perform either transpupillary photocoagulation (via either a slit-lamp microscope, or an indirect ophthalmoscope), endophotocoagulation in vitreoretinal surgery, and transscleral retinal and ciliary body photocoagulation (Fig. 5-1). Several histologic and clinical studies have demonstrated the efficacy of each of these modalities [19–24]. In view of their ergonomic and biophysical advantages, it is likely that diode lasers will become increasingly more widely used in ophthalmologic procedures. Tables 5-1 and 5-2 show the comparison between the most commonly used laser, the argon laser, and the diode laser.

RATIONALE FOR USING PHOTOCOAGULATION TO TREAT PROLIFERATIVE RETINOPATHIES

Neovascularization is a complex response of retinal vessels precipitated by an imbalance between stimulators and inhibitors of angiogenesis that occurs in the presence of large areas of ischemic retina. The presence of an angiogenic factor was postulated as early as 1948 [25]. Since then, advances in cell biology—in particular, the development of cell culture work—has shown that there are several angiogenic factors that are liberated mostly by vascular cells but also by the retinal pigment epithelium and glial cells [26–31]. Other inhibitors of cell proliferation have also been identified [32]. The normal cell–cell interaction is disrupted by ischemia and hypoxia, resulting in new vessel formation.

Panretinal photocoagulation (PRP) has been found to be effective in causing regression of neovascularization [33,34]. Although the exact mechanism for this regression is not known, several hypotheses have been advanced.

TABLE 5-1	COMPARISON OF ERGONOMIC FEATURES OF DIODE AND ARGON LASERS	
	Diode	**Argon**
Emission	810 mm	488–514.4 mm
Power	3 W	3 W
Energy requirement	Single-phase	Single/3-phase
Cooling requirement	1 A	25–50 A
	Ambient air	Air/water
Electric/optic conversion efficacy	25%	0.05%
Weight	10 kg	Not portable
Color safety filter	None	Yes
Delivery system	Slit lamp/indirect	Slit lamp/indirect
	Endo/transscleral	Endo
Micromanipulator	Absent	Available

1. Destruction of ischemic areas. Because proliferation is induced by ischemic retina, elimination of this ischemia will result in regression of new vessels [35]. Indeed, lack of response to photocoagulation can be eliminated if all nonperfused areas are treated.

2. Increasing oxygen availability. The supply of oxygen to the retina comes from the retinal and choroidal vessels. In normal circumstances, most of the choroidal oxygen supply is to the photoreceptors, which are very actively metabolizing cells. The retinal circulation can maintain adequate supply for the inner retina, provided the blood supply is normal. In the presence of vascular occlusion, hypoxia and ischemia result. Destruction of the photoreceptors and pigment epithelium allows adequate oxygen to reach the retina from the choroidal circulation [36,37].

3. Release of inhibitors of neovascularization derived from the pigment epithelium or from plasma [38].

Although the biologic mechanisms of action have not been clearly established, since Aiello's report on panretinal photocoagulation for diabetic retinopathy, several clinical trials have demonstrated the efficacy of photocoagulation in the treatment of proliferative retinopathies [3]. The largest and most important of these trials was conducted by the Diabetic Retinopathy Study Group in the United States, which reported on 1758 patients with diabetic retinopathy [39].

TREATMENT OF PROLIFERATIVE RETINOPATHIES

Diabetic retinopathy

Diabetic retinopathy remains the most common cause of blindness in the working-age population in developed countries, and it is occurring with increased frequency in the developing world. Although the argon laser is the most commonly used laser in the treatment of diabetic retinopathy, other lasers are also effective. In recent years there has been increased use of the diode laser, which, because of its relative cheapness and portability, is preferred in the less developed countries. Its effects are similar to those of the argon laser [40•]. Although there is no argument about the need for panretinal photocoagulation, the extent of treatment, intensity of treatment, and burn size have not been firmly and uniformly established.

Number of burns

The Diabetic Retinopathy Study Group study suggested 1200 burns for the treatment of proliferative retinopathy. Today, few ophthalmologists would use such a low number of burns for panretinal photocoagulation. In any one session 800 to 1200 burns should be used, and the patients should be reassessed 1 to 3 weeks later (in the case of severe neovascularization, no longer than 1 week later); further treatment should be given depending on the response of the new vessels. The ideal amount of treatment is that which gets rid of all new vessels or leaves just some inactive vestiges behind. Whereas in most patients this effect can be achieved with 2000 to 4000 burns, in some, many more are required. Aylward and coworkers [41] reported on a study in which 28 patients had proliferative retinopathy refractory to treatment and found that 89% of the patients responded when an increased number of burns (up to 11,513) was used (Fig. 5-2).

Extent of treatment

Although it is accepted that panretinal treatment is required for disc neovascularization, there is some dispute regarding the extent of treatment necessary in patients with peripheral new vessels in one or two quadrants. Our view is that panretinal photocoagulation should be used in all patients with new vessels.

TABLE 5-2	COMPARISON OF BIOPHYSICAL FEATURES OF DIODE AND ARGON LASERS		
		Diode	**Argon**
	Pigment epithelial absorption	10%	40%–50%
	Luteal pigment absorption	Less than 1%	70% blue-green
	Blood transmission	High	15% green
			Low
	Transscleral transmission	High	Absent
	Discomfort	Variable/common	Low
	Visible treatment beam	No	Yes
	Burn appearance	Delayed evolution, grey	White
	Risk for choroidal hemorrhage	Low	Very low

Fluorescein angiography will confirm that ischemia is widely distributed throughout the mid and far periphery of the retina in patients with new vessels, even if they are seen in one quadrant only. The work of Turner and coworkers [42] confirmed that within 3 years of the appearance of first peripheral new vessels, almost all patients required panretinal photocoagulation. Early treatment, even if light, is likely to prevent the formation of neovascularization in ischemic preproliferative eyes.

Intensity of treatment

The radiant exposure required to produce a given lesion primarily depends on the concentration of melanin within the retinal pigment epithelium. It is generally believed that it is only necessary to induce a burn with threshold (greyish-white) intensity. More intense burns are likely to result with more complications—nerve fiber damage and visual field loss in particular [43,44]. Although in patients with preproliferative retinopathy and in those with early new vessels light treatment is usually sufficient, in some patients with severe proliferative lesions, especially if they are apparently refractory to treatment, heavy burns resulting in xenon-arc-like, through-and-through burns that destroy retina are required (Fig. 5-3). Whether such

heavy burns can be obviated by timely vitrectomy has not been established. In young patients with very severe rapidly progressing retinopathy in whom the vitreous is not completely detached, such an operation is not without hazards.

Size and duration of burns

The number of burns applied will depend on the size of the burns. In the past it has been suggested that 200-μm burns should be applied at and near the posterior pole, and larger (300–500 μm or even larger) burns, in the periphery. The advantage of such large burns is that fewer are required, and thus the treatment time is reduced, with advantage to both physician and patient. However, with the introduction of more strict definitions of visual fields required for obtaining driving licenses in some countries (notably the United Kingdom) it has been suggested that burn sizes should not exceed 200 μm except in the very far periphery [45•].

Although most treatment is with short laser exposures of pulse duration (0.05–0.1 second), in a recent article Wade and Blankenship [46] compared 0.1- and 0.5-second argon laser burns. They found that more patients who received the shorter duration of burns lost two or more lines in visual acuity and they also suffered from more hemorrhages. However, 0.5-sec-

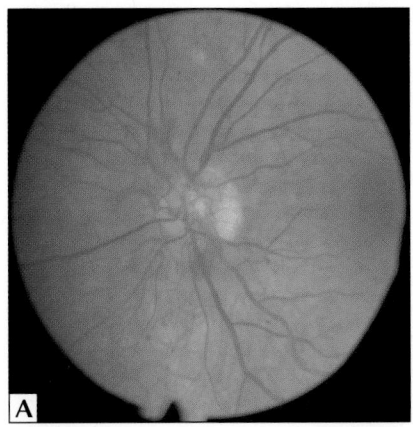 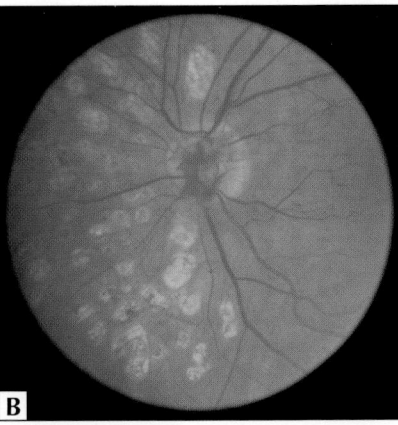 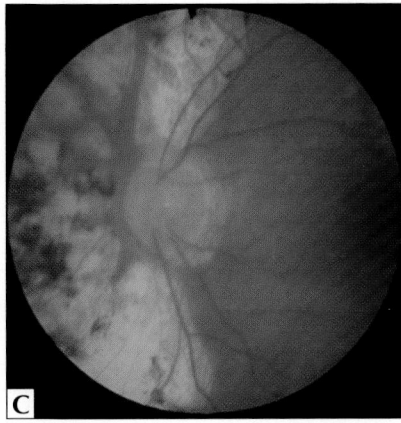

FIGURE 5-2 A, Patient with disc neovascularization before treatment. **B**, Inadequate argon laser treatment does not eliminate new vessel formation. **C**, Adequate treatment causes complete regression of new vessels.

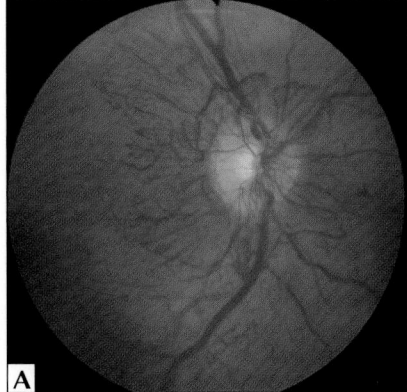 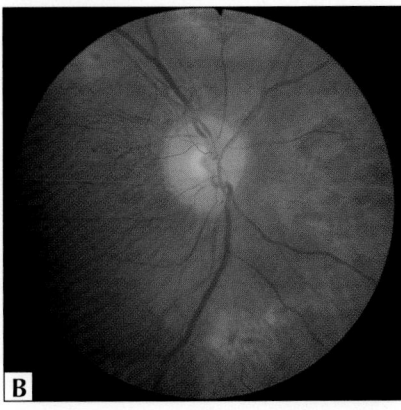

FIGURE 5-3 A, Florid disc neovascularization. **B**, Same area 3 weeks after heavy argon laser burns; new vessels show marked regression.

ond burns were more commonly associated with extension of traction detachment. Regression of new vessels was similar in the two groups.

Panretinal photocoagulation with the diode laser has been associated with discomfort because of the deeper choroidal penetration of the infrared wavelength. This symptom may be minimized by using a pulse duration of 100 ms, which will limit thermal spread into the choroid (Fig. 5-4).

Complications of diabetic retinopathy

Acute complications The most common acute complications of diabetic retinopathy are well recognized. They include the most devastating—foveal burn—which is very uncommon and is usually caused by movement of the eye. Choroidal detachment after treatment was common after heavy xenon arc photocoagulation and is only seen occasionally when very heavy treatment is required. Choroidal hemorrhage is also uncommon but is seen occasionally when krypton laser treatment is used.

The most important of the acute complications is macular edema. Although a mild degree of macular edema is not uncommon in insulin-dependent diabetic patients with extensive neovascularization, post-treatment macular edema may occur. This condition may persist and occasionally result in permanent reduction of vision. The Diabetic Retinopathy Study Group study found that 10% of patients lost two or more lines of visual acuity after treatment [39]. In a large study of 175 patients treated by panretinal photocoagulation, 47 developed increasing macular edema [47]. In 26 it was still present at 3 to 12 months, and in seven it persisted for more than 2 years. This persistence occurred despite the treatment being delivered in several sessions, although one could fault the treatment, which started near the posterior pole and was continued by concentric ring treatment more peripherally. Because of the frequency of post-treatment macular edema, our practice is to do a perifoveal grid before panretinal photocoagulation at least in those patients who are older than 50 years (in our experience they are more likely to develop macular edema, with poor recovery). This treatment is also applied in those who are younger but who have macular edema as well as new vessels.

Chronic complications The most common chronic complications of diabetic retinopathy are visual field loss and some difficulty with dark adaptation. Three articles examining field defects have been published recently. Buckley and coworkers [48] reported failures in four of five patients who had xenon light coagulation, compared with 11 of 25 patients treated by laser. A subsequent report compared diode and argon panretinal photocoagulation in 15 eyes with proliferative diabetic

retinopathy [49]. Through the use of an elegant technique they treated one hemisphere (upper or lower) with diode, the other with argon laser. Eyes that had received panretinal photocoagulation had significantly decreased fields compared with untreated eyes of diabetic patients. They found no statistically significant difference in field loss between the diode- and argon-treated hemispheres, but because they do not report the statistical power of the study, it is not possible to draw any conclusion from this finding.

Hulbert and Vernon [45•] reported failures in two of 19 patients treated by argon laser and in two of two patients treated with xenon light coagulation. They attribute their low rate of failure to the sparing use of large burns, having a local policy of using a 200-µm spot size through a nonpanfundus lens.

Our clinical experience suggests that diode laser burns tend to spread more than do argon burns of the same apparent intensity, and it would be very interesting to see a 12- to 24-month review of field loss after the use of diode panretinal photocoagulation.

A late cause of visual loss in patients with extensive photocoagulation is pigment epithelial atrophy in the perifoveal or foveal region. This complication has not been studied in detail, but now that many patients have been followed for 10 or more years, it is being seen with increasing frequency. This complication would be expected with treatment in the macular area, but it is seen even in patients who did not have any treatment between the temporal arcades. Its cause is not known.

Retinal vein occlusion

The risk for neovascularization after retinal vein occlusion seems to be positively correlated to the degree of retinal ischemia. Branch and hemisphere

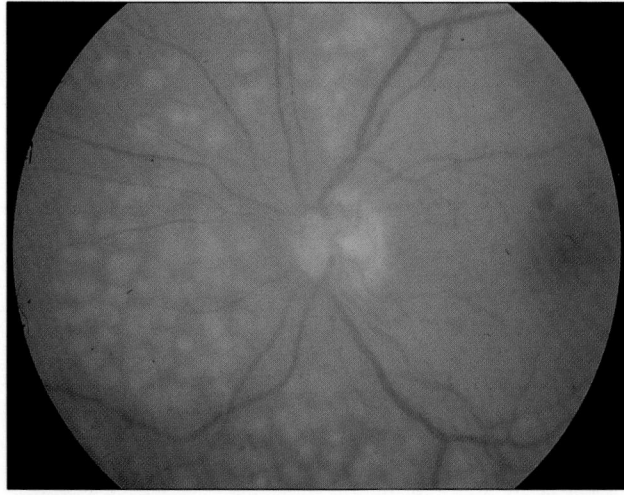

FIGURE 5-4 Diode laser panretinal photocoagulation for proliferative diabetic retinopathy. Note typical grey-white appearance of burns.

retinal vein occlusion (BRVO) tends to be complicated by preretinal or papillary new vessel formation (Fig.5-5*A* and *B*) [50]. Central retinal vein occlusion (CRVO) is complicated by rubeosis iridis and secondary glaucoma. Posterior segment neovascularization is relatively uncommon after CRVO [51].

The beneficial effects of photocoagulation in treating neovascularization complicating BRVO have been firmly established. The Branch Vein Occlusion Study Group [50] noted that photocoagulation reduced the risk for neovascularization in affected eyes and that treatment would reduce the risk for vitreous hemorrhage in eyes with established neovascularization. Magargal and coworkers [52] performed argon laser therapy in 75 cases of proliferative BRVO and caused neovascular regression in the majority of eyes treated, with an 89% success rate in preventing vitreous hemorrhage. Archer and Michalopoulos [53] carried out argon laser treatment on 50 eyes with branch vein thrombosis complicated by preretinal or papillary neovascularization. They reported total neovascular regression in 42 of 48 eyes with preretinal new vessels and in 17 of 21 eyes with papillary neovascularization.

A similar success rate has also been demonstrated in relation to red laser light from krypton lasers. In one study, total regression of neovascularization was observed in all the eyes treated [54].

Successful diode laser therapy for proliferative retinopathy after BRVO has also been reported [55•]. Eleven eyes of 11 patients were treated. Four eyes had optic disc new vessels and seven had peripheral new vessels. Closure of new vessels was observed in all (Fig. 5-5).

These studies have all demonstrated that regression usually begins within a few weeks after laser treatment and that there is a low incidence of recurrence. The efficacy of prophylactic panretinal photocoagulation in the treatment of CRVO is well documented. Margargal and coworkers [56] treated 100 eyes with ischemic CRVO with argon laser panretinal ablation. Only three eyes developed early iris neovascularization and none of the eyes developed neovascular glaucoma. Laatikainen and coworkers [57] have successfully treated established rubeosis with photocoagulation therapy. A pilot study of the treatment of six eyes has indicated the efficacy of using diode laser photocoagulation to treat CRVO complicated by both rubeosis and optic disc neovascularization [55•].

Treatment guidelines

Photocoagulation is indicated for both BRVO and CRVO in the presence of significant retinal ischemia with either threatened or established neovascularization. Ischemia is indicated by the presence of "cotton-wool" spots, deep or confluent retinal hemorrhages, and fluorescein angiographic evidence of capillary nonperfusion. The timing of treatment in BRVO will depend on the clinical features of the condition. With an ischemic CRVO, treatment should be performed within 90 days of onset because this is the typical time course for development of rubeosis.

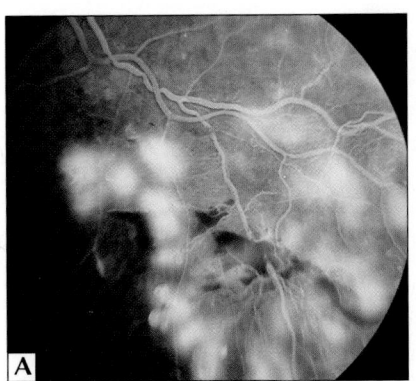
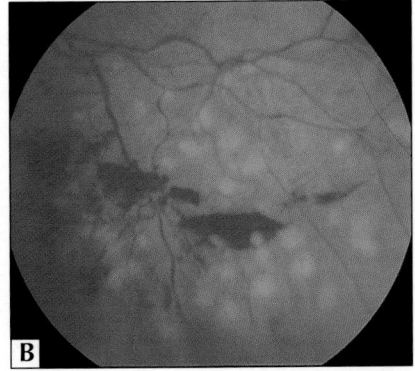
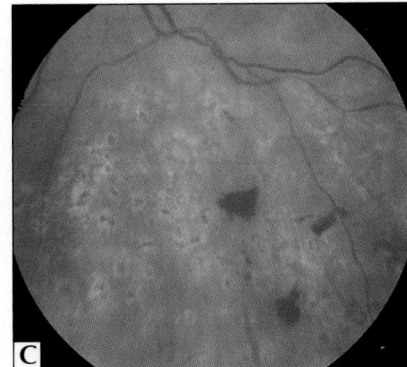
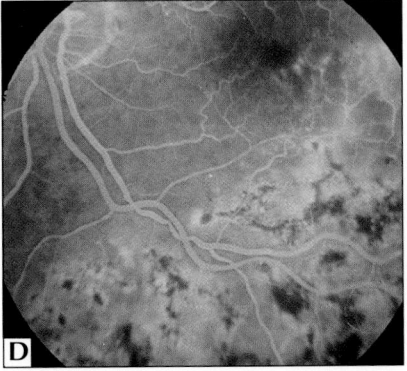

FIGURE 5-5 Diode laser treatment of branch retinal vein occlusion (BRVO). **A**, Pretreatment fluorescein angiogram of a left inferotemporal BRVO with retinal neovascularization, which demonstrates several areas of leakage from the neovascular complexes. **B**, Fundus photograph in the same patient, immediately after diode laser sector ablation. Areas of neovascularization are indicated by arrows. **C**, Eight weeks after laser therapy, the new vessels have regressed and the laser burns have become pigmented scars. **D**, Closure of the retinal new vessels is confirmed by fluorescein angiography.

Branch and hemisphere vein occlusion are treated with a scatter pattern of burns applied to the sector drained by the affected tributary (Fig. 5-6). Central retinal vein thrombosis requires panretinal photocoagulation to all four retinal quadrants. Treatment is similar to that suggested in diabetic retinopathy, but usually less treatment is required and new vessels will regress after the delivery of 1000 to 2000 burns. In CRVO the size of burns or their confluence is usually immaterial because in most patients both central and peripheral vision are already reduced significantly.

Sickle cell disease

Sickle cell disease can lead to peripheral retinal ischemia that is followed by characteristic peripheral "sea fan" (so called because of the resemblance to a type of seaweed) proliferative retinopathy. The natural course of the condition, although benign in comparison with proliferative diabetic retinopathy, is of repeated vitreous hemorrhage, autoinfarction of the involved retina, and occasional retinal detachment. Few studies have been done on proliferative sickle retinopathy, but we have at least had the first prospective study on scatter treatment of proliferative sickle retinopathy.

Treatment guidelines

Two types of treatment have been used for proliferative sickle retinopathy. Feeder-vessel treatment aims to block the large vessels that feed into a sea fan in a manner analogous to the autoinfarction of feeder vessels, which is part of the natural course of proliferative sickle retinopathy. Scatter treatment aims to decrease the amount of retinal tissue present as a stimulus to neovascularization, analogous to scatter treatment for diabetic retinopathy or after a CRVO.

The long-term effects of feeder-vessel treatment as reported after a 10-year review of cases of patients in Chicago are a clear decrease in the number of vitreous hemorrhages associated with visual loss in the treat-

ment group [58]. A complication of feeder-vessel treatment is choroidal neovascularization, probably occurring secondary to breaks in Bruch's membrane. This complication had occurred in five eyes after treatment, but was not associated with a worse outcome [59].

In Kingston, Jamaica scatter treatment was compared with no treatment in 99 treated and 75 untreated eyes [60•]. The treated eyes received scatter argon laser radiation around but not within the areas of neovascularization. Over a review period of 80 months, a reduction of visual acuity occurred in 57 of treated eyes, compared with 20 of untreated eyes. Severe visual loss in either group was associated with more than 60° of neovascularization at presentation.

In a study of sickle cell disease, treated eyes showed more regression than control eyes only in patients under age 25. Infarction of individual lesions was also more common in those treated [61].

In treating sickle cell disease, in contrast with treating CRVO and diabetic retinopathy, sector panretinal photocoagulation usually suffices. Jampol and coworkers [62•] suggest that in patients in whom regular checkups cannot be ensured, 360° circumferential scatter treatment should be applied.

Retinopathy of prematurity

With improvements in the care of low-birth-weight infants, retinopathy of prematurity continues to be an important problem for neonatologists and ophthalmologists. The Cryotherapy for Retinopathy of Prematurity Cooperative Group demonstrated that cryotherapy was effective in reducing the rate of unfavorable outcome (retinal detachment or posterior pole folds) in infants who met treatment criteria by 50%. We have no personal experience in treating this condition and therefore restrict ourselves to literature survey.

Landers and coworkers [63] and McNamara and coworkers [64] showed that indirect laser treatment applied in a similar manner to cryotherapy was as

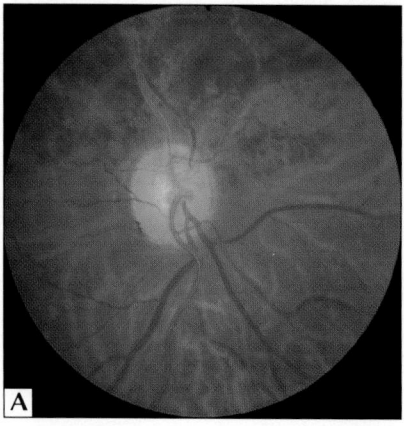
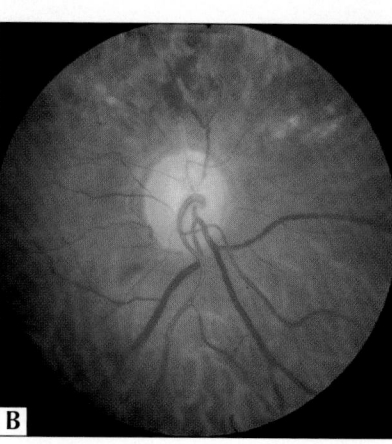

Figure 5-6 A, Hemisphere vein occlusion with disc new vessel neovascularization. **B**, Regression of new vessels after segmental treatment.

effective in reducing the rate of unfavorable outcome as was cryotherapy, albeit in smaller numbers than in the cryotherapy trials. McNamara and coworkers [65] have since reported on the use of the diode laser in stage 3+ retinopathy of prematurity. Twenty-five of 28 eyes that were treated with the diode laser showed regression at 3 months, and seven of seven followed up at 1 year showed regression. This outcome was similar to that in the fellow eyes that were treated with cryotherapy—20 of 24 showing regression at 3 months and seven of seven at 1 year. The most interesting result was the decreased incidence of systemic side effects during laser therapy, in contrast with cryotherapy, following which apneic spells or cardiopulmonary distress required intubation in two infants. Post-treatment inflammation was also less in the laser-treated group, with almost no external signs of inflammation after laser therapy compared with 2 or 3 days of lid edema, chemosis, and hyperemia after cryotherapy. The authors conclude that they would "...prefer to treat with laser because of the ease of treatment and the lower incidence of pain."

An extension of the indications for laser treatment of retinopathy of prematurity has been described by Fleming and coworkers [66••]. In common with others, they are not content with the results of treatment of posterior disease [67]. Cryotherapy at stage 3 threshold in eyes with posterior disease leaves 75% of zone 1 and 22% of zone 2 eyes with an unfavorable outcome.

Laser treatment was used in an uncontrolled trial to treat 18 eyes with posterior plus disease. The diode laser was used and treatment given using an indirect ophthalmoscope through a 28-diopter lens. At 24

weeks after treatment no eye had neovascularization or an unfavorable outcome. One eye developed transient neovascularization 3 to 4 weeks after treatment, but this condition regressed without further intervention. In all eyes the plus disease had regressed at 24 weeks (Fig. 5-7).

This protocol represents an improvement over treatment of threshold disease in this high-risk group. It still needs a prospective study to compare early treatment with treatment at threshold to confirm that the newer protocol does not achieve its success by treating eyes that may never have reached threshold even if only observed. Despite these developments in the treatment of retinopathy of prematurity, we must exercise caution because cryotherapy is still the only therapy for which the benefits have been confirmed in a large prospective trial.

CONCLUSIONS

There is now a wide choice of lasers available for the treatment of proliferative retinopathies. Within the wave band of 488/514.5 nm (argon blue-green) to 810 nm and 1064 nm (diode and Nd:YAG) there is similar clinical efficacy. The essential requirement for a therapeutic effect is the production of a retinal burn.

There are, however, other factors that may influence laser selection. The majority of patients can be effectively treated at a slit-lamp microscope. However, it may be more appropriate to use a laser-indirect ophthalmoscope if the patient is infirm or very young. In the presence of media opacities, eg, preretinal or vitreous blood, or nuclear sclerosis, the use of a long wavelength (krypton red or diode infrared) will enhance

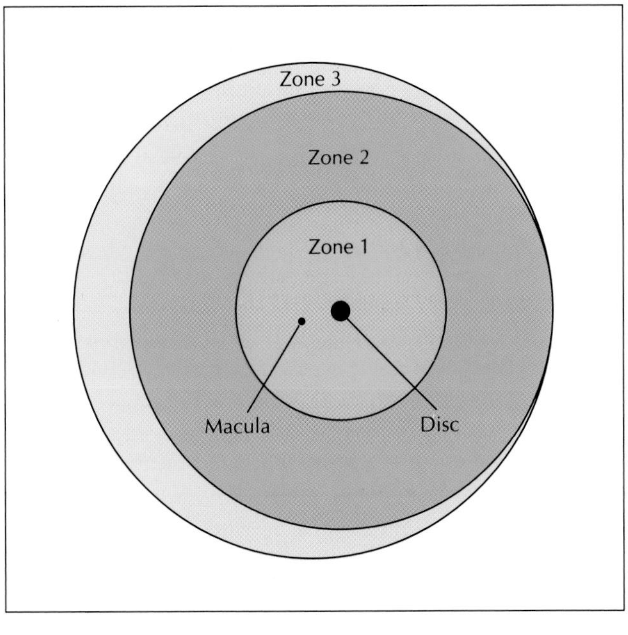

FIGURE 5-7 Treatment criteria for retinopathy of prematurity. The cryotherapy study initiated treatment of at least 5 continuous or 8 total clock hours were involved in neovascularization in zone 1, or in zone 2 with plus disease (stage 3 retinopathy of prematurity). Fleming and coworkers [66••] initiated treatment if there was "plus disease" in zone 1 or posterior zone 2. "Plus disease" is defined as progressive vascular incompetence seen as increasing dilation and tortuosity of peripheral retinal vessels, iris vessel engorgement, pupil rigidity, and vitreous haze. Eyes identified as having posterior zone 2 disease had vessels that crossed the border of zone 1 to zone 2 but that did not extend into the anterior half of zone 2.

transmission of the incident energy to the retina. Dense media opacities will require their removal with a vitreoretinal procedure, followed by endophotocoagulation, or indirect laser treatment. Alternatively, transscleral photocoagulation with a diode laser may be performed.

Regardless of the laser use, effective treatment depends on early identification of the requirement for therapy and the application of a sufficient pattern of photocoagulation. Regular follow-up of the patient will permit one to monitor the clinical response and perform re-treatment if it is indicated.

REFERENCES AND RECOMMENDED READING

Recently published papers of particular interest have been highlighted as:
• Of interest
•• Of outstanding interest

1. Meyer-Schwickerath G: *Light coagulation*. St Louis, CV Mosby; 1960.

2. British Multicentre Study Group: Photocoagulation for proliferative diabetic retinopathy. *Diabetologia* 1984, 26:109–115.

3. Aiello L, Beetham MC, Balodimos BI, *et al*.: Ruby laser photocoagulation in the treatment of diabetic proliferative retinopathy. In *Treatment of Diabetic Retinopathy*. Edited by Goldberg MF, Fine SL. Washington DC: US Department of Health Education & Welfare; 1969:437–464.

4. L'Esperance FA: An ophthalmic laser photocoagulation system: design, construction and laboratory investigations. *Trans Am Ophthalmol Soc* 1968, 66:827–904.

5. Diabetic Retinopathy Research Group: Photocoagulation treatment of proliferative diabetic retinopathy: the second report of diabetic retinopathy study findings. *Ophthalmology* 1978, 85:82–105.

6. Diabetic Retinopathy Research Group: Photocoagulation treatment of proliferative diabetic retinopathy: DRS report No 8. *Ophthalmology* 1981, 88:583–600.

7. Macular Photocoagulation Study Group: Argon laser photocoagulation for senile macular degeneration: results of a randomized clinical trial. *Arch Ophthalmol* 1982, 100:912–918.

8. Blankenship GW: Red krypton and blue-green argon panretinal laser photocoagulation for proliferative diabetic retinopathy: a laboratory and clinical comparison. *Trans Am Ophthalmol Soc* 1986, 84:967–1003.

9. Marshall J, Bird AC: A comparative histological study of argon and krypton laser irradiations of the human retina. *Br J Ophthalmol* 1979, 63:657–668.

10. L'Esperence FA: Clinical applications of the organic dye laser. *Ophthalmology* 1985, 92:1592–1600.

11. Fankhauser F, Roussel P, Steffen J, *et al*.: Clinical studies on the efficacy of high power radiation upon some structures of the anterior segment of the eye: first experiences of the treatment of some pathological conditions of the anterior segment of the human eye by means of a Q-switched laser system. *Int Ophthalmol* 1981, 3:129–139.

12. Jagger JD, Hamilton P, Polkinghorne P: Q-switched neodymium YAG laser vitreolysis in the therapy of posterior segment disease. *Graefe's Arch Clin Exp Ophthalmol* 1990, 228:222–225.

13. Okisaka S, Kashima K, Kimura T, *et al*.: Retinal photocoagulation using the Nd HAG laser. In *Docum Ophthal Proc Series 36*. Edited by Birngruber R, Gabel P. The Hague:Dr W Junk Publishers; 1984:71–80.

14.• Brancato R, Bandello F, Trabucchi G, *et al*.: Frequency doubled Nd:YAG laser versus argon-green laser photocoagulation in proliferative diabetic retinopathy: a preliminary report. *Lasers Light Ophthalmol* 1991, 4:97–102.
The green Nd:YAG laser may be the laser of the future.

15. Horeckler BL: The absorption spectra of haemoglobin and its derivatives in the visible and near infrared region. *J Biol Chem* 1943, 148:173–178.

16. Nussbaum JJ, Pruett RC, Delori FC: Macular yellow pigment: the first 200 years. *Retina* 1981, 1:296–310.

17. Rol P, Niederer P, Durr U, *et al*.: Experimental investigations on the light scattering properties of the human sclera. *Lasers Light Ophthalmol* 1990, 3:201–212.

18. Berninger TA, Canning CR, Gunduz K, *et al*.: Using argon blue light reduces ophthalmologist's color contrast sensitivity. *Arch Ophthalmol* 1989, 107:1435–1458.

19. McHugh JDA, Marshall J, Capon M, *et al*.: Transpupillary photocoagulation in the eyes of rabbit and human using a diode laser. *Lasers Light Ophthalmol* 1988, 2:125–143.

20. McHugh JDA: An investigation into the clinical potential and application of ophthalmic diode lasers. [MD Thesis] London: University of London; 1990.

21. Brancato R, Pratesi R, Leoni G, *et al*.: Retinal photocoagulation with diode laser operating from a slit lamp microscope. *Lasers Light Ophthalmol* 1988, 2:73–78.

22. McNamara A, Tasman W, Vander J, *et al*.: Diode laser photocoagulation for retinopathy of prematurity. *Arch Ophthalmol* 1992, 110:1714–1716.

23. Smiddy WE, Patz A, Quigley H, *et al*.: Histopathology of the effects of tuneable dye laser on monkey retina. *Ophthalmology* 1988, 95:957–963.

24. Haller JA, Lim JI, Goldberg MF: Pilot trial of transscleral diode laser retinopexy in retinal detachment surgery. *Arch Ophthalmol* 1993, 111:952–956.

25. Michaelson IC: The mode of development of the vascular system of the retina, with some observations of its significance for certain retinal diseases. *Trans Ophthalmol Soc UK* 1948, 68:137–180.

26. Boulton ME, McLeod D, Garner A: Vasoproliferative retinopathies: clinical, morphogenetic and modulatory aspects. *Eye* 1988, 2(suppl):S124–S139.

27. D'Amore PA, Klagsburn M: Endothelial cell mitogens derived from retina and hypothalamus biochemical and biological stimulants. *J Cell Biol* 1984, 99:545–549.

28. Gospodarowicz D, Massoglia S, Cheng J, *et al.*: Effect of retinal derived basic and acidic fibroblast growth factor and lipoproteins on the proliferation of retina derived capillary endothelial cells. *Exp Eye Res* 1986, 43:459–476.

29. Schwiegerer J, Neufeld G, Friedman J, *et al.*: Capillary endothelial cells express fibroblast growth factor, a mitogen that promotes their growth. *Nature* 1987, 325:257–259.

30. Grant M, Russel B, Fitzgerald C, *et al.*: Insulin like growth factors in vitreous. *Diabetes* 1986, 35:416–420.

31. Folkman J, Klagsburn M: Angionic factors. *Science* 1987, 235:442–447.

32. Boulton M, Lane C, Singh A, *et al.*: Effects of vitreous from microvascular cells in culture. *Curr Eye Res* 1988, 7:465–470.

33. Hercules BL, Gayed II, Lucas SB, *et al.*: Peripheral ablation in the treatment of proliferative diabetic retinopathy: a three year interim report of a randomised, controlled study using the argon laser. *Br J Ophthalmol* 1977, 61:555–563.

34. Stenkula S: Photocoagulation in diabetic retinopathy: a multicentre study in Sweden. *Acta Ophthalmol* 1984, 162(suppl):1–100.

35. Patz A: Clinical and experimental studies on retinal neovascularization. *Am J Ophthalmol* 1982, 94:715–743.

36. Wolbarsht ML, Landers MB: The rationale of photocoagulation therapy for proliferative diabetic retinopathy: a review and a model. *Ophthalmic Surg* 1980, 11:235–245.

37. Pournaras CJ, Tsacopoulos M, Strommer K, *et al.*: Scatter photocoagulation restores tissue hypoxia in experimental vasoproliferative microangiopathy in miniature pigs. *Ophthalmology* 1990, 97:1329–1333.

38. Glaser BM, Campochiaro PA, Davis JL, *et al.*: Retinal pigment epithelial cells release an inhibitor of neovascularisation. *Arch Ophthalmol* 1985, 103:1870–1875.

39. Diabetic Retinopathy Research Group: Preliminary report: the effects of photocoagulation. *Am J Ophthalmol* 1976, 81:383–394.

40.• Brancato R, Bandello F, Trabucchi G, *et al.*: Argon and diode laser photocoagulation in proliferative diabetic retinopathy: a preliminary report *Lasers Light Ophthalmol* 1990, 3:233–237.
An indication that all laser treatment of diabetic retinopathy can achieve similar results.

41. Aylward GW, Pearson RV, Jagger JD, *et al.*: Extensive argon laser photocoagulation in the treatment of proliferative diabetic retinopathy. *Br J Ophthalmol* 1989, 73:197–201.

42. Turner GS, Inglesby DV, Shariff SB, *et al.*: Natural history of peripheral neovascularisation in diabetic retinopathy. *Br J Ophthalmol* 1985, 69:420–424.

43. Seiberth V, Alexandridis E: Function of the diabetic retina after panretinal argon laser photocoagulation: influence of the intensity of the coagulation spots. *Ophthalmologica* 1991, 202:10–17.

44. Theodossiades GP, Boudouri A, Georgopoulos G, *et al.*: Central visual changes after panretinal photocoagulation in proliferative diabetic retinopathy. *Ophthalmologica* 1990, 201:71–78.

45.• Hulbert MF, Vernon SA: Passing the DVLC field regulations following bilateral panretinal photocoagulation in diabetics. *Eye* 1992, 6:456–460.
The advantage of a 200-μm spot size leading to less field loss is emphasized.

46. Wade EC, Blankenship GW: Short versus long exposure times of argon laser panretinal photocoagulation on proliferative diabetic retinopathy. *Graefe's Arch Clin Exp Ophthalmol* 1990, 228:226–231.

47. McDonald HR, Schatz H: Macular oedema following panretinal photocoagulation. *Retina* 1985, 5:5–10.

48. Buckley SA, Jenkins L, Benjamin L, *et al.*: DVLC and panretinal photocoagulation. *Eye* 1992, 6:623–625.

49. Buckley SA, Jenkins L, Benjamin L: Field loss after panretinal photocoagulation with diode and argon lasers. *Doc Ophthalmol* 1992, 82:317–322.

50. Branch Vein Occlusion Study Group: Argon laser scatter photocoagulation for prevention of neovascularization and vitreous hemorrhage in branch vein occlusion. *Arch Ophthalmol* 1986, 104:34–41.

51. Magargal LE, Donoso LA, Sanborn GE: Retinal ischemia and risk of neovascularization following central retinal vein obstruction. *Ophthalmology* 1982, 89:1241–1245.

52. Magargal LE, Brown GC, Augsburger JJ, *et al.*: Efficacy of panretinal photocoagulation in preventing neovascular glaucoma following ischemic central retinal vein occlusion. *Ophthalmology* 1982, 89:780–784.

53. Archer DB, Michalopoulos N: Treatment of neovascularisation secondary to branch retinal vein obstruction. *Int Ophthalmol* 1981, 3:141–153.

54. Roseman RL, Olk J: Krypton red laser photocoagulation for branch retinal vein occlusion. *Ophthalmology* 1987, 94:1120–1125.

55.• McHugh JDA, Marshal J, ffytche TJ, *et al.*: Initial clinical experience using a diode laser in the treatment of retinal vascular disease. *Eye* 1989, 3:516–527.
This is the first authoritative text on diode laser use in proliferative retinopathy.

56. Magargal LE, Brown GC, Ausburger JJ, *et al.*: Neovascular glaucoma following central retinal vein occlusion. *Ophthalmology* 1981, 88:1095–1101.

57. Laatikainen L, Kohner EM, Khoury D, *et al.*: Panretinal photocoagulation in central retinal vein occlusion: a randomised controlled clinical study. *Br J Ophthalmol* 1977, 61:741–753.

58. Jacobson MS, Gagliano DA, Cohen SB, *et al.*: A randomized clinical trial of feeder vessel photocoagulation of sickle cell retinopathy: a long term follow up. *Ophthalmology* 1991, 98:581–585.

59. Acheson RW, Fox PD, Chuang EL, *et al.*: Treatment of iatrogenic choriovitreal neovascularisation in sickle cell disease. *Br J Ophthalmol* 1991, 75:729–730.

60.• Farber MD, Jampol LM, Fox P, *et al.*: A randomized clinical trial of scatter photocoagulation of proliferative sickle cell retinopathy. *Arch Ophthalmol* 1991, 109:363–367.

A clear demonstration that when treatment is needed scatter photocoagulation is currently the best treatment for sea fan proliferative retinopathy.

61. Fox PD, Minninger K, Forshaw ML, *et al.*: Laser photocoagulation for proliferative retinopathy of SC disease. *Eye* 1993, 7;703–706.

62.• Jampol LM, Farber M, Rabb MF, *et al.*: An update on techniques of photocoagulation treatment of proliferative sickle cell retinopathy. *Eye* 1991, 5:260–263.

A useful review of present and past treatment.

63. Landers MB, Toth CA, Semple HC, *et al.*: Treatment of retinopathy of prematurity with argon laser photocoagulation. *Arch Ophthalmol* 1992, 110:44–47.

64. McNamara JA, Tasman W, Brown GC, *et al.*: Laser photocoagulation for stage 3+ retinopathy of prematurity. *Ophthalmology* 1991, 98:576–580.

65. McNamara JA, Tasman W, Vander JF, *et al.*: Diode laser photocoagulation for retinopathy of prematurity: preliminary results. *Arch Ophthalmol* 1992, 110:1714–1716.

66.•• Fleming TN, Runge PE, Charles ST: Diode laser photocoagulation for prethreshold, posterior retinopathy of prematurity. *Am J Ophthalmol* 1992, 114:589–592.

Earlier treatment of retinopathy of prematurity may give better results.

67. Sternberg PJ, Lopez PF, Lambert HM, *et al.*: Controversies in the management of retinopathy of prematurity. *Am J Ophthalmol* 1992, 113:198–202.

SELECT BIBLIOGRAPHY

Bloom SM, Brucker AJ: *Laser Surgery of the Posterior Segment.* Philadelphia: JB Lippincott; 1991.

Olk RJ, Lee CM: *Diabetic Retinopathy: Practical Management.* Philadelphia: JB Lippincott; 1993.

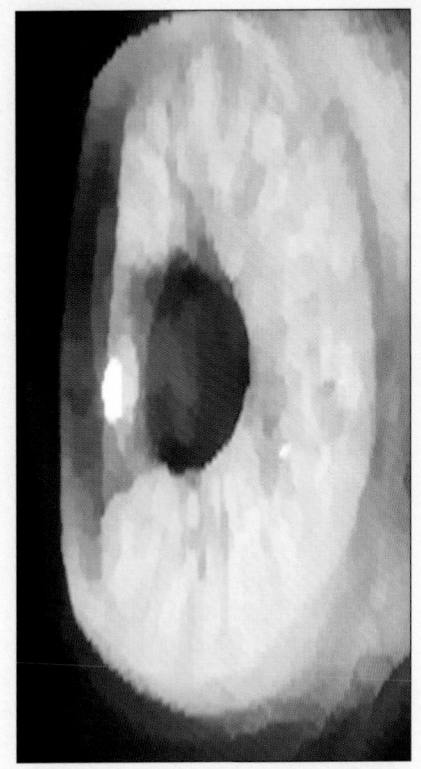

CHAPTER 6

LASER TREATMENT OF CHOROIDAL NEOVASCULAR MEMBRANE IN AGE-RELATED MACULOPATHY

GISÈLE SOUBRANE
GABRIEL COSCAS

In developed countries, age-related macular maculopathy (ARM) is the leading cause of severe and irreversible central visual loss in persons aged more than 50 years. Although the neovascular form of ARM is estimated to develop in approximately 14% of patients with ARM, this form accounts for 88% of the legal blindness associated with this condition.

The neovascular form of ARM often occurs as sudden or recent subacute visual loss with a relative central or paracentral scotoma and accompanying metamorphopsia. Ophthalmoscopic signs of choroidal neovascular membrane (CNV) include the presence of subretinal fluid; retinal, subretinal or sub–retinal pigment epithelial (RPE) blood; subretinal lipid; elevation of the RPE; cystic changes in the sensory retina; and visualization of a grayish-green subretinal lesion. Fluorescence angiography has been the standard imaging modality used in the evaluation and treatment of CNV. At present, indocyanine green (ICG) angiography can provide additional clues.

Stereoangiographic interpretation of neovascular ARM is invaluable in evaluating the type, location, and extent of CNV. Information obtained in long-term follow-ups and with stereoscopic fluorescein angiographic sequences constitute the foundation for photocoagulation treatment guidance. Recognition of the different lesion components has been an evolving process as a result of refinement of our knowledge [1••]. Choroidal neovascularization associated with ARM may have various complex angiographic appearances. CNV can be classified into two major types: classic (well-defined) CNV and occult (ill-defined) CNV. At presentation 18% of patients present with classic CNV and 82%, with occult CNV [2]. The boundaries of CNV can be obscured by different components: pigment epithelium detachment (PED), a thick layer of blood or other material, and elevated blocked fluorescence. According to this classification, different treatment approaches may be considered, but only some of them have demonstrated efficacy.

TREATMENT OF CLASSIC CHOROIDAL NEOVASCULAR MEMBRANES

Treatment guidelines

The location of classic CNV and, therefore, the treatment approaches are defined in relation to the fovea. The fovea is considered to be the anatomic center of both the xanthophyll pigment area and the foveal avascular zone [3,4]. To judge the exact location of the fovea, xanthophyll pigment is delineated on a blue light frame (shot before injection, without the barrier filter) and its geometric center is defined as the fovea. The foveal avascular zone is most visible on an early frame from the stereoangiogram. In addition, the exact location and the extent of the CNV in relation to the fovea is determined on a frame from the arteriovenous phase in which the neovascularization is best delineated but has not yet begun to leak. These landmarks are drawn either directly on a transparent paper or with the help of a viewer (Documentor D1-2 microfilm reader [Zeiss, Iena, Germany] in the Macular Photocoagulation Study) [4,5•]. At present, digitized imaging allows an automatic mapping of these landmarks (Fig. 6-1) [6,7].

Classic CNV is characterized on fluorescein angiograms by early bright choroidal hyperfluorescence with well-demarcated boundaries. In contrast to classic CNV associated with other disease, it is uncommon in ARM to observe a lacy or vascular pattern in these areas of fluorescence. With progressive dye transit, the boundaries of classic CNV become obscured by the rapid and extensive leakage of dye. During the late stages, the dye progressively pools into the overlying subsensory retinal space and into the cystic retinal spaces.

Three categories of classic CNV are distinguished: extrafoveal, juxtafoveal, and subfoveal. Extrafoveal CNV is located 200 μm or more from the center of the xanthophyll pigment and foveal avascular zone. The posterior boundary of juxtafoveal CNV falls within 1 and 199 μm from the fovea. Subfoveal CNV involves the center of the fovea.

The extent of classic CNV has been shown after surgical excision to be much larger than that seen on fluorescein angiograms [8]. Recently, a clinical, angiographic, and ultrastructural correlation of five such excised membranes showed that the central core contained new vessels that extended into a larger avascular fibrin rim [9••]. The hyperpigmented ring of elevated blocked fluorescence commonly seen around classic membranes contains the peripheral growth edge of the neovascular tissue. This area needs therefore to be included in the photocoagulation treatment area, as was recommended by the Macular Photocoagulation Study [4].

Results of photocoagulation in the treatment of classic choroidal neovascular membrane

The treatment modality that has been evaluated recently in the various studies is the complete destruction of the neovascular net with confluent, overlapping, intense laser burns. Argon green laser photocoagulation of extrafoveal CNV has been reported to influence favorably visual outcome even 3 and 5 years after treatment. The Canadian Ophthalmology Study Group [10] has shown that krypton red photocoagulation is similar to argon green treatment regarding visual acuity outcome at 1 year and the rate of recurrence.

Krypton red laser photocoagulation has been shown to be efficient for juxtafoveal (parafoveal) CNV [11].

Studies comparing the results obtained with the use of different wavelengths are still in progress (Coscas, Cascella, and Soubrane, Paper presented at the International Symposium on Fluorescein Angiography, Venice, 1990).

Recently, direct laser treatment of subfoveal CNV (new or recurrent lesions) has been demonstrated to result in less severe visual loss when compared with the natural course of this disease. The Macular Photocoagulation Study subfoveal trials studied eyes with new or recurrent subfoveal new vessels of a maximum of 3.5 and 6 disc areas, respectively. The lesion had to have classic CNV as one of its components and well-demarcated boundaries. Baseline visual acuity had to be between 20/40 and 20/320.

The Macular Photocoagulation Study New Subfoveal Trial [12] found that laser treatment was effective in reducing severe visual loss in treated eyes through 42 months of follow-up study. Persons with treated eyes also retained a stable level of contrast threshold scores and had greater reading speeds than did those who did not receive treatment; those with laser-treated eyes experienced an immediate decline in visual acuity, however. Treatment benefit was dependent on the size of the membrane and the initial acuity. Eyes with small or intermediate membranes and poor initial visual acuity had a greater treatment bene-

fit. No significant difference in any of the visual outcomes or the frequency of persistent or recurrent CNV was found in eyes treated with the argon green versus the krypton red laser.

Treatment for recurrent subfoveal CNV also showed positive results with respect to severe visual acuity loss, average visual acuity, and average change in visual acuity at a 2-year follow-up visit [12,13]. Reading speed and contrast threshold levels supported the use of treatment.

Complete treatment, as performed in the Macular Photocoagulation Study, requires extensive patient education to prepare these patients for an immediate and possibly sizable drop in visual acuity in exchange for a better long-term level of visual function. Thus, close monitoring could be undertaken until visual acuity spontaneously declines before direct photocoagulation is applied.

Reluctance to ablate the foveal center that results in an immediate and permanent decline in visual acuity has led to consideration of the use of an alternative technique of laser photocoagulation. The technique of perifoveal laser photocoagulation of Créteil of subfoveal CNV consists of a "donut" of confluent burns to the periphery of a choroidal neovascular lesion with sparing of the central foveal avascular zone (400 μm in diameter) [14]. In a randomized clinical trial, our tech-

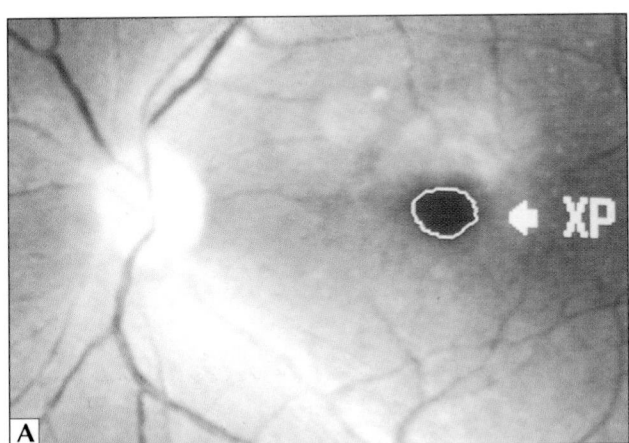

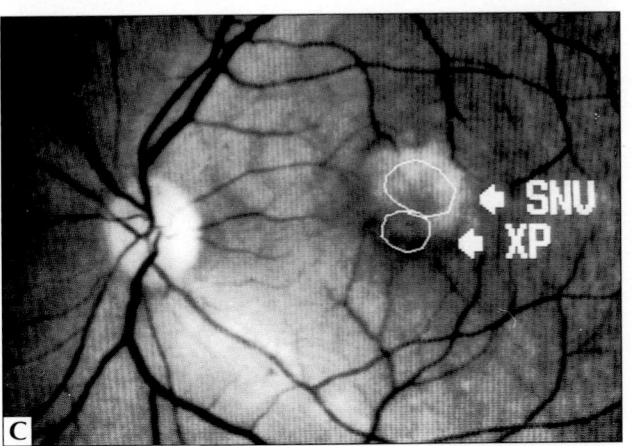

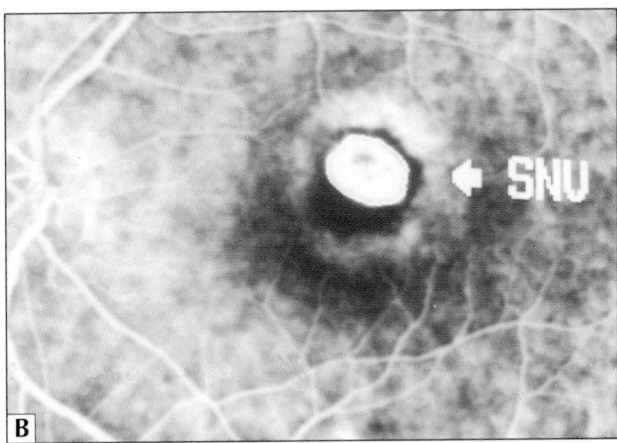

FIGURE 6-1 Automatic mapping of digitized pretreatment fluorescein angiography to locate the choroidal new vessels in relation to the fovea. A, Frame in blue light: the xanthophyll area shows as a dark central zone. B, Automatic detection of the well-defined network, best visible on this early frame of fluorescein angiography. C, Automatic overlay of both images, allowing the exact location and limits of the area to treat and the area to avoid. (Courtesy G. Mimoun.)

nique of perifoveal laser treatment was applied to well-defined and ill-defined CNV (Fig. 6-2A). A lifetable analysis demonstrated a six-line loss of vision in 17% of the treated eyes compared with 48% of untreated eyes at the 2-year visit. A final-reading visual acuity of J4 or better was attained with the assistance of low-vision aids in 73% of the treated eyes and in 47% of the untreated eyes. Finally, morphologic success, defined as resolution of fluorescein leakage in the area ablated by laser treatment, was achieved in 53 of 68 treated eyes compared with 19 of 59 untreated eyes progressing to an atrophic scar (Fig. 6-2B). Persistent subretinal fluid and fluorescein leakage inside the foveal avascular zone, which resolved with time, was common in treated eyes because this area was not photocoagulated. This study suggests that perifoveal treatment may be helpful in preserving visual acuity and in providing superior low-vision rehabilitation, particularly for near-vision tasks.

Postoperative evaluation and management

Laser treatment is performed with the objective of destroying the CNV and preventing the eye from developing recurrences. The high rate of recurrences after photocoagulation in eyes with ARM necessitates that complete treatment of the membrane be performed. The Macular Photocoagulation Study concluded that incomplete treatment of well-defined CNV is associated with poorer visual prognosis than is no treatment. Therefore, preoperative and postoperative laser fundus photographs must be carefully compared to ensure that complete treatment of subretinal neovascular membranes is performed. Manual tracing techniques have been used to ensure that laser burns photographically documented in the early postoperative period have covered the preoperative angiographically visible membranes [4]. This process requires time for photographic processing and relies on images that have been taken with the same camera at the same image magnification and with the same field definition. The recent availability of digital acquisition of fundus angiograms has led to the development of different software programs to digitally overlay sequential fluorescein angiograms and red-free images of eyes with CNV. Post-treatment digitized images can be obtained immediately or at short intervals after surgery and rapidly compared with the digitized preoperative angiogram frame that most clearly defines the neovascular membrane (Fig. 6-3) [15•]. Imaging systems internally compensate for differences in magnification and centering. It remains to be demonstrated that regular use of this technique assessing the adequacy of treatment reduces the high rate of recurrence.

Approximately 60% of the treated eyes will experience recurrent CNV within the first 3 months after

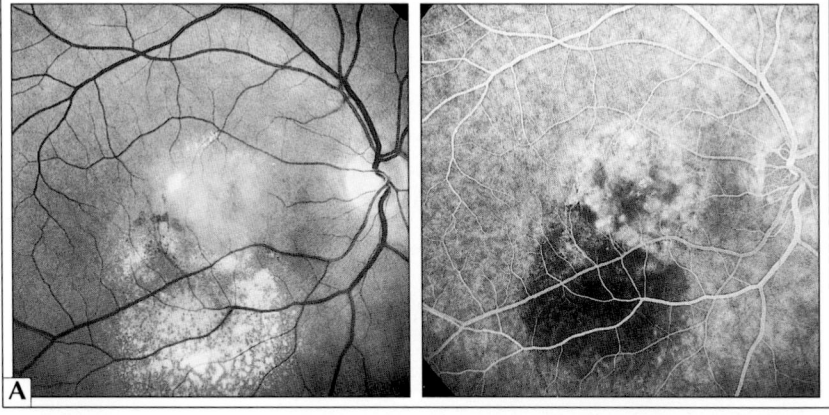

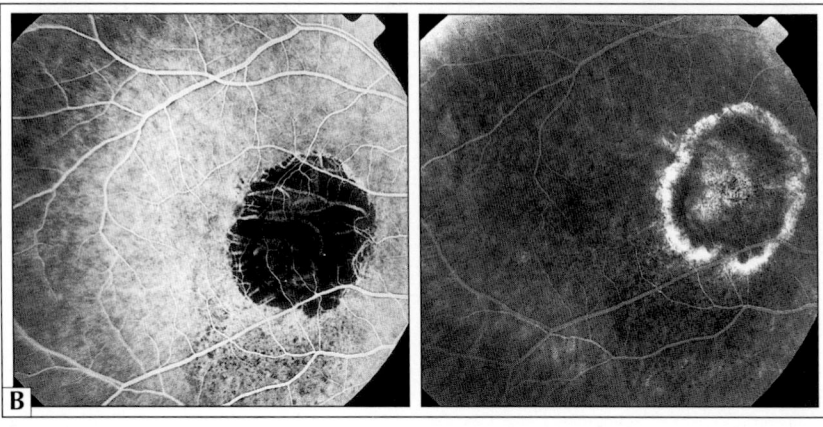

FIGURE 6-2 Perifoveal laser treatment. A, Pretreatment angiogram discloses an ill-defined subfoveal membrane with accumulation of hard exudates inferiorly. B, Post-treatment angiogram: laser burns have been applied to the entire neovascular membrane but sparing the whole avascular zone. Burns have resulted in an atrophic central scar. No residual neovascularization nor leakage of dye is visible even on the late frame.

treatment, but will also have recurrences after that time. Post-treatment visits are concentrated in the period in which recurrences are at high risk to occur. A biomicroscopic and an angiographic examination are performed at 2 weeks to rule out any persistence. Earlier evaluation with fluorescein angiography does not identify persistent CNV because of profuse leakage of the dye within the photocoagulation scar. It was recently suggested that ICG angiography performed 3 to 5 days after treatment was able to image persistent CNV precisely [16]. We are at present conducting a study to evaluate at what time after krypton photocoagulation ICG angiography is most helpful in identifying persistences: immediately after treatment, at 3 days, or at 2 weeks. Follow-up visits must be performed at 1, 2, and 3 months postoperatively and every trimester thenafter to identify recurrences. Re-treatment of any classic CNV recurrence is recommended especially when sparing the fovea.

In experimental models, the formation of new choroidal vessels after laser photocoagulation could explain the high recurrence rate observed in clinical experience [17]. An ultrastructure study of the choroidal vascular repair following krypton laser injury in rats showed that three processes occurred—initial recanalization of the damaged vessels and neovascular-

ization at the periphery of large lesions, followed at 2 weeks by atrophy of both recanalized and newly formed capillaries [18]. This observation is in agreement with the timing and the location of recurrences following laser photocoagulation in patients. However, the factors playing a role in determining the progression to atrophy of the new vessels in these models are still unknown.

Randomized clinical trials have demonstrated the efficacy of using laser photocoagulation to treat classic well-defined CNV in any location compared with allowing the disease to pursue its natural course. The resulting visual function is related to the location of the membrane, the quality of the initial photocoagulation treatment, and the absence of associated occult new vessels.

TREATMENT OF OCCULT CHOROIDAL NEOVASCULAR MEMBRANE

Features of occult CNV may be subdivided into isolated occult CNV or vascularized PEDs [1••]. In the first type of occult CNV, isolated CNV (or late leakage of undetermined source), the early phase of the angiogram does not identify a discrete and discernible source of

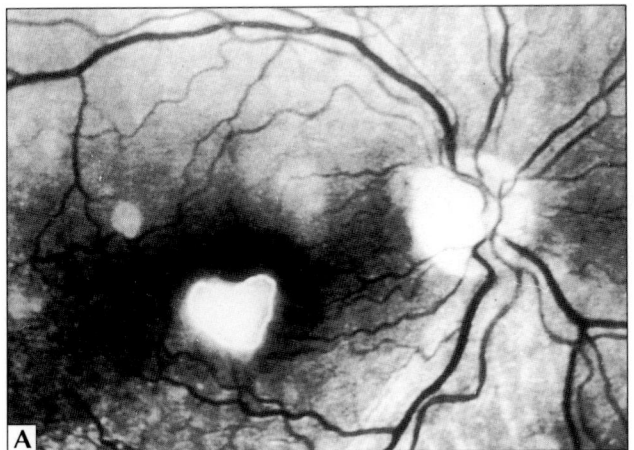

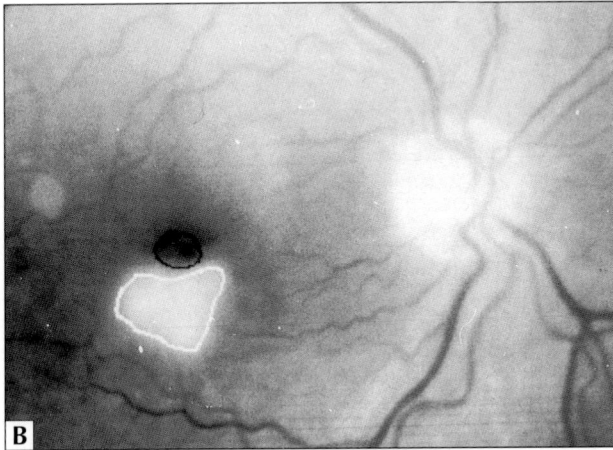

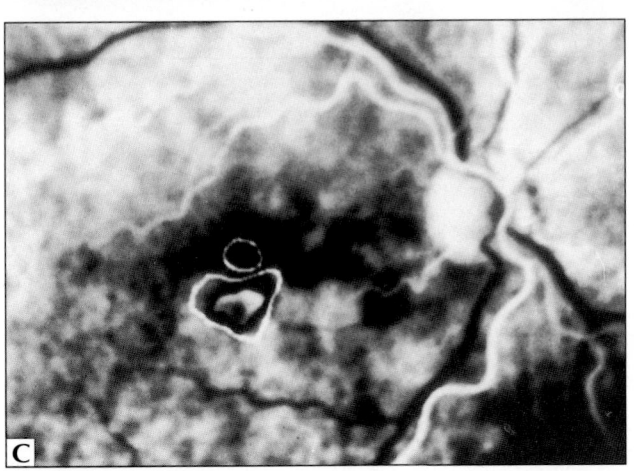

FIGURE 6-3 Automatic overlay of the post-treatment red-free frame on the pretreatment angiogram. **A,** Post-treatment red free frame. **B,** Blue light frame with no delineation of the xantrophyll pigment and the laser burns. **C,** Superposition of the treated area on the pretreatment angiogram. (Courtesy of G. Mimoun.)

leakage (Fig. 6-4A and B). On the other hand, frames from the mid and late phases show diffuse leakage into the overlying subsensory retinal space, often with punctate or stippled hyperfluorescence in the outer retina (Fig. 6-4C and D). The boundaries of this form of occult CNV are always poorly demarcated.

In contrast to the serous PED, which typically presents an early, homogenous, intense progressive hyperfluorescence of its entire extent, a vascularized PED (fibrovascular) is uneven with areas of bullous hyperfluorescent detachment and areas of delayed and uneven filling (Fig. 6-5). Presence of CNV is suggested by an area of early localized and accentuated hyperfluorescence. These areas can be small (focal) or extensive (plaque), and unique or multiple within or at the border of the PED (Fig. 6-5). CNV can be located within a notch with ill-defined stippled hyperfluo-

rescent points. These forms of CNV were excluded from all randomized clinical trials because the boundaries of the neovascular membrane cannot precisely be determined.

Treatment of vascularized pigment epithelial detachment

Treatment of PEDs in elderly persons is controversial. The results of the Moorfields clinical trial, which showed a greater visual loss in persons with treated as opposed to untreated avascular PED, discouraged many ophthalmologists. In 1982, subpigment epithelial new vessels were not known and not identified. A reassessment of the entry angiograms of this trial as to the presence or absence of new vessels beneath the PED has been performed based on the acquired knowledge in the past 10 years [19]. The analysis indi-

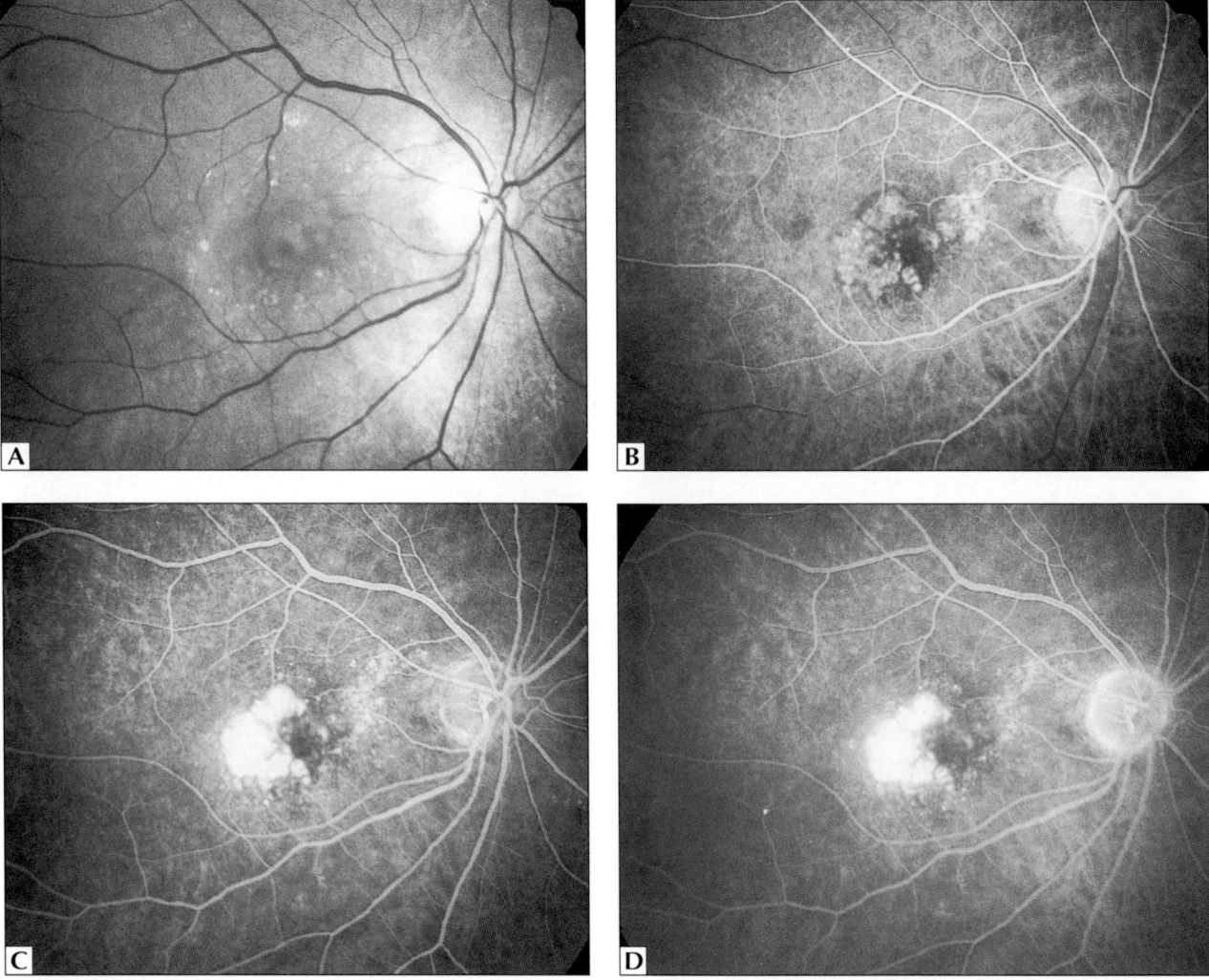

FIGURE 6-4 Isolated occult choroidal neovascular membrane imaged with fluorescein angiography. **A**, Red-free frame: serous drusen only visible at the periphery of the macular retinal detachment. **B**, Arterial phase: uneven early hyperfluorescence predominantly located temporal to the avascular zone but also nasally. **C**, Mid phase: increase of the temporal hyperfluorescence. **D**, Late phase: intense staining of the temporal zone. The nasal lesion exhibits only stippled fluorescence. Faint hyperfluorescence of the retinal detachment can be seen.

cates that a heterogeneous group of eyes were recruited into the study [20]. There is no indication after review to modify the original conclusion that grid laser photocoagulation does not improve the visual prognosis in "avascular" retinal PEDs. However, these results do not apply to "vascularized" PEDs. Notches at the edge of PEDs on fluorescein angiograms are believed to indicate the site of choroidal new vessels. Treatment directed to the ill-defined hyperfluorescence and the contiguous edge of the PED induced resolution or decrease of PED in eight of the 14 eyes treated [21].

The problem of delineating the new vessel complex within the PED may be resolved by the development of ICG angiography. ICG dye has a peak absorption (805 nm) and fluorescence (835 nm) in the near infrared range, theoretically allowing visualization through

overlying fluid hemorrhage, lipid, and pigment that may otherwise limit or prevent detection of underlying CNV by fluorescein angiography [22]. The technique has been available for several years, but clinical value was limited until recently. It has not been until the recent technologic advance of combining digital imaging systems or scanning laser ophthalmoscopes with ICG cameras that the advantages of ICG dye have been realized [23,24••,25].

As a result of their work, Yannuzzi and coworkers [24••] have shown that new blood vessels associated with RPE detachments may be defined by ICG angiography in patients in whom fluorescein angiography has not been helpful. On fluorescein angiograms the leakage and staining of fluorescein of the PED partially obscures the origin of the dye, or the CNV (Fig. 6-5). Presumed CNV can manifest on ICG

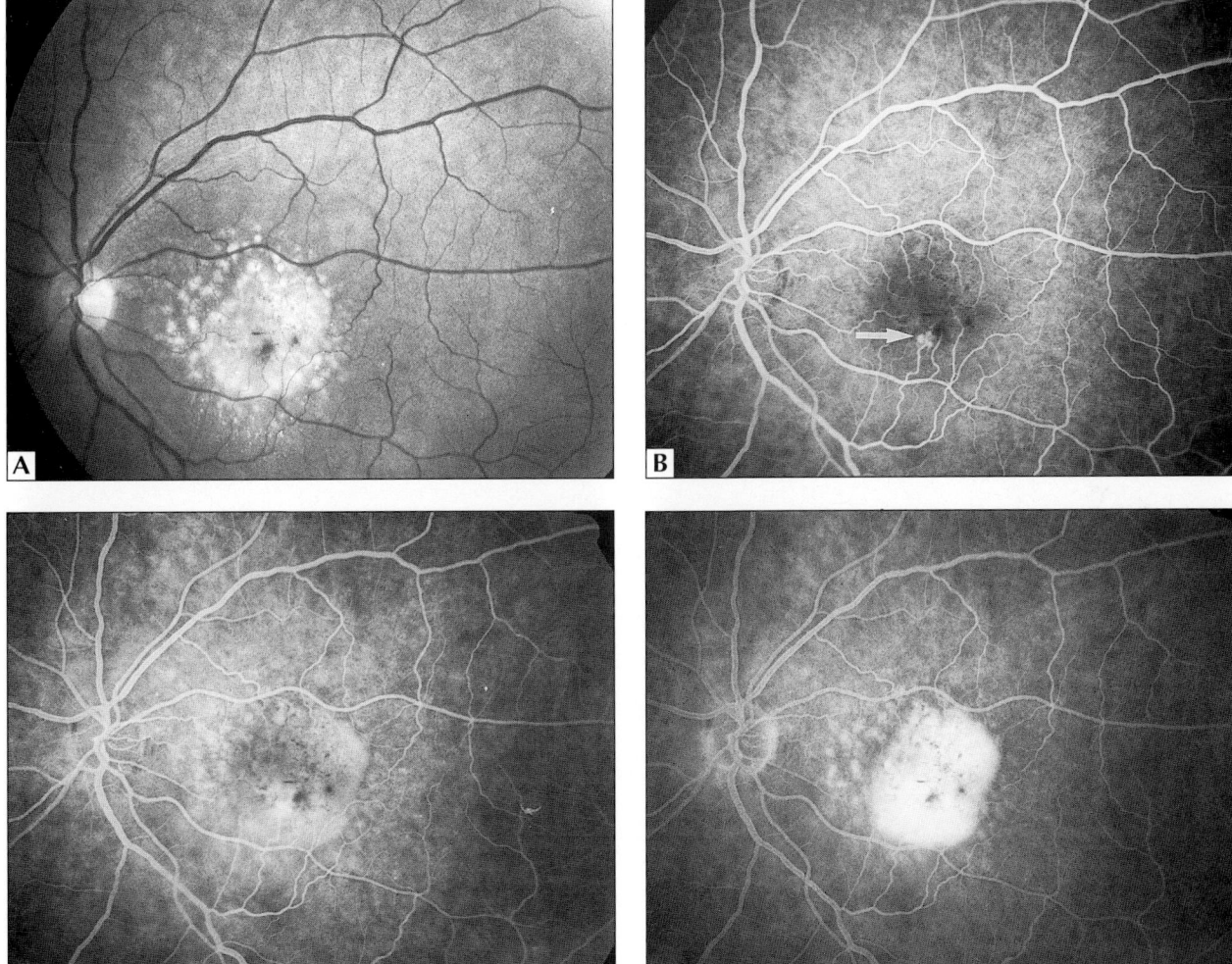

FIGURE 6-5 Vascularized pigment epithelium detachment (PED) imaged with fluorescein angiography. **A,** Red-free frame: macular PED with three retinal hemorrhages surrounded by serous drusen. **B,** Arteriovenous phase: the PED is not filled with fluorescein. A focal area is hyperfluorescent (*arrow*). **C,** Mid phase: the early hyperfluorescent area is less prominent as the temporal part of the PED begins to fill with the dye. **D,** Late phase: the irregular PED is completely hyperfluorescent; the early hyperfluorescent area is no longer visible; and the serous drusen are staining.

angiograms as a focal, well-defined area of hyperfluorescence contrasting the blockage of the detached pigment epithelium (Fig. 6-6). In Yannuzzi and coworkers' study [24••], a conversion to well-defined CNV was noted in 45% of the cases of vascularized PED (17 of 38 eyes).

This well-circumscribed focus must be precisely located in relation to the fovea and to the retinal vessels used as landmarks for photocoagulation treatment. A small reinjection of ICG will fill the retinal vessels in the late phase [26]. A determination of the location of the "hot-spot" to the fovea mapping of the digitized scanning laser ophthalmoscope images of the early-phase fluorescein and of the late-phase ICG angiography with the reinjection was found to be very helpful in our clinic.

Indocyanine green has not yet proven value in the management of vascularized PEDs. A preliminary study on ICG-guided laser photocoagulation has been performed, which successfully eliminated the occult CNV in nearly half of the cases of vascularized PED, resulting in stabilized or improved vision (Slakter and coworkers, Unpublished data). However, ICG angiographic identification of hyperfluorescent areas that are not detected on fluorescein angiograms, despite the absence of significant blood or pigment, raises questions as to what is being defined on the ICG study. Only clinicopathologic correlation will determine whether ICG angiography can visualize the presence and full extent of CNV and whether it offers practical advantage over fluorescein angiography. However, ICG angiography may represent a

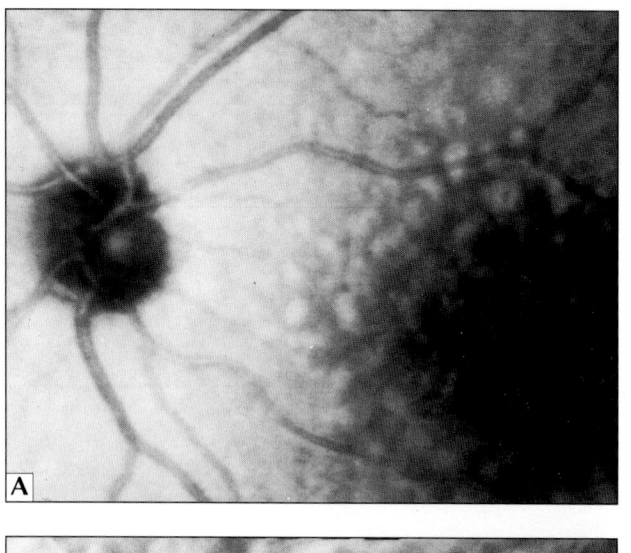
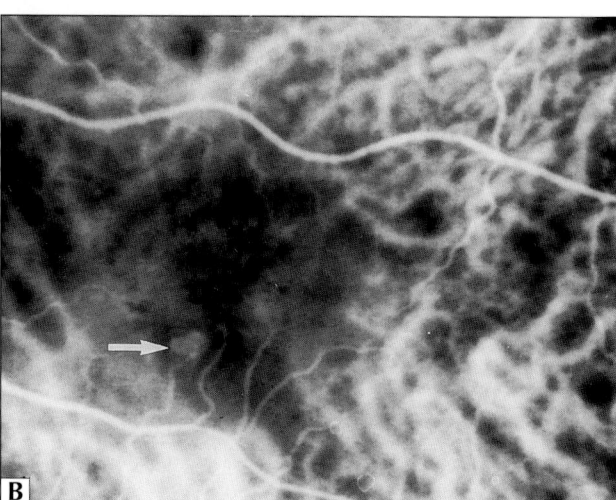
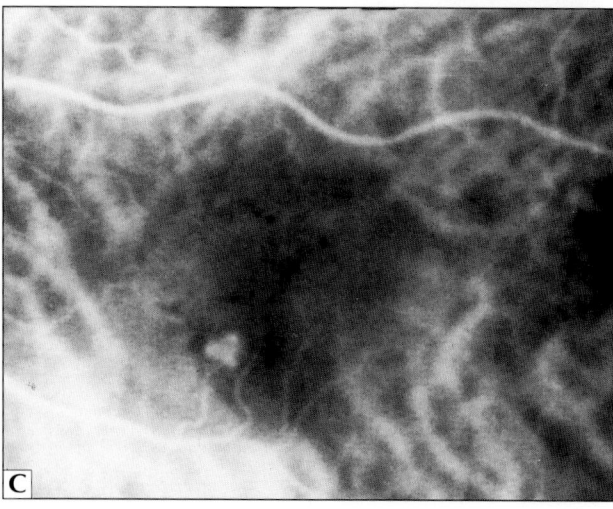
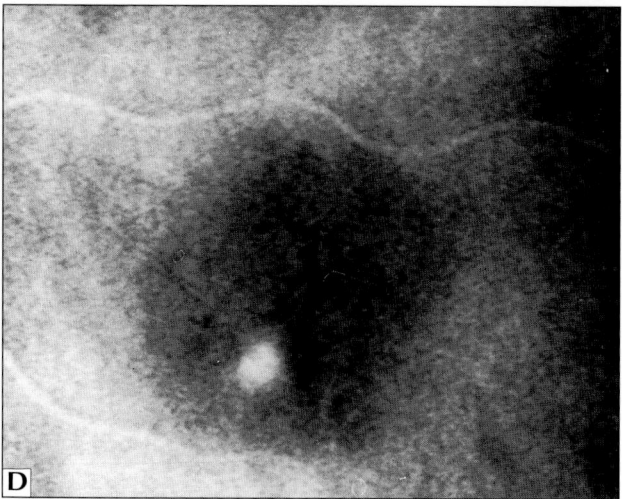

FIGURE 6-6 Vascularized pigment epithelium detachment (PED) imaged with indocyanine green (ICG) angiography (same case as Fig. 6-5). **A**, Infrared frame: the serous drusen are more prominent than on the red-free frame. **B**, Early phase: choroidal arteries and veins are already filled with the dye. A small hyperfluorescent net is clearly identified (*arrow*). **C**, Mid-phase: the neovascular membrane is outlined with a hyperfluorecent ring. The PED remains hypofluorescent. **D**, Late phase: the dark PED has well-defined borders. Some leakage of ICG occurs from the new vessels.

major advance in the definition of vascularized and nonvascularized PEDs.

Treatment of isolated occult choroidal neovascular membrane

The treatment of isolated occult CNV based on fluorescein angiography has been shown to be successful in only one third of eyes and therefore cannot be recommended [27]. Failure of treatment is clearly related to the unprecise delineation of the boundaries of the membrane.

Digital ICG angiography may provide better definition and accurate location of occult CNV. A conversion of isolated occult CNV into well-defined CNV was noted in 17 of 65 eyes (26%) in one study (Fig. 6-7) [28]. ICG overcomes the shielding effect of xanthophyll

which, in fluorescein angiography, gives a false impression of being spared by the CNV. This phenomenon might explain the unfavorable results obtained by fluorescein-guided photocoagulation of occult CNV. ICG-guided laser photocoagulation eliminated successfully the occult CNV in 29 of 44 such eyes in one report, resulting in stabilized or improved vision (Slakter and coauthors, Unpublished data).

Yannuzzi and coworkers [24••] emphasize the necessity of obtaining late-phase ICG angiograms (30 to 40 minutes) to visualize the neovascularization adequately (Fig. 6-7D). One of these late frames, a large area of faint fluorescence with well-delineated borders, supposedly represents the isolated occult membrane. However, the large extent of this ICG fluorescence, mostly involving the whole macular area, in our expe-

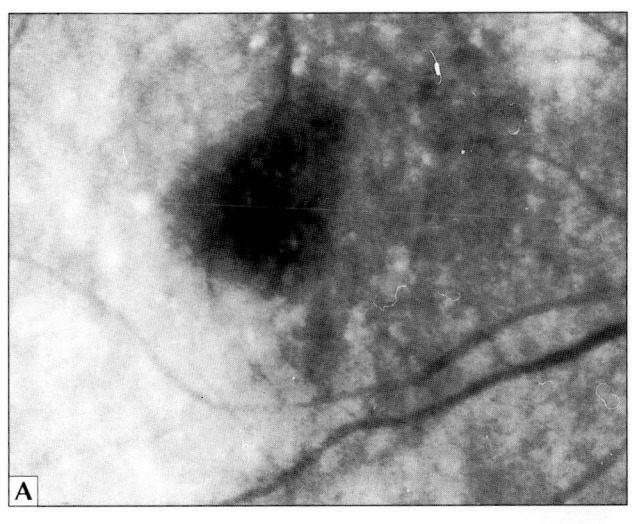

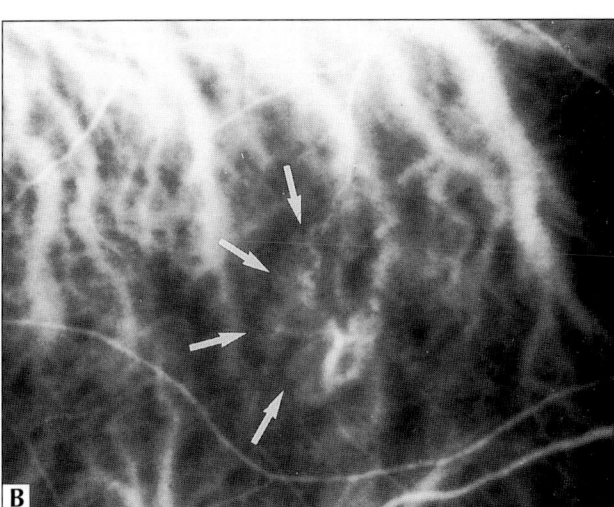

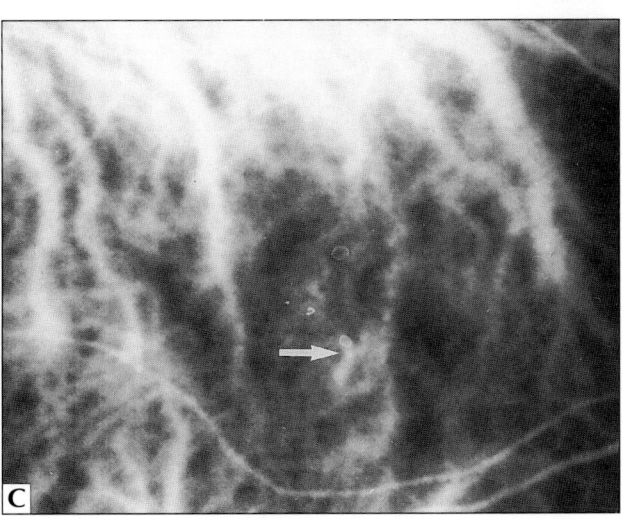

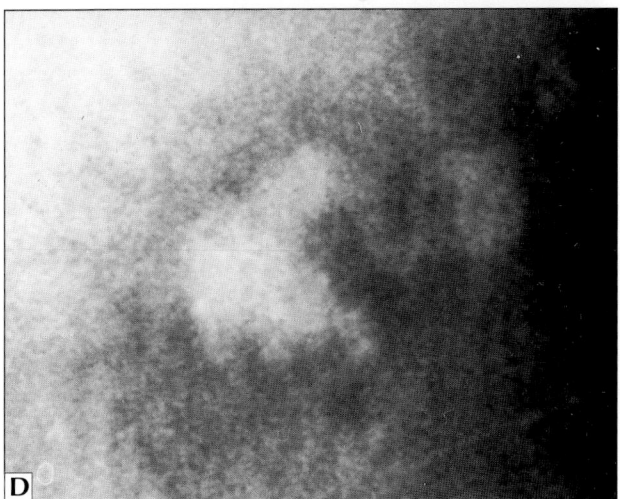

FIGURE 6-7 Isolated occult new vessels imaged with indocyanine green angiography (same case as in Fig. 6-4). **A,** Infrared frame: visibility of the retinal detachment. **B,** Early phase: hyperfluorescence of a central feeder-vessel resolving into faint capillaries (*arrows*) surrounded by a hypofluorescent ring. **C,** Mid phase: persistence of the visibility of the feeder vessel (*arrow*). **D,** Late phase: staining of both parts of the neovascular membrane, more prominent temporally than nasally.

rience, could be the staining of the fibrous tissue, located histopathologically within the thickened and detached Bruch's membrane—without choroidal neovascularization [29]. Thus, we rely more on ICG angiography performed with the laser scanning ophthalmoscope, as introduced by Scheider and coworkers [30]. The continuous recording of the ICG videoangiogram often allows the identification in the early first passage of a definite neovascular net, the only component requiring treatment; it also sometimes allows visualization of the actual feeding vessels. This rapid filling can only be seen by chance on single images.

TREATMENT OF OBSCURED CHOROIDAL NEOVASCULAR MEMBRANE

Three components can block the angiographic detection of CNV: thick blood, elevated blocked fluorescence, and accumulation of whitish material. Thus, the type of CNV present cannot be identified.

Hemorrhagic disciform

Thick blood that is contiguous or overlying an area of classic or occult CNV may obscure fluorescence from the choroid and from CNV directly beneath it. In fluorescein angiography, late leakage of dye may be observed within the blockage of subretinal blood, probably corresponding to a part of the CNV located more anteriorly. However, photocoagulation treatment limited to this area was never reported to be successful.

Hayashi and DeLaey [31] were the first to demonstrate that ICG videoangiography was better at delineating neovascularization under this condition. Destro and Puliafito [32] also noted that ICG videoangiography was useful in the study of CNV if there was hemorrhage overlying the neovascularization. Both studies reported isolated results of photocoagulation guided by videoangiography.

Because the presence of a large hemorrhage beneath the macula leads to rapid degeneration of the overlying retina and to permanent structural damage, eyes with thick hemorrhages rarely recover much vision spontaneously. Because of this poor natural history, several investigators have reported on the possible role of surgical removal of the blood through the use of modern vitrectomy techniques [33,34]. The visual results with this type of surgery, however, are usually disappointing because the underlying disease process is progressive, and extensive CNV and recurrent hemorrhages are common. One other factor in visual loss caused by subretinal hemorrhage is related to the presence of fibrin [35]. The fibrin-mediated photoreceptor damage can experimentally be avoided by the addition of tissue plasminogen activator. The use of fibrinolytic drugs, tissue

plasminogen activator most recently, has been evaluated during surgical evacuation of subretinal hemorrhage and so has been used as an adjunct to the surgical evacuation of subretinal hemorrhage [36]. However, several studies have reported that vision improved significantly in none of the eyes with ARM [37,38,39••]. The indications for this evolving surgical procedure are at present uncertain, although there is agreement that, in general, the sooner the subretinal hemorrage is removed, the better (less than 8 days).

Blocked choroidal fluorescence

Another lesion component that can block the boundaries of CNV is an area of elevated blocked fluorescence on stereofluorescein angiograms [1••]. This feature is always a component of a complex lesion usually involving the two major types of CNV—classic and occult—and eventually a PED. These areas are often well demarcated by their elevation in addition to the dense obscuration of the choroidal fluorescence. Clinically, they probably correspond to areas of fibrous tissue or hyperplastic pigment epithelium [9••]. Until now, their imaging in ICG angiography has not been described.

Accumulation of material

In addition to blood, white-yellowish material can mask the underlying CNV on fluorescein angiograms. Fibrin resulting from a subretinal hemorrhage, hard exudates, and pseudovitelliform material totally hide the leakage of dye. In addition, on ICG angiograms they also block the underlying choroidal fluorescence. However, our experience has shown that ICG videoangiography allows identification of the associated CNV in pseudovitelliform macular lesions.

ALTERNATIVE PHOTOCOAGULATION TECHNIQUES

Complete laser treatment of CNV is performed with the objective of destroying the CNV and preventing the eye from developing recurrent CNV. Despite the widespread use of laser photocoagulation, the mechanism by which it clinically eradicates CNV in successfully treated eyes is not completely understood. Although the directly visible thermal effects of laser energy are believed to play a fundamental role in coagulating neovascular tissue, there may be other secondary effects that induce closure or regression of CNV.

Scatter macular photocoagulation

Extrafoveal scatter macular photocoagulation could, indirectly, by a laser–tissue interaction, enhance involution of the subfoveal neovascular tissue. The observation that RPE cells release inhibitors of neovascularization *in vitro*, combined with evidence that proliferation of RPE after laser treatment of experimentally induced CNV may envelop the CNV and help absorb subretinal fluid, indicates that laser-treated RPE may have an important role in the sequestering and closure of choroidal neovascular tissue. Alternately, laser photocoagulation may act by ablating areas of choroidal vascular insufficiency, as observed in ICG angiography [24••,36]. In this theory, laser treatment might convert hypoxic watershed zones to an anoxic state, thereby terminating or reversing angiogenic factors and simultaneously inducing a regression of CNV. Furthermore, this technique, by minimizing destruction of foveal photoreceptors, could allow a better visual acuity.

Based on these hypotheses, two studies were performed. Tornambe and coworkers [40•] conducted a pilot study evaluating the effects of scatter macular photocoagulation in eyes with subfoveal CNV. Well-demarcated subfoveal lesions of up to 3500 μm were treated with yellow laser in a scatter pattern of 350 to 700 spots measuring 200 to 500 μm. In half of the eyes (18 eyes), treatment was applied to the extrafoveal macular retina beyond the perimeter of the classic CNV, with sparse applications in the nasal macula. In the remaining 22 eyes, confluent treatment was also applied to the extrafoveal portion of the classic CNV because these eyes had at least 50% of the well-defined component outside the foveal area. Eighty percent of the patients had visual acuity of 20/200 or better, compared with 53% after an average follow-up period of 28 months (range, 1 to 4 years). Treatment was successful at stopping angiographic leakage in

approximately 50% of the patients. The lack of control subjects is a pitfall of this study.

Based on the same rationale, a randomized pilot study was conducted on subfoveal isolated occult CNV, for which no treatment modality is presently available (Soubrane, Algan, and Nounou, Paper presented at the International Symposium on Fluorescein Angiography, Venice, 1990). These subfoveal membranes are usually very extensive and often compatible, with a useful visual acuity precluding the use of subfoveal or perifoveal laser photocoagulation. Twenty-nine eyes with an initial acuity of between 20/20 and 20/100 were randomly assigned to treatment (15 eyes) and observation (14 eyes). Treated eyes received 300 to 500 very mild laser burns of 200-μm size and 0.2 second duration, applied outside the area of fluorescein leakage of the serous retinal detachment (Fig. 6-8). After a mean follow-up period of 30 months (range, 15 to 35 months), no difference was noted between treated and observed eyes regarding final visual acuity and angiographic features. Although this approach is very attractive, no positive results are presently available requiring a longer period of follow-up to substantiate the previous hypothesis.

Reduction of photoreceptor damage

Focal treatment of choroidal neovascularization demands measures that can be taken to minimize retinal damage to preserve central visual function. The continuous-wave neodymium-yttrium aluminum garnet (Nd:YAG) laser had been studied to determine whether CNV could be successfully treated with this technique while attempting to minimize overlying photoreceptor damage [41•]. Continuous-

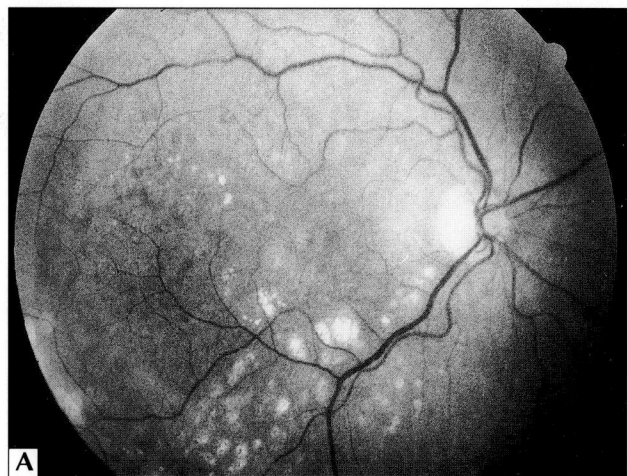

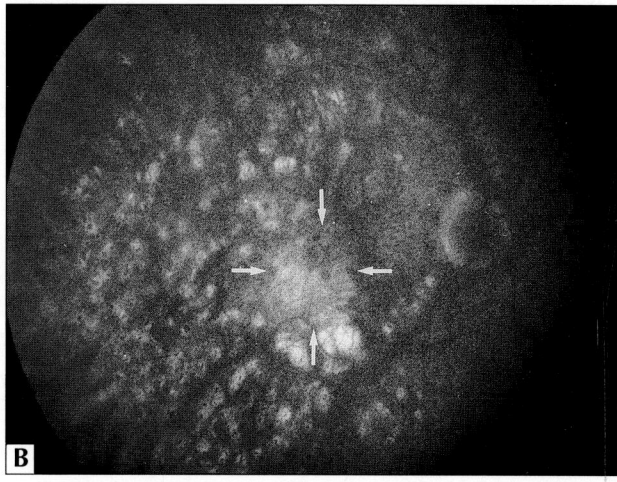

FIGURE 6-8 Scattered laser photocoagulation for subfoveal occult choroidal neovascular membrane (CNV) with fair visual acuity. **A**, Red-free frames: atrophic scars of laser burns are identifiable in the inferior part of the posterior pole. **B**, Late fluorescein angiogram: numerous mild laser scars are distributed in the posterior pole sparing the area of CNV (*arrows*). Neovascular activity is minimal.

wave Nd:YAG laser application induces sufficient coagulation in the choroid while causing only mild damage to the RPE and retina because of its longer wavelength (1064 nm). In 17 of 19 eyes with ARM and juxtafoveal classic CNV, the Nd:YAG laser obliterated the membrane, and visual acuity remained stable or improved. However, these results concern only a small sample size with a lack of control subjects and a limited follow-up period.

The extent of retinal damage is related to the passage of temperature transients away from the RPE. Among the different schemas of biophysical factors that might be exploited to localize damage, repetitive-pulse photocoagulation seems to be the most promising technique [42]. In one study, multiple short argon laser pulses applied to the rabbit retina resulted in the healing of the pigment epithelium in a single sheet of cells, showing clear signs of viability, and the photoreceptors were not damaged [43•].

Dye-enhanced photocoagulation (photocoagulation enhanced with supravital dyes) has been suggested for use since 1984. The light absorption characteristics of the vital tissues can be modified by exogenous dyes. Three dyes (fluorescein, ICG, and patent blue violet) have a relative high absorption coefficient at wavelengths within the range attained by available laser sources (argon blue-green, diode [810 nm], and red dye [630 nm] laser, respectively), and their maximal permissible doses are high in humans [44]. Experimental work in pigmented rabbits has shown that only ICG–enhanced photocoagulation produced a choroidal damage throughout the full thickness of the choroid, whereas patent blue violet–enhanced photocoagulation damaged only the inner layer of the choroid.

The diode laser, which has an emission peak similar to the absorption peak of ICG, was applied in a pilot study to six eyes with classic subfoveal CNV presumed secondary to pseudohistoplasmosis (three eyes), idiopathy (two eyes), and myopia (one eye) [45]. Stabilization of visual acuity was obtained in all eyes as well as closure of CNV.

ALTERNATIVE TREATMENT MODALITIES

Although three randomized trials have established the superiority of laser treatment over observation for subfoveal CNV, patients could expect no improvement in vision or return of reading or driving ability. Because macular photocoagulation is not a panacea, other ways, surgical or medical, were sought to manage this condition.

Surgical management of choroidal neovascular membrane

The surgical approach to subfoveal lesions was introduced by De Juan and Machemer [34]. Large-flap techniques were followed by small retinotomy techniques [37,46]. Different authors published the result of surgical excision of subfoveal CNV [38,39••,47,48]. Despite refinements in the surgical technique, the published results do not show convincing positive results in the treatment of ARM (Table 6-1). It must be emphasized that current studies are not uniform in their inclusion criteria.

It would seem appropriate to use this surgical technique for CNV only in cases of occult or obscured CNV in which no other therapeutic option exists. Experience with the technique is at present gained by extending patient follow-up periods, improving instrumentation and, even more, by refining patient selection to identify groups of patients for whom a randomized, prospective clinical trial would be appropriate (such a trial is presently underway). Research in RPE and photoreceptor regeneration and transplantation may further refine these surgical techniques and improve visual outcome.

TABLE 6-1	RESULTS OF STUDIES ON THE SURGICAL REMOVAL OF SUBFOVEAL CHOROIDAL NEOVASCULAR MEMBRANE IN EYES WITH AGE-RELATED MACULAR MACULOPATHY							
Study	**Eyes, n**	**Type of choroidal neovascular membrane**	**Initial visual acuity**	**Postoperative visual acuity**			**Follow-up, mo**	**Complications**
				↑	NC	↓		
Lambert and coworkers [37]	10	Classic	20/200 - CF	7	—	3	6	0 Recurrences 2 RD
Thomas and coworkers [38••]	33	Classic and occult	20/30 - CF	8	15	10	3–16	12 Recurrences 2 RD 4 Macular puckers
Berger and coworkers [47]	19	Classic and occult	20/80 - CF	4	10	5	0.25–10	3 Recurrences 0 RD

↑—improved; NC—no change; ↓—worsened; RD—retinal detachment.

Radiation treatment

Recent experimental studies have shown that low doses of radiation significantly reduce the neovascular component of ocular wound healing. Patients receiving cephalic teletherapy are unlikely to develop significant retinopathy when exposed to low doses of radiation. A pilot study was designed to evaluate the effects of teletherapy on age-related subfoveal CNV [49]. In 11 of 19 such eyes (63%) treated with 10 or 15 Gy of 6-MV photons, visual acuity was maintained or improved at a 12-month follow-up examination. Neovascular membrane regression, measured by image analysis, was observed in 77% of the eyes at 12 months after radiation treatment.

This study is very stimulating. However, the type of new vessels treated was not precisely analyzed. In a complex neovascular lesion, it is very challenging to measure and determine the exact limits of the membrane. The authors compared these results of teletherapy with results in a group of patients (seven patients) who declined treatment, which does not constitute a correct control group. The radiation technique must obviously be refined because the optic nerve is presently interested by the radiation.

Pharmacologic management for choroidal neovascular membrane

Angiogenesis describes the generation of new blood capillaries and is a key element in ocular neovascularization modulated by both inhibitory and stimulatory factors, in which only some factors implicated are presently known. Pharmacologic treatment constitutes a promising alternative or adjunct approach to the treatment of CNV. The rationale behind using a pharmacologic approach to treat choroidal neovascularization is to use direct inhibitors of angiogenesis or to suppress some of its initiators.

In histopathology, macrophage infiltration is frequent in the early stage of choroidal neovascularization. Macrophages have been implicated in vascular endothelial cell proliferation *in vitro* as well as in new vessel formation *in vivo*. The majority of mononuclear leukocytes that accumulated at the sites of laser lesions in an animal model of laser-induced choroidal neovascularization were derived from the systemic circulation [50]. This finding suggests that the initial stage of choroidal neovascularization may possibly be susceptible to systemic drugs that interfere with macrophage activation or chemotaxis.

Interferon alfa, interferon beta, and to a lesser extent, interferon gamma were shown to inhibit angiogenesis in experimental models. Interferon alfa-2a and alfa-2b caused regression of new blood vessels in an *in vivo* primate model of neovascularization of the iris [51•]. Antiangiogenic effects of interferon were demonstrated in a clinical setting of life-threatening hemangiomas in children.

As a result of the first case report, Fung [52] investigated the potential use of interferon in seven patients with CNV secondary to ARM. In these patients, the neovascular membranes were either completely within, or encroached on the foveal avascular zone. Fung found that successful outcome was limited to those patients with small, recent subretinal neovascular membranes. Subsequent to this publication, reports have stated that interferon alfa was of no benefit for neovascularization secondary to ARM in small groups with controls [53,54]. However, the 6- to 12-week treatment periods in the previously mentioned studies would not be expected to be of sufficient duration because the usual time to clinical response for interferon alfa in other indications is 3 to 12 months. The most recent report states an objective improvement in visual acuity in three out of five patients [55]. At present, large randomized controlled trials are underway.

CONCLUSIONS

The biomicroscopic and stereofluorescein angiographic features of neovascular ARM have complex appearances. Our knowledge of and our therapeutic approach to ARM choroidal neovascularization has tremendously improved in the last 10 years. Recognition of the various types of CNV is crucial in determining eligibility to laser photocoagulation use. Randomized, prospective clinical trials with long-term follow-ups have demonstrated that laser treatment is beneficial in terms of visual acuity in classic, well-defined extrafoveal, and juxtafoveal CNV. For classic subfoveal CNV, two techniques are used— complete ablation or perifoveal treatment of Créteil.

In our approach, the choice of treatment is guided by the published results. Complete ablation, as recommended by the Macular Photocoagulation Study, showed more rapid and stable benefit in small and intermediate subfoveal CNV with low initial visual acuity. For larger lesions, the perifoveal technique of Créteil seems more appropriate because the patients do not experience an immediate and definitive visual loss, but benefit from treatment—especially for near-vision tasks. This difficult choice of treatment techniques should decrease with education of both the ophthalmologists and of the patients because most of the subfoveal lesions are initially extrafoveal.

Immediate post-laser photographic control and overlay will help to ensure adequate coverage and reduce the incidence of recurrences and persistence. The results of this complete and heavy photocoagulation could be improved with the use of other wavelengths or other techniques of photocoagulation.

Occult, obscured, or complex ARM lesions, which constitute the majority of lesions in patients at presentation, should be the prime candidates for alternative treatment techniques with photocoagulation, drugs, or surgery. These other treatment approaches must be evaluated in prospective studies carefully designed with strict inclusion criteria based on fluorescein and ICG angiographic features, with both long-term follow-up and appropriate control groups. The natural history of neovascular ARM is well known in its late stages, both clinically and histopathologically, but the knowledge of the early stages needs to be refined to identify high-risk characteristics and to prevent the ingrowth of new vessels.

REFERENCES AND RECOMMENDED READING

Recently published papers of particular interest have been highlighted as:
• Of interest
•• Of outstanding interest

1.•• Macular photocoagulation study group: subfoveal neovascular lesions in age-related macular degeneration: guidelines for evaluation and treatment in the macular photocoagulation study. *Arch Ophthalmol* 1991, 109:1242–1257.
This article provides detailed angiographic analysis of all components of the neovascular lesions in ARM.

2. Freund KB, Yannuzzi LA, Sorenson JA: Age-related macular degeneration and choroidal neovascularization. *Am J Ophthalmol* 1993, 115:786–791.

3. Quentel G, Coscas G: Intérét des rétinographies en lumière monochromatique (verte, rouge et bleue) lors de la photocoagulation des membranes néovasculaires juxtafovéolaires. *Bull Mem Soc Fr Ophthalmol* 1981, 81:1047–1050.

4. Chamberlain JA, Bressler NM, Bressler SB, *et al.*: Photographs and fluorescein angiograms in the identification and treatment of choroidal neovascularization in the Macular Photocoagulation Study. *Ophthalmology* 1989, 96:1526–1534.

5.• Coscas G: Dégénérescence maculaires acquises Liées à l'age et néovaisseaux sous-rétiniens. In *Rapport à la Société Française d'Ophtalmologie.* Masson: Paris; 1991:486.
Analytic synthesis of the literature published on ARM until 1990 considering pathogenesis, clinical features, and treatment approaches.

6. Clark FM, Freeman WR, Goldbaum MH: Digital overlay of fluorescein angiograms and fundus images for treatment of subretinal neovascularization. *Retina* 1992, 12:118–126.

7. Mimoun G, Soubrane G, Bunel P, *et al.*: Calque automatique des néovaisseaux sous-rétiniens: un nouvel outil pour la photocoagulation maculaire. *Ophtalmologie* 1991, 5:29–32.

8. Grossniklaus HE, Martinez JA, Brown VB, *et al.*: Immunohistochemical and histochemical properties of surgically excised subretinal neovascular membrane in age-related macular degeneration. *Am J Ophthalmol* 1992, 114:464–472.

9.•• Lopez PF, Lambert HM, Grossniklaus HE, *et al.*: Well defined subfoveal choroidal neovascular membranes in age-related macular degeneration. *Ophthalmology* 1993, 100:415–422.
This article correlates the angiographic, clinical, and histologic characteristics of five surgically excised well-defined CNVs in eyes with ARM. The central core of neovascularization is surrounded with a dark rim found to be fibrin.

10. The Canadian Ophthalmology Study Group: Argon green vs krypton red laser photocoagulation of extrafoveal choroidal neovascular lesion: one year results in age-related macular degeneration. *Arch Ophthalmol* 1993, 11:181–185.

11. Macular Photocoagulation Study Group: Krypton laser photocoagulation for neovascular lesions of age-related macular degeneration: results of a randomized clinical trial. *Arch Ophthalmol* 1990, 108:816–824.

12. Macular Photocoagulation Study Group: Laser photocoagulation of subfoveal neovascular lesions in age-related macular degeneration: results of a randomized clinical trial. *Arch Ophthalmol* 1991, 109:1220–1241.

13. Macular Photocoagulation Study Group: Laser photocoagulation of subfoveal recurrent neovascular lesions in age-related macular degeneration: results of a randomized clinical trial. *Arch Ophthalmol* 1991, 109:1232–1241.

14. Coscas G, Soubrane G, Ramahefasolo C, *et al.*: Perifoveal laser treatment for subfoveal choroidal new vessels in age-related macular degeneration: results of a randomized clinical trial. *Arch Ophthalmol* 1991, 109:1253–1265.

15.• Mimoun G, Bunel P, Soubrane G, *et al.*: A new algorithm for automatic detection of subretinal new vessels using digital fluorescein angiography. *Invest Ophthalmol Vis Sci* 1992, 33(suppl):723.
Automatic detection of the location of the CNV to the fovea by digital imaging systems with overlay techniques.

16. Wolf S, Wald KJ: Detection of persistent choroidal neovascularisation using indocyanine green choroidal angiography. *Retina* 1993, 13:81–82.

17. Ryan SJ: Subretinal neovascularization after argon laser photocoagulation. *Graefes Arch Klin Exp Ophthalmol* 1980, 215:29–42.

18. Pollak A, Korte GE: Vascular remodeling after laser photocoagulation: concurrent regeneration and atrophy. *Acta Anatomica* 1992, 143:151–159.

19. Barondes MJ, Pagliarini S, Chisholm IH, *et al.*: Controlled trial of laser photocoagulation of pigment epithelial detachments in the elderly: a four-year review. *Br J Ophthalmol* 1992, 76:5–7.

20. Pagliarini S, Barondes MJ, Chisholm IH, *et al.*: Detection of subpigment epithelial neovascularization in cases of retinal pigment epithelial detachments: a review of the Moorfields Treatment Trial. *Br J Ophthalmol* 1992, 76:8–10.

21. Maguire JI, Benson WE, Brown GC: Treatment of foveal pigment epithelial detachments with contiguous extrafoveal choroidal neovascular membanes. *Am J Ophthalmol* 1989, 109:523–529.

22. Flower RW, Hochheimer BF: Infrared absorption angiography of the choroid and some observations on the effects of high intraocular pressure. *Am J Ophthalmol* 1973, 74:600–614.

23. Guyer DR, Puliafito CP, Mones JM, *et al.*: Digital indocyanine green angiography in chorioretinal disorders. *Ophthalmology* 1992, 99:287–290.

24.•• Yannuzzi LA, Slakter JS, Sorenson JA, *et al.*: Digital indocyanine green videoangiography and choroidal neovascularization. *Retina* 1992, 12:191–223.

First large clinical study describing the results of digital ICG angiography in 129 eyes with ARM. This article summarizes the current status of ICG evaluation of CNV.

25. Scheider A, Schroedel C: High resolution indocyanine green angiography with scanning laser ophthalmoscope. *Am J Ophthalmol* 1989, 108:458–459.

26. Brucker AJ, Brant A, Nyberg W: "Landmark injection" for localization of choroidal lesions using indocyanine green angiography. *Retina* 1993, 13:169–171.

27. Soubrane G, Coscas G, Francais C, *et al.*: Occult subretinal new vessels in age-related macular degeneration: natural history and early laser treatment. *Ophthalmology* 1990, 97:649–657.

28. Krott R, Quaranta M, Coscas G: Choroidal circulation and indocyanine green videoangiography in eyes presenting occult subretinal neovascularization. *Invest Ophthalmol Vis Sci* 1993, 34(suppl):1164.

29. Bressler SB, Silva JC, Bressler NM, *et al.*: Clinicopathologic correlation of occult choroidal neovascularisation in age-related macular degeneration. *Arch Ophthalmol* 1992, 110:827–832.

30. Scheider A, Kaboth A, Neuhauser L: Detection of subretinal neovascularization membranes with indocyanine green and infrared scanning laser ophthalmoscope. *Am J Ophthalmol* 1992, 113:45–51.

31. Hayashi K, De Laey JJ: Indocyanine green angiography of neovascular membranes. *Ophthalmologica* 1985, 190:30–39.

32. Destro M, Puliafito CA: Indocyanine green videoangiography of choroidal neovascularization. *Ophthalmology* 1989, 96:846–853.

33. Vander JF, Federman JL, Greven C, *et al.*: Surgical removal of massive subretinal hemorrhage associated with age-related macular degeneration. *Ophthalmology* 1991, 98:23–27.

34. De Juan E Jr, Machemer R: Vitreous surgery for hemorrhagic and fibrous complications of age-related macular degeneration. *Am J Ophthalmol* 1988, 105:25–29.

35. Toth CA, Morse LS, Hjelmeland LM, *et al.*: Fibrin directs early retinal damage after experimental subretinal hemorrhage. *Arch Ophthalmol* 1991, 109:723–729.

36. Sternberg P, Aguilar HE, Drews C, *et al.*: The effect of tissue plasminogen activator on retinal bleeding. *Arch Ophthalmol* 1990, 108:720–722.

37. Thomas MA: The use of vitreoretinal surgical techniques in subfoveal choroidal neovascularization. *Curr Opin Ophthalmol* 1992, 3:349–356.

38. Lambert HM, Capone A Jr, Aaberg TM, *et al.*: Surgical excision of subfoveal neovascular membranes in age-related macular degeneration. *Am J Ophthalmol* 1992, 113:257–262.

39.•• Thomas MA, Grand GM, Williams DF, *et al.*: Surgical management of subfoveal choroidal neovascularization. *Ophthalmology* 1992, 99:952–968.

Results of a large series of surgical excision of CNV in patients with ARM, presumed ocular histoplasmosis syndrome, and miscellaneous diagnosis.

40.• Tornambe PE, Poliner LS, Hovey LJ, *et al.*: Scatter macular photocoagulation for subfoveal neovascular membranes in age-related macular degeneration: a pilot study. *Retina* 1992, 12:305–314.

This is a nonrandomized, uncontrolled study of 40 ARM eyes with various types of subfoveal CNV. Scatter macular photocoagulation was applied outside of the CNV with or without focal extrafoveal ablation of CNV.

41.• Nishikawa S, Okisaka S: Photocoagulation with continuous wave Nd:YAG laser for neovascular maculopathy. *Jpn J Ophthalmol* 1992, 36:44–55.

Continuous-wave Nd:YAG laser photocoagulation was used to treat 19 juxtafoveal CNVs successfully in 17 eyes.

42. Sliney DH, Marshall J: Tissue specific damage to the retinal pigment epithelium: mechanisms and therapeutic implications. *Lasers Light Ophthalmol* 1992, 5:17–28.

43.• Roider J, Michaud NA, Flotte TJ, *et al.*: Response of the retinal pigment epithelium to selective photocoagulation. *Arch Ophthalmol* 1992, 110:1786–1792.

Multiple short argon laser pulses were shown to coagulate selectively the RPE while sparing the directly adjacent neural retina and choroid in rabbits.

44. Matsumoto M, Miki T, Obana A, *et al.*: Choroidal damage in dye-enhanced photocoagulation. *Lasers Light Ophthalmol* 1993, 5:157–165.

45. Reichel E, Puliafito CA: Indocyanine green dye enhanced diode laser photocoagulation of well-defined subfoveal choroidal neovascular membranes. *Invest Ophthalmol Vis Sci* 1993, 34(suppl):1164.

46. Blinder KJ, Peyman GA, Paris CL, *et al.*: Submacular scar excision in age-related macular degeneration. *Int Ophthalmol* 1991, 15:215–222.

47. Lopez PF, Aaberg TM, Lambert HM, *et al.*: Choroidal neovascularization occurring within a demarcation line. *Am J Ophthalmol*, 1992, 114:101–102.

48. Berger AS, Kaplan HJ: Clinical experience with the surgical removal of subfoveal neovascular membranes. *Ophthalmology* 1992, 99:969–976.

49. Chakravarthy U, Houstan RF, Archer DB: Treatment of age-related subfoveal neovascular membranes by teletherapy: a pilot study. *Br J Ophthalmol* 1993, 77:265–273.

50. Martini B, Ryan SJ: Argon laser lesions of the retina, occurrence and origin of macrophages. *Eur J Ophthalmol* 1992, 2:51–57.

51.• Stinson WG, Miller JW, Puliafito CA, *et al.*: Alpha interferon treatment of experimental iris neovascularization. *Invest Ophthalmol Vis Sci* 1991, 32(suppl):1046.

Regression of experimental iris neovascularization was observed in nonhuman primates after treatment with interferon alfa. None of the controls showed a similar evolution.

52. Fung WE: Interferon alpha 2a for treatment of age-related macular degeneration. *Am J Ophthalmol* 1991, 112:349–350.

53. Poliner LS, Tornamble PE, Michelson PE, *et al.*: A randomized trial of interferon alpha 2a for subfoveal neovascularization in age-related macular degeneration. *Ophthalmology* 1993, 100:1417–1424.

54. Thomas MA, Ibanez HE: Interferon alfa-2a in the treatment of subfoveal choroidal neovascularization. *Am J Ophthalmol* 1993, 115:563–568.

55. Engler CB, Sander B, Krofoed P, *et al.*: Interferon alpha 2a treatment of patients with subfoveal neovascular macular degeneration: a pilot investigation. *Acta Scand Ophthalmol* 1993, 71:27–31.

SELECT BIBLIOGRAPHY

Coscas G, Soubrane G: Photocoagulation des néovaisseaux sous-retiniens dans la dégénérescence maculaire sénile par laser à argon: résultats d'une etude randomisée de 60 cas. *Bull Mem Soc Fr Ophtalmol* 1982, 94:149–154.

Macular Photocoagulation Study Group: Argon laser photocoagulation for neovascular maculopathy: five-year results from randomized clinical trials. *Arch Ophthalmol* 1991, 109:1109–1114.

Macular Photocoagulation Study Group: Argon laser photocoagulation for senile macular degeneration: results of randomized clinical trial. *Arch Ophthalmol* 1982, 100:912–918.

Moorfields Macular Study Group: Treatment of senile macular degeneration: a single blind randomized trial by argon laser photocoagulation. *Br J Ophthalmol* 1982, 66:745–753.

Soubrane G, Coscas G, Baudouin C, *et al.*: Long term follow-up of randomized argon blue-green trial. *Graefes Arch* 1984, 8:132.

CHAPTER 7

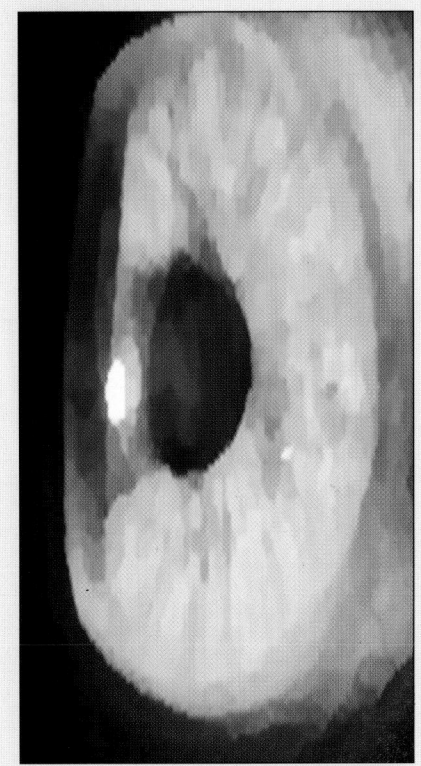

PHOTOCOAGULATION TREATMENT OF PIGMENTED INTRAOCULAR TUMORS

LEONIDAS ZOGRAFOS

At present, laser photocoagulation often is used in the conservative treatment of pigmented choroidal tumors. However, photocoagulation is rarely the sole or primary therapeutic modality. More often, photocoagulation is applied in conjunction with radiotherapy or is used for management of the side effects of irradiation. The use of new infrared lasers, the light of which penetrates deeply into tissue, and the use of laser light in photodynamic therapy, open up interesting new possibilities for the conservative treatment of uveal melanomas.

Laser photocoagulation is a commonly used treatment in ocular oncology and is used most often with other therapeutic modalities. One of the first applications of xenon photocoagulation, described by G. Meyer-Schwickerath in 1952, was the treatment of choroidal melanomas. This application was soon followed by photocoagulation treatment of retinoblastomas, choroidal hemangiomas, and vascular tumors of the retina. Soon after its introduction, laser photocoagulation supplanted xenon photocoagulation for most ophthalmic applications. Nevertheless, laser photocoagulation's implementation in ocular oncology was slower, and xenon photocoagulation is used even today for some indications.

Although photocoagulation is widely used, there are few reports in the ophthalmic literature regarding photocoagulation treatment of intraocular tumors, and there are even fewer reports of large series of patients with sufficiently long follow-up to allow sound evaluation of the results. The few reports are in contrast to the wide range of clinical and experimental applications for which the numerous new lasers are being used. Possible new uses of

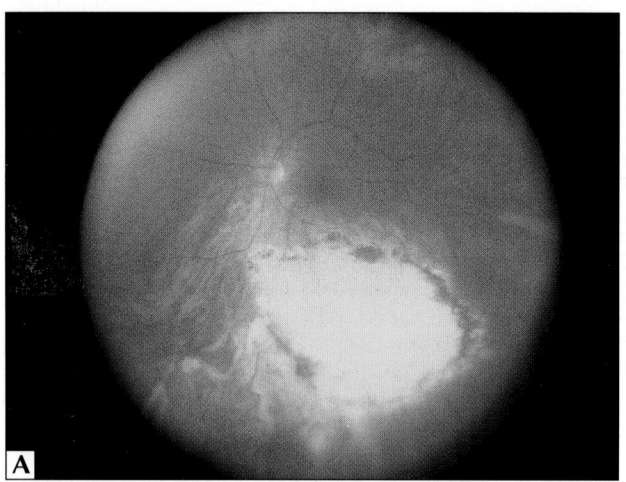

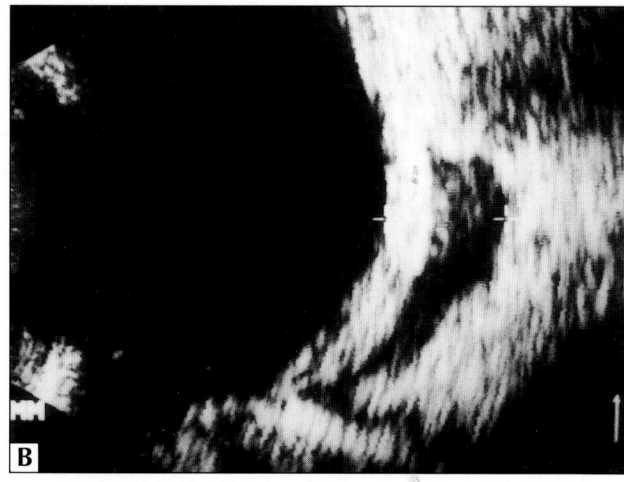

FIGURE 7-1 A, Wide-angle photograph of a chorioretinal scar 5 years after xenon photocoagulation of an uveal melanoma.

B, Ultrasound of a large extraocular extension of tumor behind the atrophic chorioretinal scar.

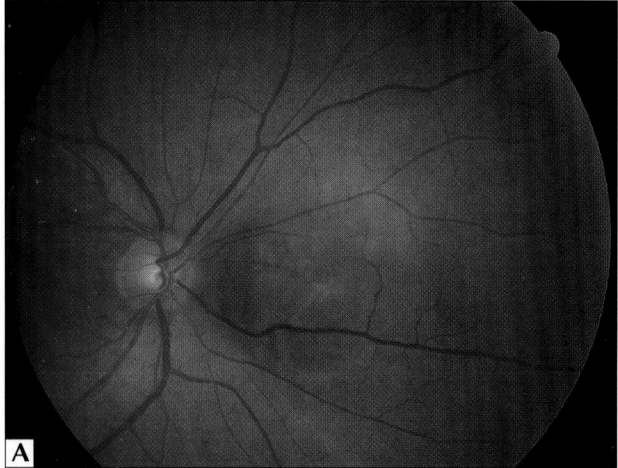

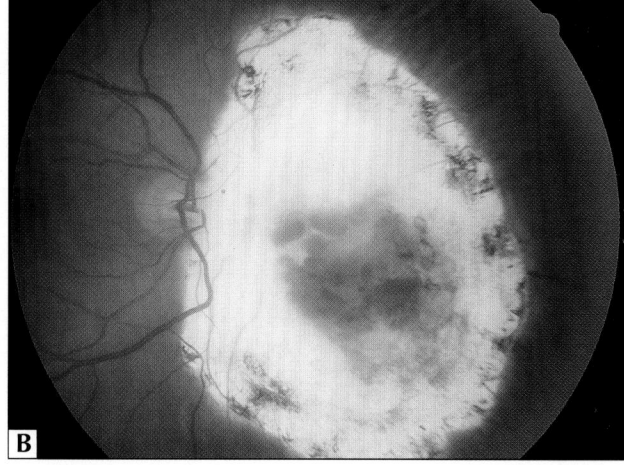

FIGURE 7-2 A, Small uveal melanoma localized in the nasal part of the disc and treated by a combination of krypton laser and xenon photocoagulation. **B**, Two years

after treatment, there is an atrophic chorioretinal scar containing a focus of pigmentation in its center. Visual acuity was 20/20.

the new lasers also offer interesting possibilities in the treatment of intraocular tumors.

PHOTOCOAGULATION TREATMENT OF CHOROIDAL MELANOMAS

The bulk of our knowledge on photocoagulation treatment of uveal melanomas is derived from the statistical analyses of two series of cases treated by xenon photocoagulation. The first of these series, reported by G. Meyer-Schwickerath [1], consists of 164 cases; the second series, reported by Jules Francois [2], consists of 122 cases. In these two series, the same photocoagulation technique was used. First, a circular atrophic photocoagulation scar was produced by a double row of confluent photocoagulation spots, after which an attempt was made to isolate the tumor from the choroidal circulation. In the second stage, progressive photoablation of the tumor was carried out in two to five sessions.

Reevaluation of the second series of cases by independent observers demonstrated that after a follow-up period of at least 5 years, 43.75% of the cases were considered as clinically cured. The tumor-related mortality was 12.5% and 50% of the treated eyes were ultimately enucleated [3]. Late local recurrences, as long as 16 years after the treatment, did occur. Scleral invasion was present in 55% of the enucleated eyes, extrascleral extension was present in 35% of the cases, and invasion of the optic nerve was identified in 70% of the cases.

In addition, in the short term, in spite of some positive results, numerous complications that led to partial or total functional loss were described. The most common of these were tractional retinal detachment, preretinal fibrosis, vitreous hemorrhage, retinal vascular occlusion, cystic macular edema, and pigment dispersion into the vitreous body, as well as persistent inflammatory reaction and complicated cataract.

L'Esperance [4] and Shields et al. [5] have proposed a photocoagulation technique using the argon laser with the same therapeutic protocol introduced by Meyer-Schwickerath for xenon photocoagulation of melanomas. In a small series of cases, after a follow-up ranging only from 58 to 150 months, the local recurrence rate was much higher in cases treated with the argon laser (64%) than in cases treated by xenon photocoagulation (14%) [5]. Less penetration of the blue-green argon light into the tumor mass behind the pigment epithelium, where most of the light is absorbed, may partly explain this difference. In addition, laser photocoagulation may cause microexplosions on the surface of the tumor, which could lead to hemorrhages, as well as to a dispersion of viable tumor cells in the vitreous cavity. In an attempt to reduce the risk of the latter, Foulds and Damato [6] proposed the use of argon or krypton laser with low energy and long exposures. It is interesting to note the short-term results for small melanomas treated in this manner, as well as for recurrent melanomas similarly treated, following local surgical excision.

Treatment of uveal melanomas by various forms of radiotherapy, such as brachytherapy or external beam irradiation with charged particles, presently offers greater security than does photocoagulation for the control of localized tumors (Fig. 7-1). For this reason, radiotherapy is almost always the treatment of choice, even in those situations where a small tumor is located in the nasal part of the optic disc and photocoagulation presents less potential risk for functional loss (Fig. 7-2).

Currently, the use of laser photocoagulation is widespread for the treatment of some side effects of ocular radiotherapy and for more conservative management of uveal melanomas. In cases of irradiation-induced retinal ischemia, sectorial or panretinal photocoagulation is quite effective in preventing neovascular glaucoma as well as vitreous hemorrhage from epipapillary or preretinal new vessels (Fig. 7-3).

Laser photocoagulation of the surface of the tumor may effectively reduce the exudative reaction that originates from the altered retinal vessels that overlie the tumor, as well as from the vessels within the tumoral mass, thereby contributing to a more

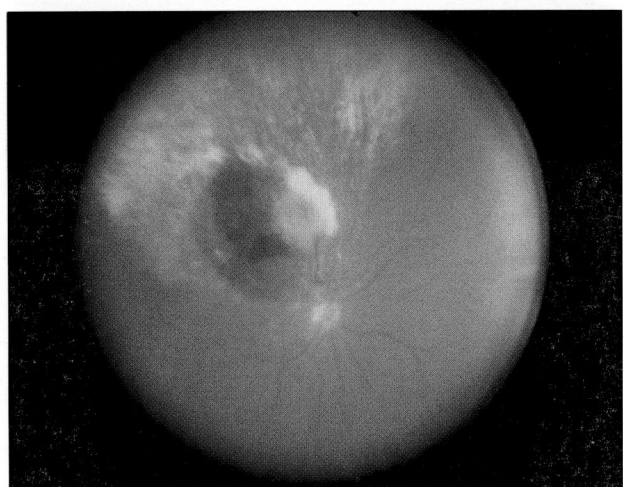

FIGURE 7-3 Sectorial photocoagulation of ischemic zones resulting from arteriovenous occlusion following proton beam irradiation of a uveal melanoma localized in the upper temporal quadrant. The retina overlying the tumor, as well as the entire upper temporal quadrant, are treated with confluent laser burns.

rapid reattachment of the secondary exudative retinal detachment and to absorption of the lipid deposits that often surround the tumor. The creation of a barrage of laser photocoagulation spots between the macula and the tumor may, in some cases, protect the macula from secondary detachment and preserve vision (Fig. 7-4). Laser photocoagulation may also, in some cases, eliminate small recurrences of the tumor following conservative treatment with either irradiation or local excision.

The systematic use of argon laser or xenon photocoagulation combined with radiotherapy has been reported (Fig. 7-5) [7–10]. In these various series, combined therapy resulted in a more rapid and complete regression of the tumor, a more rapid reabsorption of the secondary exudative detachment of the retina, and a decrease in the percentage of cases in which vitreous

hemorrhages occurred. However, the combination of these two therapeutic modalities did not have any beneficial effect on visual function during either short- or mid-term follow-up.

More recently, Lee *et al.* [11] reported a more rapid tumor regression after photocoagulation with a diode laser (630–680 nm) used in conjunction with application of radioactive iodine plaques. This rapid tumor regression may be related to deeper penetration of the tissue by the longer wavelengths. We can expect an even greater efficiency of the diode laser as units capable of even longer wavelength become available. The diode laser can be used also in transscleral treatment of the tumor basis. Furthermore, the efficacy of this laser can be amplified by injection of indocyanine green, which increases the absorption of its light. The efficacy of this technique was demonstrated in an

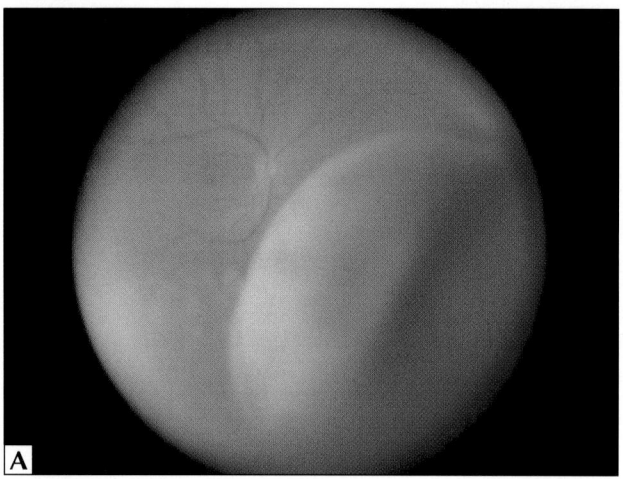

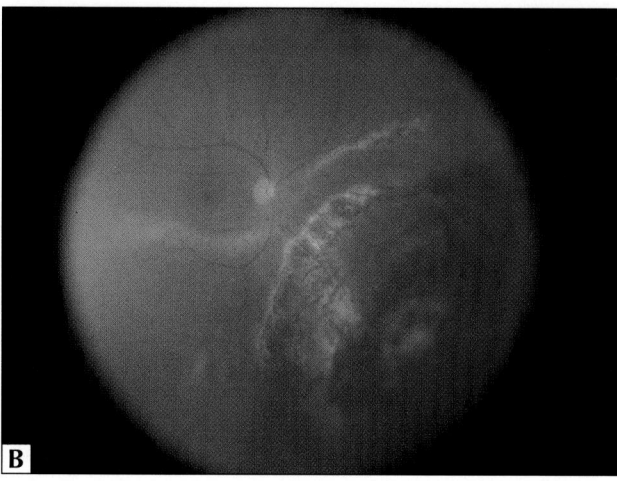

FIGURE 7-4 A, Large uveal melanoma localized in the inferior nasal quadrant accompanied by an inferior, bullous, exudative segmentary retinal detachment that is progressing toward the macula. **B**, Fundus picture of the melanoma 1.5 years

after treatment with accelerated proton beam combined with a double barrage of laser photocoagulation. The tumor is markedly reduced in size and the retina is flat; visual acuity was 20/40.

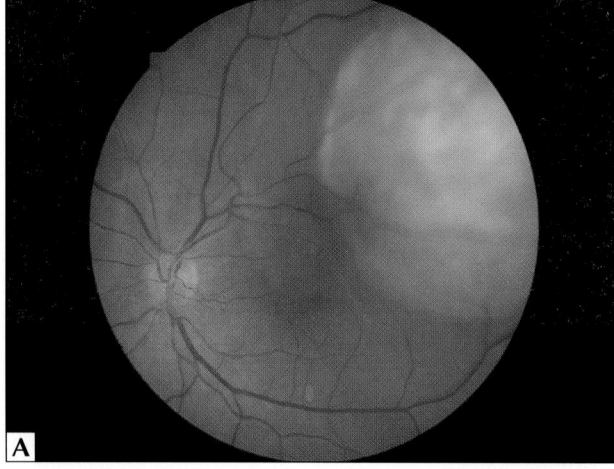

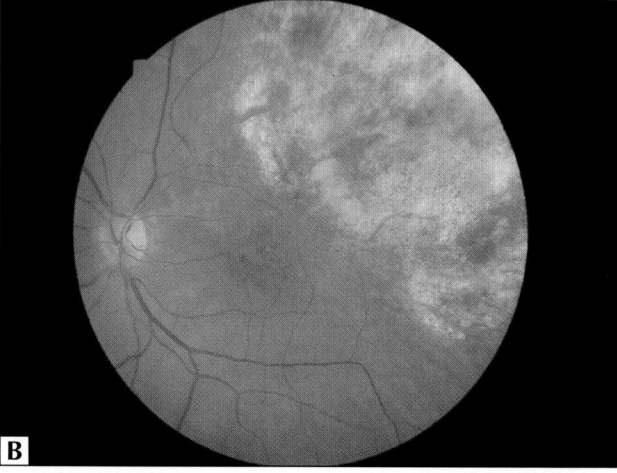

FIGURE 7-5 A, Paramacular uveal melanoma treated by a combination of proton beam irradiation and surface photocoagulation with the argon laser. **B**, Treatment resulted in

rapid regression of the tumor, which, 1 year after treatment, is seen as a flat, partially pigmented chorioretinal scar.

animal experiment, in which extensive necrosis was produced [12,13].

Diode lasers can be used also at a low energy setting to cause an increase in intratumor temperature, such as in transpupillary hyperthermia, which is a new therapeutic approach under investigation for the treatment of uveal melanomas. Another therapeutic approach under investigation is photodynamic therapy. This technique is based on the concept that some molecules may serve as photosensitizers. Concentration of these photosensitizers within tumor cells would thus make the cells sensitive to wavelengths absorbed by the chromophores. Until now, the only substances tested for the treatment of uveal melanomas have been a hematoporphyrin derivative, chloroaluminum sulfonated phthalocyanine and Bacteriochlorin a [14–22]. Preliminary results, although variable, are interesting.

PHOTOCOAGULATION TREATMENT OF NEVI AND ATYPICAL MELANOCYTIC TUMORS OF THE CHOROID

In cases of choroidal nevi, laser photocoagulation may be used to treat neovascular membranes that sometimes develop on the surface of these lesions (Fig. 7-6). The proliferation of a neovascular membrane on the surface of pigmented choroidal tumors is a rare phenomenon, and in most cases is associated with a choroidal nevus, that makes localized contact with the optic disc or that infiltrates the macula. The presence of such a neovascular membrane is not prognostic of evolution of the lesion or of malignant transformation of the choroidal nevus. The functional prognosis of these eyes is excellent if the neovascular membrane is in an extrafoveal location and if it can be eliminated com-

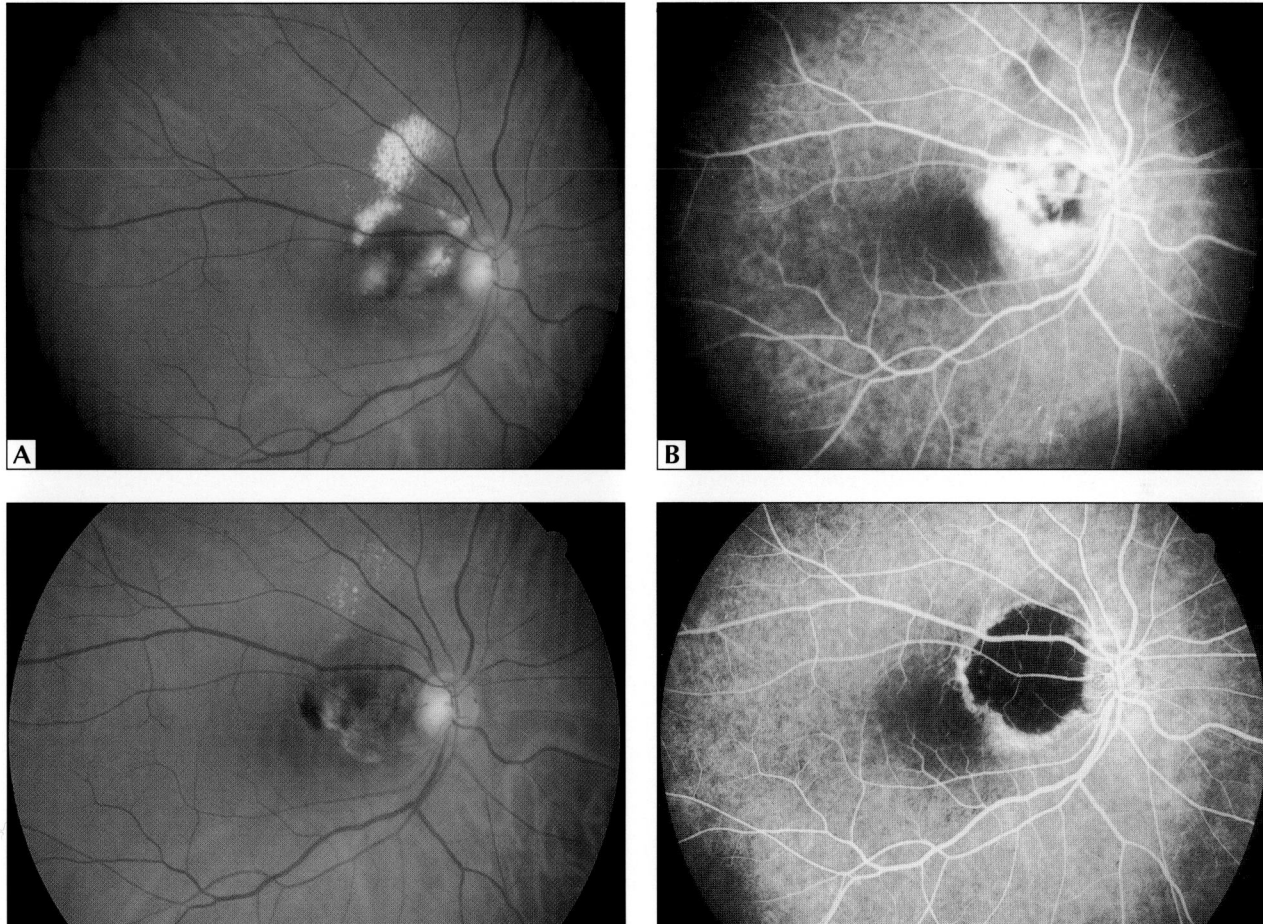

FIGURE 7-6 A and **B**, Clinical and angiographic photographs of an extrafoveal neovascular membrane on the surface of a localized choroidal nevus that is in contact with the optic disc. Note lipid deposits and serous detachment of the macula. Visual acuity was reduced to 20/200.

C and **D**, Clinical and angiographic photographs 1 year after laser photocoagulation of the neovascular membrane. The retina is reattached and the lipid deposits have been reabsorbed. Visual acuity at this time had improved to 20/25.

pletely by photocoagulation [23]. In contrast, functional prognosis is unfavorable if the neovascular membrane infiltrates the macular region and cannot be completely destroyed by laser photocoagulation. In rare instances, a spontaneous regression of the neovascular membrane may occur. This eventuality must be taken into account before performing photocoagulation treatment of a neovascular membrane close to the fovea.

In most cases of atypical choroidal melanocytic tumors, an observation period is used to document the presence or absence of tumor growth before a treatment course is started. Some tumors present with a limited exudative retinal detachment that involves the macula, which can affect central vision. In these cases, a photocoagulation treatment may be applied to the surface of the tumor. Treatment has to be limited to the central part of the tumor. The tumor borders must not be treated by photocoagulation as the creation of photocoagulation scars may mask possible tumor growth. Close follow-up of patients is extremely important as tumor growth may extend through photocoagulation-induced ruptures of Bruch's membrane, resulting in a mushroom-shaped lesion [24, 25].

CONCLUSIONS

Laser photocoagulation alone is rarely used in ocular oncology. Rather, laser photocoagulation is most often used as a complementary treatment, mainly to manage the side effects of ocular irradiation and to prevent serious loss of vision. Although at present there are not any concrete statistical data on the effects of new lasers in the treatment of intraocular pigmented tumors, preliminary clinical and experimental results are very promising.

REFERENCES AND RECOMMENDED READING

Recently published papers of particular interest have been highlighted as:
* Of interest
** Of outstanding interest

1. Meyer-Schwickerath G, Bornfeld N: Photocoagulation of choroidal melanomas: thirty years experience. In Intraocular tumors. Edited by Lommatzsch PK, Blodi FC. Berlin: Akademie-Verl; 1983:269–276.

2. François J: Treatment of malignant choroidal melanomas by xenon photocoagulation. In *Intraocular Tumors*. Edited by Lommatzsch PK, Blodi FC. Berlin: Akademie-Verl; 1983:277–285.

3. De Laey JJ, Hanssens M, Ryckaert S: Photocoagulation of malignant melanomas of the choroid, a reappraisal. *Bull Soc Belge Ophthalmol* 1986, 213:9-18.

4. L'Esperance FA Jr.: *Ocular Photocoagulation, A Stereoscopic Atlas*. St. Louis: CIV Mosby Co.; 1975:157–162.

5.• Shields JA, Glazer LC, Mieler WF, *et al.*: Comparison of xenon arc and argon laser, photocoagulation in the treatment of choroidal melanomas. *Am J Ophthalmol* 1990, 109:647–655.

This is a review of 38 cases of selected choroidal melanomas that were treated by photocoagulation. Xenon arc photocoagulation was used in 22 patients and argon laser was used in 16 patients. Although all treated tumors were initially eradicated, there was subsequent regrowth in three of the 22 patients treated with xenon photocoagulation and in 10 of the 16 patients treated with argon laser.

6. Foulds WS, Damato BE: Low-energy long-exposure laser therapy in the management of choroidal melanoma. *Graefe's Arch Clin Exp Ophthalmol* 1986, 224:26–31.

7. Zygoulska-Mach H, Maciejewski Z, Link E: Conservative treatment of choroidal melanomas combined use of cobalt plaques and photocoagulation. In *Intraocular Tumors*. Edited by Lommatzsch PK, Blodi FC. Berlin: Akademie-Verl; 1983:417–423.

8. Zografos L, Gailloud CI: Traitement conservateur des melanomes de la chorolde avec les applicateurs de cobalt 60 radioactifs. *Klin Monatsbl Augenheilkd* 1983, 182:499–501.

9. Moura RA, McPherson AR, Easley J: Malignant melanoma of the choroid: treatment with episcleral 198Au plaque and xenon-arc photocoagulation. *Ann Ophthalmol* 1985, 17:114–125.

10.• Ausburger JJ, Kleineidam M, Mullen D: Combined iodine-125 plaque irradiation and indirect ophthalmoscope laser therapy of choroidal malignant melanomas: comparison with iodine-l25 and cobalt-60 plaque radiotherapy alone. *Graefe's Arch Clin Exp Ophthalmol* 1993, 500–507.

This is a report on the short-term impact of combined episcleral iodine-125 plaque radiotherapy and argon laser treatment in a series of 24 patients with choroidal melanoma. The endpoint of laser therapy was a well-defined atrophic chorioretinal scar, and complete or nearly complete nonfluorescence of the lesion on fluorescein angiography. In a case-by-case matched comparison, the tumor treated with supplemental laser regressed substantially faster and more completely that did those treated by either type of plaque therapy alone. However, short-term visual loss was greater in eyes treated by the combined therapy.

11.• Lee KY, Sabates FN, Ziemianski MC, *et al.*: Combined iodine-125 plaque irradiation and laser photocoagulation in the treatment of choroidal malignant melanoma. In *Tumors of the Eye*. Edited by Bornfeld N, Gragoudas ES, Hopping W, Lommatzsch PK, Wessing A, Zografos L. Amsterdam: Kugler; 1991:441–447.

This is a retrospective study of 22 choroidal nevi with overlying neovascularization follow-up for a mean of 6.5 years. Fifteen of these patients had a final visual acuity in the affected eye of

20/200 or better. Five of six patients treated with laser had visual improvement of two or more lines. Laser treatment, when indicated, if effective and may be safely performed.

12. Damato BE: An approach to the management of patients with uveal melanoma. *Eye* 1993, 7:388–397.

13. Chong LP, Ozler SA, De Queiroz JM, *et al.*: Indocyanine green-enhanced diode laser treatment of melanoma in a rabbit model. *Retina* 1993, 13:251–259.

14. Liu LHS, Ni C: Hematoporphyrin phototherapy for experimental intraocular malignant melanoma. *Arch Ophthalmol* 1983, 101:901–903.

15. Tse DT, Dutton JJ, Weingeist TA, *et al.*: Hematoporphyrin photoradiation therapy for intraocular and orbital malignant melanoma. *Arch Ophthalmol* 1984, 102:833–838.

16. Phillips AMR, Browne BH, Allan D, *et al.*: Haematoporphyrin photosensitisation treatment of experimental choroidal melanoma. *Eye* 1987, 1:680–685.

17. Favilla I, Barry WR, Gosbell A, *et al.*: Phototherapy of posterior uveal melanomas. *Br J Ophthalmol* 1991, 75:718–721.

18. Miller JW, Stinson WG, Gregory WA, *et al.*: Phthalocyanine photodynamic therapy of experimental iris neovascularization. *Ophthalmology* 1991, 98:1711–1719.

19. Panagopoulos JA, Svitra PP, Puliafito CA, *et al.*: Photodynamic therapy for experimental intraocular melanoma using chloroaluminum sulfonated phthalocyanine. *Arch Ophthalmol* 1989, 107:886–890.

20. Ozler SA, Nelson JS, Liggett PE, *et al.*: Photodynamic therapy of experimental subchoroidal melanoma using chloroaluminum sulfonated phthalocyanine. *Arch Ophthalmol* 1992, 110:555-561.

21. Schuitmaker JJ, Van Best JA, Van Delft JL, *et al.*: Bacteriochlorin a, a new photosensitizer in photodynamic therapy: in vivo results. *Invest Ophthalmol Vis Sci* 1990, 31:1444–1450.

22. Schuitmaker JJ, Vrensen GFJM, Van Delft JL, *et al.*: Morphologic effects of bacteriochlorin a and light in vivo on intraocular melanoma. *Invest Ophthalmol Vis Sci* 1991, 32:2683–2688.

23.• Callanan DG, Lewis ML, Byrne SF, *et al.*: Choroidal neovascularization associated with choroidal nevi. *Arch Ophthalmol* 1993, 111:789–794.

This is a retrospective study of 22 choroidal nevi with overlying neovascularization followed-up for a mean of 6.5 years. Fifteen of these patients had a final visual acuity in the affected eye of 20/200 or better. Five of six patients treated with laser had visual improvement of two or more lines. Laser treatment, when indicated, is effective and may be safely performed.

24. Folk JC, Weingeist TA, Coonan P, *et al.*: The treatment of serous macular detachment secondary to choroidal melanomas and nevi. *Ophthalmology* 1989, 96:547–551.

25.• Erie JC, Robertson DM, Mieler WF: Presumed small choroidal melanomas with serous macular detachments with and without surface laser photocoagulation treatment. *Am J Ophthalmol* 1990, 109:259–264.

A review of 22 patients who had presumed small choroidal melanomas associated with a serious macular detachment. In 13 eyes, the tumor surface was treated with laser photocoagulation to reattach the retina and improve vision. Twelve of the tumors that received surface photocoagulation grew after treatment. Seven of these tumors developed a collar-button configuration. Surface photocoagulation applied to a growing melanoma appears to increase the likelihood of tumor extension through Bruch's membrane.

SELECT BIBLIOGRAPHY

Bornfeld N, Gragoudas ES, Höpping W, *et al.*, eds: Tumors of the eye. In *Proceedings of the International Symposiums in Geneva, Switzerland, November 23–27, 1987, and Essen, FRG, September 21–23, 1989.* Amsterdam: Kugler; 1991.

Shields JA, Shields CL: *Intraocular Tumors: A Text and Atlas.* Philadelphia: WB Saunders; 1992.

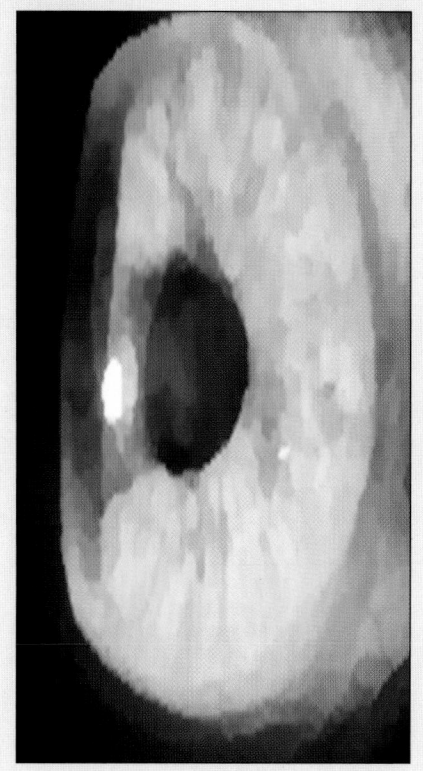

CHAPTER 8

LASER MANAGEMENT OF BRANCH AND CENTRAL RETINAL VEIN OCCLUSION

DANIEL FINKELSTEIN

Branch and central retinal vein occlusion (CRVO) are common retinal vascular disturbances. Together, they are the second most frequent cause of retinal vascular disturbance, after diabetic retinopathy. They share the vision–limiting problems of macular edema and neovascularization. Guidelines for the laser management of branch retinal vein occlusion (BRVO) have been provided by the Collaborative Branch Vein Occlusion Study Group and were published in the 1980s [1,2]. Laser management of macular edema and iris neovascularization for CRVO remain controversial and are presently being studied by the Collaborative Central Vein Occlusion Study Group [3].

This article reviews recommendations for laser management of macular edema and neovascularization in BRVO as previously presented by the Branch Vein Occlusion Study Group and summarizes the considerations for laser treatment of CRVO until the results of the Collaborative Central Vein Occlusion Study become available. Summary reviews of vein occlusion are available elsewhere [4–7].

BRANCH RETINAL VEIN OCCLUSION

Macular edema

The diagnosis of macular edema in the acute phase of BRVO can be difficult because of overlying intraretinal hemorrhage that may not permit appreciation of retinal thickening, cystoid spaces, and evaluation of potential visual acuity. Hemorrhage alone can reduce visual acuity significantly, and this decreased acuity can return to normal if there is no other macular disease when the hemorrhage resorbs.

We have found it helpful to distinguish four types of macular edema because different laser management techniques apply to each type: perfused macular edema,

nonperfused (ischemic) macular edema, mixed (perfused and nonperfused) macular edema, and macular edema from a distant BRVO. The distinction among these four types of edema depends on high-quality fluorescein angiography of the macula after there is sufficient absorption of intraretinal hemorrhage so that capillary detail can be appreciated.

In perfused macular edema, one sees intact perifoveal retinal capillaries on the transit of the fluorescein angiogram with late accumulation of fluorescein dye in a central cyst involving the center of the fovea (Fig. 8-1). In nonperfused macular edema, fluorescein angiography demonstrates a loss of capillary perfusion in the macular region with no late accumulation of fluorescein dye in the center of the fovea (Fig. 8-2). In the acute phase of the BRVO that causes ischemic macular edema, however, the appearance is clinically similar to perfused edema, demonstrating a thickened fovea and macula with cystoid spaces present. When fluorescein angiography is performed in ischemic vein occlusion, there is often some fluorescein leakage at the border zone between the perfused and nonperfused retina during the acute phase (the first 6 months), but this leakage is not sufficient to produce accumulation of fluorescein in the center of the fovea.

A mixture of perfused and nonperfused edema is frequently seen in the acute phase of the BRVO. There is some dilatation and leakage from perifoveal capillaries along with nonperfusion and a suggestion of leakage of fluorescein dye from the late fluorescein angiogram into the center of the fovea. It is unclear how much of the foveal cystoid edema is from perfused edema and how much is from nonperfused edema. Therefore, wait 6 to 12 months for spontaneous involution of the nonperfused edema and then reevaluate the situation.

In distant edema where there is macular edema and a peripheral BRVO in which the blocked segment does

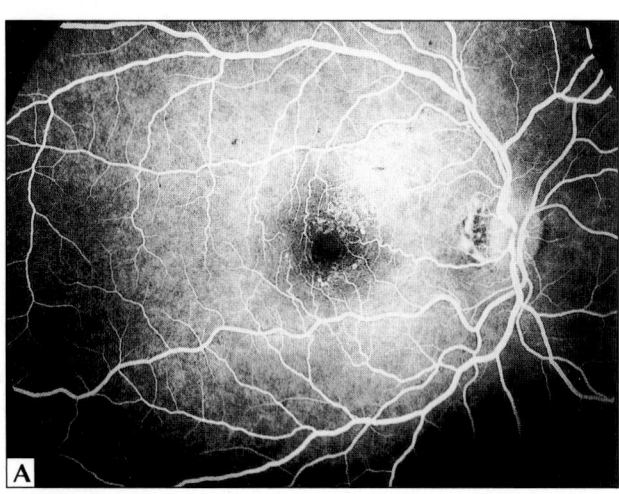

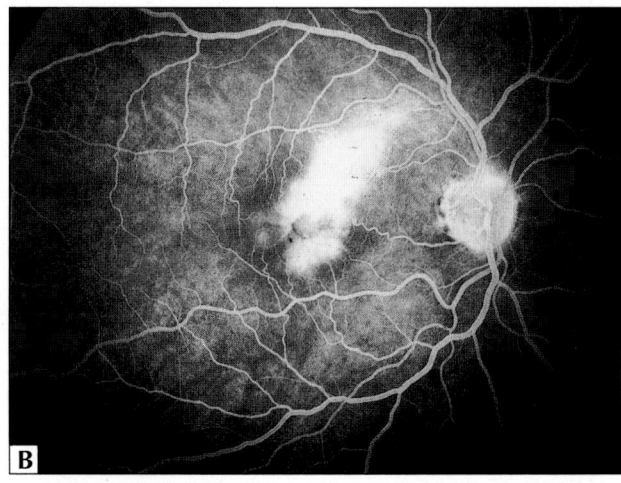

FIGURE 8-1   **A**, Fluorescein angiogram, transit phase, demonstrating perfused capillary circulation. **B**, Fluorescein angiogram, late phase, same case as Figure 8-1A, demonstrating leakage of fluorescein into central foveal cyst.

not involve the macula, the cause of the macular edema remains obscure. This is a rare type of macular edema in BRVO.

The natural history of vision change without therapy has been described to some degree. For perfused edema, the type predominantly studied in the Branch Vein Occlusion Study, about one third of patients showed spontaneous improvement without laser photocoagulation. For the nonperfused and mixed forms of macular edema, a small, pilot study suggested that the spontaneous improvement rate was far higher, about 90% [8]. Probably because the macular edema from a distant BRVO is so uncommon, there are no good natural history studies of vision loss in this form of edema. However, in our limited experience, we have seen some patients spontaneously improve [9].

Laser management

Once the acute phase of the BRVO has resolved so that there has been sufficient intraretinal hemorrhage absorption to obtain high quality fluorescein angiography, the type of macular edema may be ascertained. If the macular edema is a perfused type, with intact capillaries and leakage of fluorescein dye into the center of the fovea, one may next assess the status of visual acuity. If visual acuity has been gradually improving, the patient may fall into a group of patients who show spontaneous improvement. Laser photocoagulation should not be considered until it is clearly demonstrated that visual acuity has stabilized. If visual acuity stabilizes (at a somewhat arbitrary level of 20/40 or worse), grid laser photocoagulation may be considered. The patient must understand that statistically the likelihood of improvement is only one to two lines of visual acuity, with some patients improving far more and some patients not improving at all. Of course, the patient should be told that if the fellow eye is good, improvement in visual acuity is not likely to benefit visual function if the fellow eye remains with better acuity.

Grid laser photocoagulation includes the segment of leaking and dilated capillaries on a high quality fluorescein angiogram and may extend from the vascular arcade to the border of the foveal avascular zone, if those areas are dilated and leaking. As a general guideline, the grid laser photocoagulation is applied using 100μm spots for 0.1 second about one burn width apart, with a light to medium white burn seen at the level of the pigment epithelium (Fig. 8-3). Although the treatment is usually performed under topical anesthesia at one sitting, it seems reasonable to remain some distance from the foveal avascular zone at the first sitting, particularly if the foveal landmarks are unclear. In such a circumstance, if a fluorescein angiogram is performed 2 months after the treatment, a better evaluation can be made, based on the pigmentation from the previous treatment along with any continued leakage and vision loss, whether additional laser photocoagulation is needed closer to the foveal avascular zone. Laser photocoagulation probably can be performed satisfactorily with any wavelength if the laser produces a light to medium light burn. There was no evidence from the Collaborative Branch Vein Occlusion Study that laser photocoagulation needed to be performed early in the course of macular edema [1]. Consequently, it is emphasized to wait for good resorption of intraretinal hemorrhage and a sufficient follow-up to ensure that visual acuity has stabilized and is not spontaneously improving before considering laser photocoagulation.

Complications of grid laser photocoagulation are rare when the procedure is performed by an experienced surgeon, but patients must understand complications can occur that may reduce visual acuity, including paracentral scotomas or preretinal fibrosis. Macular

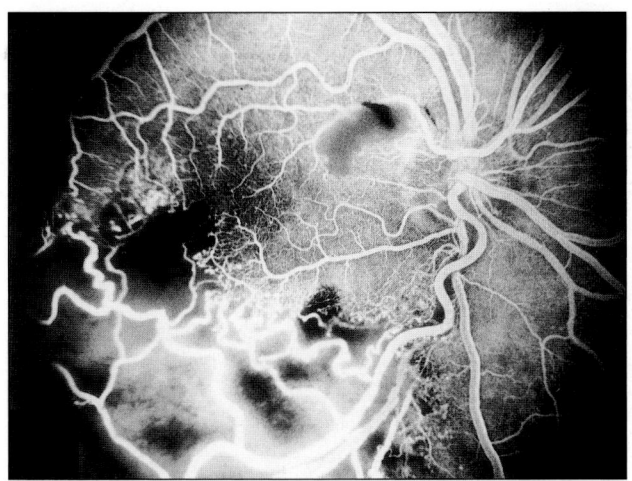

FIGURE 8-2 Fluorescein angiogram, transit phase, demonstrating partial macular nonperfusion.

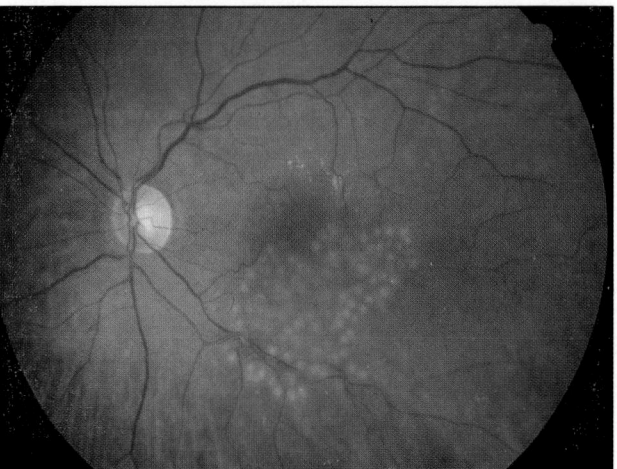

FIGURE 8-3 Post-treatment color photograph demonstrating pattern of grid laser photocoagulation for the management of macular edema secondary to branch retinal vein occlusion.

edema responds to grid laser photocoagulation within 4 to 8 weeks, although its temporal response has never been definitively studied. Visual acuity may respond quickly to grid laser photocoagulation, but may also continue to slowly improve over months to years after edema has lessened.

Neovascularization

Retinal neovascularization is a frequent complication of BRVO, occurring in about 50% of patients who have a large BRVO (about one quadrant of the fundus or more) associated with capillary nonperfusion (retinal ischemia) of significant extent (defined as 5 disc diameters in diameter or more). Because about 50% of large BRVOs are associated with ischemia, it would be expected that about 25% of large BRVOs will develop neovascularization. BRVOs that are well perfused will not develop neovascularization. (Remember that ischemic retina may be present only in the far periphery). Neovascularization may occur at the optic nerve head (neovascularization of the disc) or in the peripheral retina (neovascularization elsewhere).

Iris neovascularization is a rare complication of BRVO and seems to be associated with only very large areas of nonperfusion (greater than 1 quadrant of the fundus) and more frequent in patients with diabetes.

Retinal neovascularization usually begins to appear between 4 and 12 months after an ischemic BRVO has occurred. Infrequently, the neovascularization may be noted to develop only after the 1st year of the occlusion. Although the appearance of neovascularization is usually apparent, the appearance must be carefully distinguished from collateral vessels that can form in BRVO and that can mimic the appearance of neovascularization. If it is unclear whether abnormal blood vessels represent collateral vessels or neovascularization,

fluorescein angiography may be helpful to demonstrate profuse leakage from neovascularization or no leakage and minimal staining from collateral vessels.

About 50% of patients with neovascularization will develop significant traction or vitreous hemorrhage as vision-limiting complications. The Collaborative Branch Vein Occlusion Study demonstrated that scatter laser photocoagulation placed over the ischemic segment of the fundus from beyond the vascular arcade to the far periphery can reduce by 50% the onset of neovascularization for ischemic occlusions and can reduce by 50% the occurrence of vitreous hemorrhage in cases that already have neovascularization. Because prophylactic treatment of all ischemic BRVO would lead to twice as many treatments as necessary (because 50% of ischemic patients do not develop neovascularization) the Collaborative Branch Vein Occlusion Study suggested that laser photocoagulation be applied only after neovascularization begins to develop. However, if a patient cannot be followed every 4 months for the first 2 years after an ischemic occlusion to watch for development of neovascularization, then one could consider scatter laser photocoagulation before the development of neovascularization.

Scatter laser photocoagulation is applied in the same general manner as it is for the management of proliferative diabetic retinopathy, with 200 to 500 μm medium white burns at 0.1 to 0.2 second, absorbed at the level of the retinal pigment epithelium (Fig. 8-4). One should not attempt to directly close the neovascularization with focal treatment either on the disc or in the peripheral retina. Although topical anesthesia is often adequate, some patients suffer significant discomfort and may require peribulbar or retrobulbar anesthesia.

Complications of laser photocoagulation

Laser photocoagulation is remarkably safe when performed by an experienced surgeon for both macular treatment for macular edema and peripheral scatter treatment for the management of neovascularization. However, side effects and complications can occur. Patients must be thoroughly informed of the important benefits and risks of photocoagulation when deciding with the physician if laser photocoagulation should be performed.

The patient being treated for macular edema should understand that grid laser photocoagulation will produce a noticeable scotoma pattern of a "cluster of grapes" or black dots in the region of treatment that will gradually fade over a period of weeks to months. However, some patients will find the persistence of these scotomas to be an annoying disability. If laser photocoagulation leads to confluent spots, a resulting larger scotoma could be disabling for reading vision or other fine visual tasks, even if the visual acuity is improved by the treatment. Other complications and

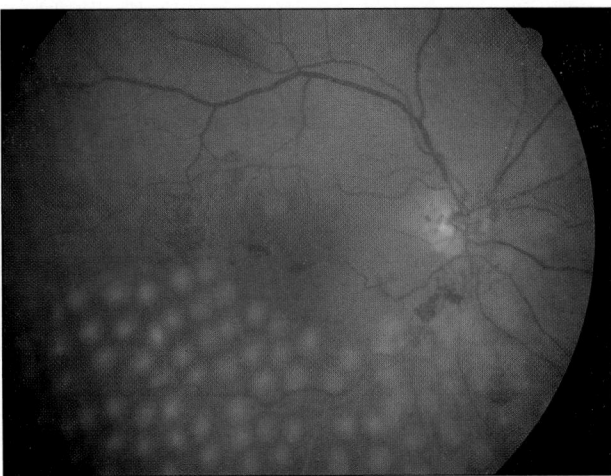

FIGURE 8-4 Post-treatment color photograph demonstrating pattern of scatter laser photocoagulation for the management of neovascularization secondary to branch retinal vein occlusion.

side effects of macular photocoagulation include inadvertent foveal treatment, preretinal fibrosis, and subretinal fibrosis. Particular care should be taken to avoid photocoagulation over sheets of intraretinal hemorrhage because the resultant heating of the retinal surface is a cause of preretinal fibrosis. In addition, laser photocoagulation with sufficient power to puncture Bruch's membrane may be expected to be associated with macular fibrosis. Laser photocoagulation for the management of neovascularization also can produce side effects and complications. Scatter photocoagulation can reduce the visual field extent in the quadrant being treated. Photocoagulation over sheets of intraretinal hemorrhage should be avoided because it can produce preretinal traction that could extend to macular distortion. Other vision-limiting complications and side effects can occur, but are less frequent.

CENTRAL RETINAL VEIN OCCLUSION

Central retinal vein occlusion is usually not difficult to diagnose when there is scattered intraretinal hemorrhage in all quadrants with dilated retinal veins. However, remember that bilateral acute disease, even if markedly asymmetric, may indicate a hyperviscosity syndrome that should be managed by caring for the hyperviscosity rather than considering management for complications of vein occlusion. In addition, situations that decrease arterial inflow to the eye, such as carotid disease, may present a fundus pattern similar to CRVO, and this also must be managed by evaluating the underlying condition.

Perfused central retinal vein occlusion with macular edema

When high quality fluorescein angiography demonstrates perfusion of the macular capillary circulation with leakage of fluorescein dye causing vision decrease, previous reports suggest edema may spontaneously lessen and patients' visual acuity will improve over the

1st months of follow-up in about one third of patients, about one third of patients may remain stable, and about one third of patients may worsen. No therapy has been proven to be beneficial if macular edema persists or worsens with persisting or worsening visual acuity loss. However, in a small series of patients, grid laser photocoagulation has been suggested as a beneficial treatment, demonstrating that a small number of patients who had documented stable edema and visual acuity loss improved immediately following laser photocoagulation (Fig. 8-5) [10]. The grid laser photocoagulation performed for macular edema in that small pilot series is under clinical research study in the Collaborative Nationwide Central Vein Occlusion Study. The study has completed follow-up of patients and is expected to report information regarding the efficacy of laser grid photocoagulation in 1994 or 1995. Until that time, one may consider grid laser photocoagulation in patients who have documented stable vision decrease with documented stable perfused macular edema as a cause of that acuity loss.

Nonperfused central retinal vein occlusion

Nonperfused CRVO usually produces a devastating loss of central acuity along with extensive nonperfusion. Occasionally, nonperfusion occurs only in the peripheral retina and this nonperfusion must be carefully searched for by high quality fluorescein angiography that "sweeps" to the periphery looking for extensive areas (10 disc areas or greater) of nonperfusion. When there is extensive ischemia, iris neovascularization (and sometimes retinal neovascularization) has been reported at rates of 20% to 80%. Be mindful that perfused vein occlusions, particularly very early in the course of the vein occlusion, can become nonperfused. Iris neovascularization usually begins to develop in the first 2 to 4 months following the ischemic vein occlusion. Iris neovascularization usually begins at the pupillary border, although rarely it is first seen in the angle by gonioscopy. Iris neovascularization, whether at the

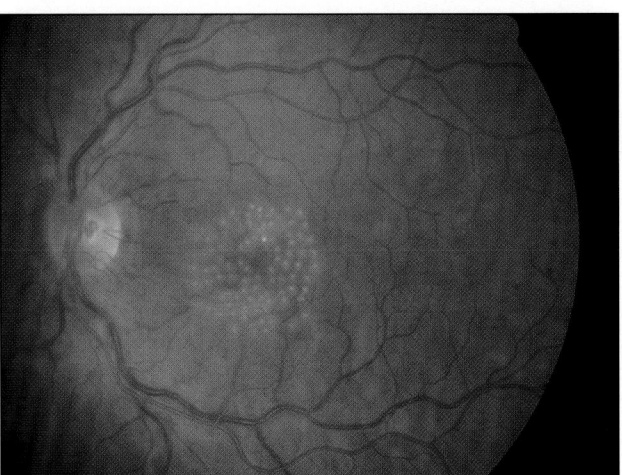

FIGURE 8-5 Post-treatment color photograph demonstrating pattern of grid laser photocoagulation for the management of macular edema secondary to central retinal vein occlusion.

pupillary border or in the angle, is far easier to recognize without pupillary dilatation.

Many clinicians believe that panretinal photocoagulation can prevent the development of iris neovascularization or cause its regression after it has appeared (Fig. 8-6). However, it has not been firmly established that panretinal photocoagulation is useful in this regard. To determine whether panretinal photocoagulation can prevent iris neovascularization, the Collaborative Nationwide Central Vein Occlusion Study is investigating the efficacy of laser photocoagulation in the prevention of iris neovascularization in ischemic vein occlusion and is expected to report these data in 1994 or 1995. Until these data become available, one may consider either prophylactic panretinal photocoagulation when ischemic CRVO has been documented or careful follow-up of such patients with scrutiny of the undilated pupil and application of panretinal photocoagulation after the development of iris neovascularization.

Diagnosis of iris neovascularization

Occasionally, vessels appear on the surface of the iris that mimic the development of iris neovascularization. Certain clues are sometimes helpful. For example, if few vessels are seen at the pupillary border of the involved eye and also the fellow eye, one might suspect the vessels represent a congenital variant or aging change rather than the true development of iris neovascularization. If prominent vessels are seen in the angle, but without peripheral anterior synechiae (PAS), or if similar vessels are seen in the angle of the fellow eye, one may also suspect they do not represent true angle neovascularization. Presently, iris angiography does not seem to be helpful in distinguishing true iris neovascularization from conditions that may mimic iris neovascularization. On occasion, it may be so diffi-

cult to determine if true iris neovascularization is present that one may wish to follow a patient closely, every few days or weekly, to watch for growth of the vessels that would indicate true iris neovascularization as a significant risk for the development of neovascular glaucoma.

Panretinal photocoagulation

Panretinal photocoagulation in ischemic vein occlusion for the prevention or control of iris neovascularization can be difficult for several reasons. First, the quantity of intraretinal hemorrhage may limit the ability to place burns at the level of the pigment epithelium. Using krypton red laser photocoagulation may be helpful in circumstances where there is moderately extensive intraretinal hemorrhage because the krypton red laser may be able to penetrate or extend under areas of hemorrhage. The previously mentioned complications from laser absorption by surface intraretinal hemorrhage are of less concern in CRVO. In CRVO there is almost always devastating loss of macular function from the permanent change of reduced vision in ischemic vein occlusion because of loss of capillary circulation to the macula.

If iris neovascularization that limits dilatation of the pupil because of posterior synechiae has already begun to appear, panretinal photocoagulation may be difficult because of inadequate pupillary dilatation. On occasion, dilatation of the pupil using the laser to break the synechiae may be possible, particularly if the synechiae are just forming.

If intraocular pressure elevates, whether or not associated with PAS or from the iris and angle neovascularization, media haze may be produced from corneal opacity as well, which limits the ability to perform panretinal photocoagulation. Under these circumstances, administration of intensive topical steroids for 1 or 2 days on an hourly basis with intensive dilatation, can be helpful.

If adequate panretinal photocoagulation is not possible, pancryocoagulation can be considered. If media opacity or vitreous hemorrhage prevents pancryocoagulation as well, vitrectomy and intraocular photocoagulation can be considered.

CONCLUSIONS

For the management of the complications of BRVO including macular edema and neovascularization, laser photocoagulation has been demonstrated as beneficial by randomized clinical trial. For CRVO, the use of laser photocoagulation for complications of macular edema and iris neovascularization are similarly now under study; suggestions for laser management are presented until the results of the randomized clinical trial become available.

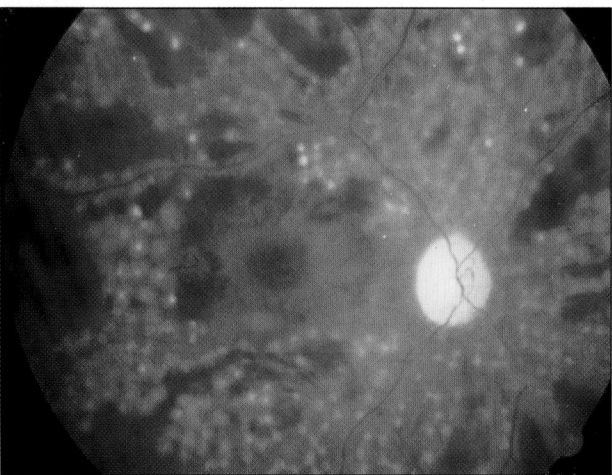

FIGURE 8-6 Post-treatment color photograph demonstrating pattern of panretinal photocoagulation for the management of iris neovascularization secondary to ischemic central retinal vein occlusion.

REFERENCES AND RECOMMENDED READING

Recently published papers of particular interest have been highlighted as:

- • Of interest
- •• Of outstanding interest

1. Branch Vein Occlusion Study Group: Argon laser photocoagulation for macular edema in branch vein occlusion. *Am J Ophthalmol* 1984, 98:271–282.

2. Branch Vein Occlusion Study Group: Argon laser scatter photocoagulation for prevention of neovascularization and vitreous hemorrhage in branch vein occlusion. *Arch Ophthalmol* 1986, 104:34–41.

3.• Central Vein Occlusion Study Group: Baseline and early natural history report. The Central Vein Occlusion Study. *Arch Ophthalmol* 1993, 111:1087–1095.

These findings confirm the importance of frequent follow-up examinations, including undilated slit-lamp examination of the iris and gonioscopy in the treatment of patients with recent onset of CRVO.

4. Gutman FA: Evaluation of a patient with central retinal vein occlusion. *Ophthalmology* 1983, 90:481–483.

5. Hayreh SS: Classification of central retinal vein occlusion. *Ophthalmology* 1983, 90:458–474.

6. Kohner EM, Laatikainen L, Oughton J: The management of central retinal vein occlusion. *Ophthalmology* 1983, 90:484–487.

7. Kearns TP: Differential diagnosis of central retinal vein obstruction. *Ophthalmology* 1983, 90:475–480.

8.• Finkelstein D: Ischemic macular edema; recognition and favorable natural history in branch vein occlusion. *Arch Ophthalmol* 1992, 110:1427–1434.

Cases evaluated as incomplete macular perfusion showed a greater frequency of improvement (91%) in visual acuity than did perfused cases (29%) ($P = 0.003$) after a mean follow-up of 39 months.

9. Finkelstein D, Patz A: Distant effect of peripheral branch vein occlusion on the macula. *Tr Am Ophthalmol Soc* 1988, LXXXVI:380–388.

10. Klein ML, Finkelstein D: Macular grid photocoagulation for macular edema in central retinal vein occlusion. *Arch Ophthalmol* 1989, 107:1297–1302.

SELECT BIBLIOGRAPHY

Coscas G, Dhermy P: Occlusions veineuses rétiniennes. In *Sociétíe Francaise D'Ophtalmologie* Paris: Masson; 1978.

Orth DH, Patz A: Retinal branch vein occlusion. *Surv Ophthalmol* 1978, 22:357–376.

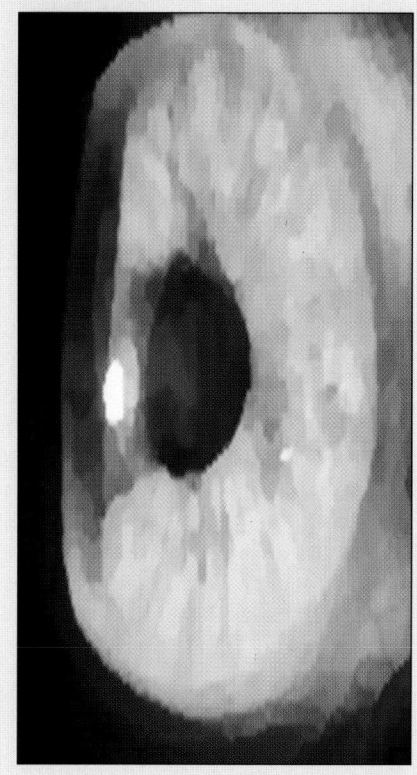

CHAPTER 9

TECHNIQUE AND INDICATIONS FOR ENDOLASER COAGULATION IN VITREOUS SURGERY

KWANG J. LEE
GHOLAM A. PEYMAN

In the 1980s, endophotocoagulation emerged as the ideal method for effecting intraoperative retinal coagulation. Its predecessors, intraocular diathermy and cryotherapy, suffered from numerous disadvantages, most of them stemming from the requirement that the diathermy tip or the cryoprobe come in contact with the retinal tissue to achieve coagulation, thereby risking injury to the retina and the choroid. These disadvantages were largely overcome with the advent of light energy for photocoagulation.

The first light source used for endophotocoagulation in humans was the xenon arc [1]. However, it soon became apparent that the coherent and monochromatic argon or krypton laser light provided a superior energy source for photocoagulation [2,3]. By using an optical fiber, a special intraocular probe, and a protective filter, a laser light can be safely delivered to the retina for scatter or focal photocoagulation during vitreous surgery (Fig. 9-1) [4]. Unlike the divergent beam of xenon arc light, the coherent laser light allows the endolaser probe to be operated at a safe working distance from the retina, thus minimizing the likelihood of the probe accidentally striking the retina during surgery. Although spot size and power density of a laser burn vary in relation to the distance between the probe and the retina surface, the variability is relatively slight in comparison with that of the xenon arc, and, therefore, complications related to excessive burns are infrequent. Most importantly, the laser probe can be used in various media, including silicone oil, perfluorocarbon liquids, and gas without incurring damage to the probe tip. In addition, rapid firing and limited excursions of the laser probe to coagulate large areas of the retina with efficiency are possible, thereby reducing operating time. In contrast, xenon arc light cannot be used in an air-filled eye, requires a close working distance from the retinal surface of less than 1 mm because of beam divergence, and does not permit rapid firing.

The ability of an intraocular endolaser system to perform retinal photocoagulation in a rapid, safe, and predictable manner has led to the development of several laser systems that operate on different wavelengths.

EQUIPMENT

Laser wavelength

The laser wavelengths that may be used for endophotocoagulation include argon blue-green, krypton red, dye, diode, and continuous-wave neodymium-yttrium aluminum garnet (Nd:YAG). Among them, the argon green is the most common wavelength used by ophthalmologists today. Both argon laser wavelengths, blue (488 nm) and green (514.5 nm), are absorbed well by melanin pigments in the choroid and the retinal pigment epithelial cells, as well as by the hemoglobin. Because of the undesirable absorption of blue-wavelength laser energy by the xanthophyllic pigment in the macula, the green wavelength is preferred for endolaser photocoagulation.

The krypton red (640 nm) and semiconductor diode (817 nm) lasers produce lights with longer wavelengths and less absorption by the melanin and hemoglobin pigments than does the argon green laser. Such characteristics make them effective lasers for retinal coagulation in the presence of intravitreal hemorrhage. However, because of less melanin absorption, krypton and diode lasers require higher amounts of energy to coagulate the retina than does the argon green laser, especially when the uvea is sparsely pigmented. Although the krypton red wavelength may be used for endophotocoagulation, its use does not provide a sig-

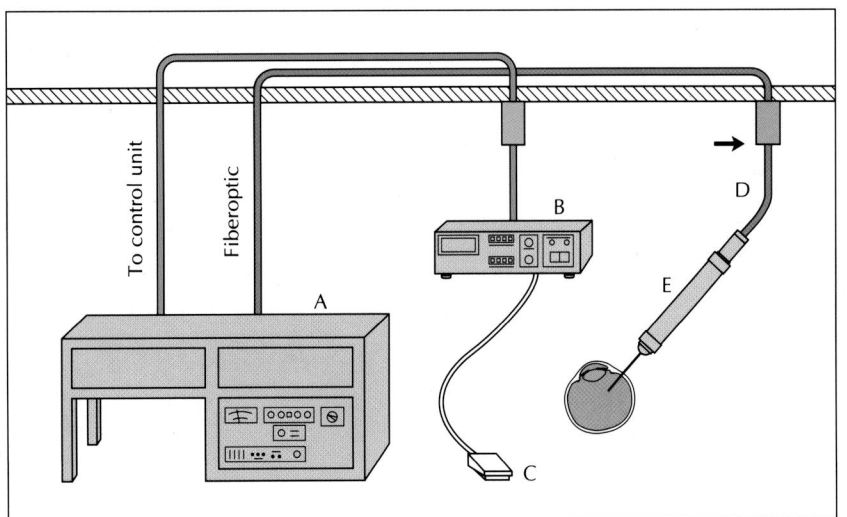

FIGURE 9-1 Schematic representation of endolaser system. (*From* Peyman and Schulman [4]; with permission.)

To control unit

Fiberoptic

A
B
C
D
E

nificant advantage over the argon green wavelength during most vitreous surgery.

The semiconductor diode laser, on the other hand, does provide some important advantages to vitreoretinal surgeons [5••,6]. It uses standard voltage for a power output of up to 1 to 2 W and can also be driven by a battery. No special delivery equipment is necessary because the laser light can be transmitted inside the eye through a commercially available endophotocoagulator probe. The solid-state–conduction diode laser does not require a water-cooling system; it can be cooled by air. These features endow the diode laser system with compact size, portability, affordability, and a long-lasting lifetime. The clinical effectiveness of the diode wavelength has been proved for the treatment of conditions such as proliferative diabetic retinopathy and proliferative vitreoretinopathy, and for retinal detachment repairs. No significant untoward effects of the wavelength have been noted.

The Nd:YAG laser uses a wavelength of 1060 nm, which results in a deeper tissue penetration than do shorter wavelengths. Its melanin absorption is less than that of shorter wavelengths, requiring five to six times the energy needed by green and red wavelengths. There is a delay of 1 to 2 minutes before the coagulated lesion becomes visible to the surgeon. Although animal experiments have proved that the continuous-wave Nd:YAG endolaser can be used to create a chorioretinal burn in a safe manner through the use of compact, inexpensive instrumentation, the clinical utility of this infrared wavelength is limited [6].

Laser delivery system

The argon laser source requires a water- or air-cooling system, as do the other gas lasers. A semiconductor diode laser, however, is air cooled. The laser console, located inside the operating room, is connected to the sterile portion of the disposable fiberoptic and the endolaser probe through a long fiberoptic cable

(Fig. 9-1). The probe is a 20-gauge cylinder that can be inserted through a conventional pars plana sclerotomy made with a microvitreoretinal blade.

Retinal view during endophotocoagulation is obtained with the use of a contact lens, an endoilluminator, and an operating microscope fitted with a protective filter. This filter blocks the laser light reflected to the eyes of both the surgeon and the assistant. Photocoagulation is achieved with the probe located approximately 3 mm from the retinal surface.

Recently, endolaser probes with the capacity to perform other functions for bimanual vitreoretinal surgery have been developed. The Peyman-D'Amico endolaser probe, with an aspiration capability, consists of a fiberoptic and an aspiration conduit inside a 20-gauge cylinder (Fig. 9-2) [8•]. The fiberoptic, connected to a laser source, delivers light energy for photocoagulation. The aspiration is achieved through a port on the tip of the probe. An opening on the probe's handle, controlled by a fingertip, allows passive egress of the intraocular fluid and therefore functions as a fluted needle. The combination probe then allows laser application immediately after the air-fluid exchange without the need to change instruments.

Another multifunction endolaser probe, developed by Peyman and Lee, has endoillumination and infusion capabilities in addition to the aspiration function [9••]. The multifunction probe completely frees the surgeon's other hand to use another vitreoretinal instrument in the bimanual technique (Fig. 9-3). Both probes allow laser photocoagulation of the retinotomy site to proceed immediately after subretinal fluid drainage without being interrupted by an exchange of instruments. The immediate coagulation overcomes repeated accumulation of subretinal fluid around the retinotomy, which can prevent adequate laser uptake. The probes are also used to clear the hemorrhage from the retinal surface, thereby allowing laser photocoagulation to proceed to the area uninterrupted. By reducing exchanges of

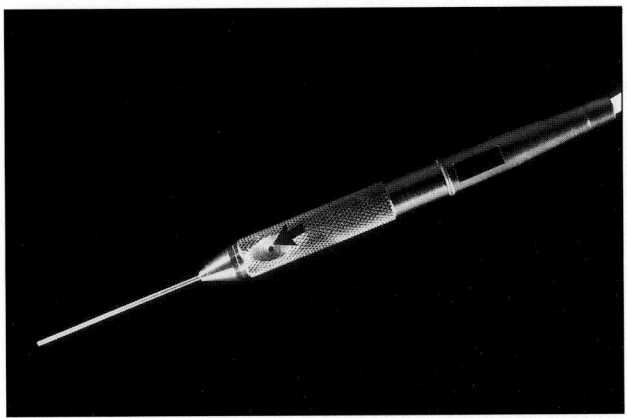

FIGURE 9-2 Endolaser probe with aspiration capability. (*From* Peyman *et al.* [8•]; with permission.)

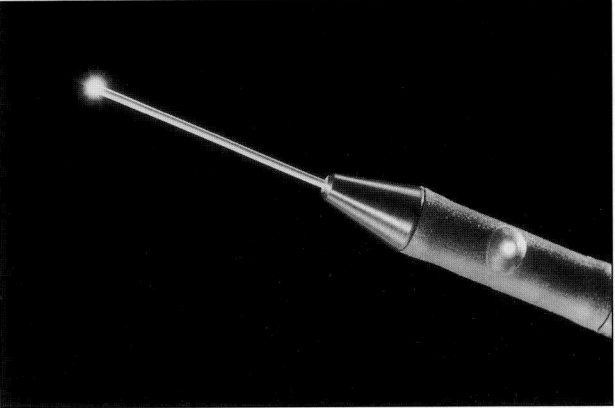

FIGURE 9-3 Multifunction endolaser probe. (*From* Peyman and Lee [9••]; with permission.)

instruments, the possibility of retinal incarceration to the sclerotomy sites as well as retinal dialysis, peripheral retinal tears, or prolonged surgery, are avoided.

The endolaser tip may be either straight or bent (Fig. 9-4) [10]. Although both tip designs allow adequate photocoagulation of the retina, the bent-tip probe allows better access to the peripheral retina, particularly near the entry site of the endolaser in the superior portion of the retina.

INDICATIONS FOR USE

Endolaser photocoagulation may be applied for three reasons: 1) to obliterate ischemic retina and reduce neovascular stimulus in proliferative retinopathy; 2) to create chorioretinal adhesion to seal retinal breaks; and 3) to destroy the ciliary body to reduce intraocular pressure [3,11,12].

Proliferative retinopathy
The purpose of endophotocoagulation is to reduce the stimulus for angiogenesis by destroying the ischemic retina. The laser is usually applied to the previously untreated area of the retina to complete the panretinal photocoagulation. Intraoperative endolaser photocoagulation following removal of vitreous opacity obviates later sessions of photocoagulation, which are more difficult to perform because of postoperative blurring of the fundus view, discomfort, and inconvenience. Endolaser photocoagulation may be performed during vitreous surgery for proliferative diabetic retinopathy, sickle cell disease, vein occlusion, ocular ischemic syndrome, lupus erythematosus, and Eales' disease.

Retinopexy
Endolaser photocoagulation is used to produce a chorioretinal adhesion around a retinal break. Various types of retinal breaks require chorioretinal adhesions during vitreous surgery to prevent postoperative retinal detachment. Examples of treatable retinal breaks include relaxing and drainage retino-

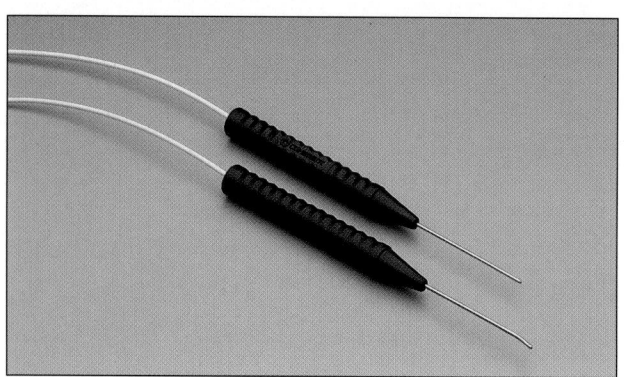

FIGURE 9-4 Endolaser probes, straight and bent tipped. (Courtesy of Coherent, Palo Alto, CA.)

tomies as well as significant retinal tears. Two to three rows of laser burns are usually placed around the retinotomy site. With the advent of macular surgery, the endolaser is also used to coagulate the retinotomy site made to extricate subfoveal membranes and hematoma. Peripherally located retinal tears may also be amenable to endolaser photocoagulation when combined with scleral depression. However, in phakic eyes, these lesions are often better treated by cryotherapy or indirect binocular laser applications. In a traumatic chorioretinal injury, the retinal perforation site is surrounded with a row of laser burns to reduce the likelihood of subsequent choroidal hemorrhage.

Glaucoma
Selective ciliary body ablation with an endolaser probe is possible in an aphakic eye when scleral depression is performed. Often, other surgical means of glaucoma management have failed in these patients.

Miscellaneous indications
Bleeding retinal vessels may be closed by using endolaser photocoagulation during vitrectomy, although endodiathermy is more effective in performing this task. Vitreous surgery for rare entities, such as retinal detachments associated with coloboma, optic pit, and internal resection of choroidal melanoma, benefit from endolaser photocoagulation. Situations other than the need for vitreous surgery may also call for the use of an endolaser. For example, the endolaser may be used to close a cyclodialysis cleft in the treatment for ocular hypotony. Choroidal perforation may be achieved with endolaser photocoagulation burns to drain subretinal fluid externally in a scleral buckling procedure.

TECHNIQUES

A desired intensity of chorioretinal burn is obtained by controlling the exposure time, power, and the distance of the endolaser probe from the retinal surface. A test burn to the peripheral retina is used to assess the degree of uptake at a given setting variable. The probe is held approximately 2.0 to 2.5 disc diameters from the retinal surface. An exposure time of between 0.3 second and 0.5 second is chosen. A good initial power level at which to begin photocoagulation is 0.4 W. The photocoagulation is then performed while adjusting the variables in small increments until a desired reaction is obtained. A green aiming beam is used to predict the size and location of each burn when using the argon laser.

COMPLICATIONS

The risk to the surgeon in performing the endophotocoagulation procedure is minimal when using the appropriate filter. All modern operating microscopes for vitreous surgery therefore come equipped with filters in front of the objective lens to protect the eyes of the surgeon and the assistant.

Although complications may occur in the eye of a patient with any laser delivery modality, some complications are specifically related to endolaser photocoagulation. The endophotocoagulation procedure requires careful attention to the distance between the probe and the retina. Unlike the slit-lamp delivery mode, the intensity of a burn could be significantly altered by an inadvertent change in the probe–retina distance, thereby resulting in excessive coagulation. The excessive burns may result in occlusion of a major retinal vessel, retinochoroidal hemorrhage, and rupture of Bruch's membrane. The formation of subretinal neovascularization may then ensue. Inadvertent strike of the retina or the lens with the endolaser probe may occur, causing retinochoroidal injury or cataract, respectively. Special caution must be exercised inside the gas-containing eye during the photocoagulation procedure. The gas–fluid interface could reflect an incident laser beam and cause coagulation of the retina at an unintended site.

CONCLUSIONS

The use of an endolaser for retinal photocoagulation is safe, easy, effective, and is associated with minimal side effects. With the benefits of laser treatments for many retinal conditions clearly proven in various clinical trials, the endolaser has become an essential tool that is used extensively in the everyday performance of vitreoretinal surgery. Despite the emergence of different wavelengths for use with endophotocoagulation, argon green remains the most widely used wavelength by vitreoretinal surgeons today. For nonvitrectomy cases or when the most anterior retina in a patient with phakic eyes needs to be photocoagulated, however, binocular indirect ophthalmoscopic laser therapy or cryotherapy is preferred.

The combination of laser photocoagulation with other functions in a single instrument has produced multifunction endolaser probes, which facilitate bimanual vitreoretinal surgery for better surgical results.

ACKNOWLEDGMENT

Supported in part by US Public Health Service grants EY07541 and EY02377 from the National Eye Institute, National Institutes of Health, Bethesda, MD.

REFERENCES AND RECOMMENDED READING

Recently published papers of particular interest have been highlighted as:

- • Of interest
- •• Of outstanding interest

1. Charles S: Endophotocoagulation. *Ophthalmol Times* 1979, 4:48–69.

2. Peyman GA, Grisolano JM, Palacio MN: Intraocular photocoagulation with the argon-krypton laser. *Arch Ophthalmol* 1980, 98:2062–2064.

3. Peyman GA, Salzano TC, Green JL Jr: Argon endolaser. *Arch Ophthalmol* 1981, 99:2037–2038.

4. Peyman GA, Schulman JA: *Intravitreal Surgery: Principles and Practice.* Norwalk, CT: Appleton-Century-Crofts, 1986.

5.•• Puliafito CA, Deutsch TF, Boll J, *et al.*: Semiconductor laser endophotocoagulation of the retina. *Arch Ophthalmol* 1987, 105:424–427.

This study demonstrated the use of diode lasers for ophthalmic photocoagulation in rabbits. The lasers evaluated emitted at 808 and 817 nm, were air cooled and portable, and produced lesions similar in appearance to those produced by argon laser photocoagulation.

6. Smiddy WE: Diode endolaser photocoagulation. *Arch Ophthalmol* 1992, 110:1172–1174.

7. Peyman GA, Conway MD, Ganti S, *et al.*: A neodymium-YAG endolaser. *Ophthalmic Surg* 1983, 14:309–313.

8.• Peyman GA, D'Amico DJ, Alturki WA: An endolaser probe with aspiration capability. *Arch Ophthalmol* 1992, 110:718.

This endolaser probe with aspiration capability can be used as a flute needle for drainage of subretinal fluid and for endolaser treatment of a retinotomy site after vitrectomy. The instrument allows removal of vitreous and subretinal fluid during air-fluid exchange and immediate endolaser photocoagulation without exchange of instruments.

9.•• Peyman GA, Lee KJ: Multifunction endolaser probe. *Am J Ophthalmol* 1992, 114:102–104.

This endolaser probe combines endolaser, fiberoptic illumination, aspiration, and infusion capabilities. In retinal detachment surgery, the need to exchange instruments between subretinal fluid drainage and endolaser application is eliminated. In surgery for diabetic retinopathy, aspiration and backflush capabilities allow clearing of blood and debris from the retinal surface, permitting endolaser application without instrument exchange.

10. Peyman GA: A bent-tipped endolaser probe. *Ophthalmic Surg* 1987, 18:185–186.

11. Fleischman JA, Swartz M, Dixon JA: Argon laser endophotocoagulation. *Arch Ophthalmol* 1981, 99:1610–1612.

12. Landers MB III, Trese MT, Stefansson E, *et al.*: Argon laser intraocular photocoagulation. *Ophthalmology* 1982, 89:785–788.

SELECT BIBLIOGRPAHY

Peyman GA, Schulman JA: *Intravitreal Surgery: Principles and Practice.* Norwalk, CT: Appleton & Lange; 1994.

Ryan SJ: *Retina,* vol III. St. Louis: CV Mosby; 1989.

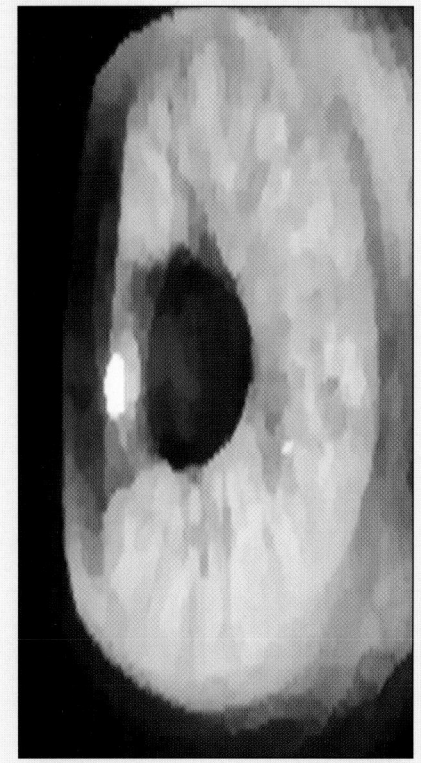

CHAPTER 10

NEW DELIVERY SYSTEMS AND NEW USES OF LASERS

JOEL M. KRAUSS
DAVID R. GUYER

Ophthalmologists were the first physicians to use lasers for medical applications, and they remain at the forefront of developments in laser technology. New instruments and techniques are continually being developed, and few go untested for potential ophthalmic use. Diode lasers represent more of an economic and ergonomic revolution than a fundamentally new laser–tissue interaction. Aided by advances in endoprobes and indirect ophthalmoscopy, diode lasers are already being used to treat a variety of vascular diseases and may become the treatment of choice for retinopathy of prematurity. The development of diode lasers at shorter wavelengths and pulse durations offers the potential for these devices to supplant many larger, more expensive ophthalmic lasers. Laser keratorefractive surgery is a rapidly evolving field, and ablation is also being studied for intraocular use. Whereas in the past decade photodisruption, and, increasingly, ablation have joined photocoagulation as established procedures, there is good reason to believe that the field of ophthalmic lasers is far from mature.

DIODE LASERS

Laser principles

Diode lasers emit radiation with exceptional electrical-to-optical efficiency (around 50%). They are much smaller, less expensive, and more portable than traditional ophthalmic lasers, only requiring a standard electrical outlet to achieve clinically necessary power levels. Such devices are constructed by joining n- and p-type semiconductors, which serve as electron donors and acceptors, respectively, creating a recombination region at their junction. The size of the band gap, across which photons jump and which thus establishes the emission wavelength, is determined by the addition (doping) of other atoms. The band gap in gallium arsenide (GaAs) semiconductors is particularly well suited to the production of light, with the application of an external electrical potential across the p–n junction creating an electron population inversion and the parallel GaAs crystal faces serving as semitransparent mirrors. Internally reflected light then stimulates further photon emission in the recombination region, ultimately resulting in output that is coherent and monochromatic, albeit very divergent (in contrast to the collimated output of the argon and many other lasers). Laser power is increased by constructing arrays of many diodes, with coupling between active zones making the total output spatially coherent.

Most diode lasers studied for ophthalmic use contain GaAs crystals doped with aluminum (GaAlAs) and emit between 780 and 850 nm (commercial versions are now generally 810 nm), although any given laser has only a single emission line and is not tunable. Radi-

ation in this range is readily transmitted by the ocular media, and, in contrast to some shorter wavelengths, only 46% incident on the retina is absorbed by the retinal pigment epithelium (RPE) (12%) and choroid (34%) [1]. However, for the diode laser to be clinically useful, this lower absorption requires higher power, which could not be achieved until recently.

Applications

Retina

Puliafito and coworkers [2•], using diode lasers at 808 and 817 nm, 50 to 130 mW, 0.2 to 1.0 second, and a 700-μm spot size, reported the first therapeutically useful diode laser lesions. Their endophotocoagulation system produced lesions in rabbit retinas that were similar to argon, krypton, and neodymium-yttrium aluminum garnet (Nd:YAG) laser damage as determined by ophthalmoscopy and fluorescein angiography, but histologic damage was limited to the outer retina. Brancato and Pratesi [3] achieved similar early experimental results and also reported the first transpupillary diode laser photocoagulation. Using a diode laser endophotocoagulation system in rabbits, Smiddy and Hernandez [4] demonstrated that retinal cell disruption was confined primarily to the outer nuclear layer in mild burns, involved the inner nuclear layer in moderate burns, and involved ganglion cell loss in severe burns. Brancato and coworkers [5] first coupled a diode laser to a slit-lamp biomicroscope, achieving retinal photocoagulation in rabbits with 120 mW, 0.3 to 1.0 second, and 200 × 500 μm; they subsequently tested this system on a human eye scheduled for enucleation [6].

Brancato and coworkers [7•] conducted a histologic comparison of diode and argon retinal lesions produced in rabbits with 120 mW at 0.1 to 1.0 second. Threshold lesions similar to clinical argon applications were created at diode exposures of 0.8 second. There were zones of coagulation necrosis and vacuolation in the RPE, whereas sensory retina damage was confined to photoreceptor cells and nuclei of the inner nuclear layer. Photoreceptor nuclei were intensely but irregularly pyknotic, with wide disc fragmentation and dispersion of cellular debris, and there was irregular obliteration of the choriocapillaris and some disorganization of the choroidal pigment. Although the basal membrane was intact, choriocapillary endothelial cells were swollen, and there were occasional capillary thromboses. The ganglion cell layer contained many intercellular lacunae, but no alterations were observed in the inner limiting membrane. These changes varied somewhat from those produced by the argon green laser, where some damage occurs in all retinal layers (Fig. 10-1). McHugh and coworkers [8] demonstrated that, as might be expected, diode laser lesions are histologically most similar to those produced with the krypton red light of 647 nm. Wallow and coworkers [9] found that moderate diode laser lesions in monkey retinas were similar to argon ones, but more intense diode laser lesions involved scarring of ciliary nerves in the choroid or sclera, with macrophage invasion and loss of myelin sheaths and axis cylinders.

Radiation at 810 nm readily traverses the sclera, and Jennings and coworkers [10] successfully performed experimental transscleral retinal photocoagulation in rabbits, transmitting the laser output via a fiberoptic. Treatment at 200 mW produced lesions after exposures of 5 to 10 seconds, reflecting a variability experienced with other transscleral wavelengths. The sclera overlying the chorioretinal lesions remained intact, and there was substantially less disruption of the blood–retinal barrier than is seen with cryotherapy, which may be important in reducing the incidence of proliferative vitreoretinopathy after retinal detachment surgery. Peyman and coworkers [11] reported achieving 810-nm transscleral retinal photocoagulation in rabbits with 200 to 500 mW and 0.5-second exposures, whereas

300 to 400 mW and 0.5-second exposures produced ciliary body destruction. However, there was again significant variability, and hence, unpredictability in the lesions, with explosive reactions encountered at some higher powers. It has been suggested that the lesion variability may be overcome by gradually titrating exposure power and duration to achieve clinically desirable levels, with an endpoint of gray or gray-white, rather than white, spots [12,13]. More recent work indicates that altering the diode laser output to bursts of microsecond pulses contained within millisecond envelopes allows more selective and reproducible retinal photocoagulation [14,15].

In early clinical trials, McHugh and coworkers [16•] and Balles and coworkers [17•] demonstrated the potential efficacy of diode laser transpupillary photocoagulation, via a slit-lamp biomicroscope, for the treatment of such retinal vascular diseases as diabetic retinopathy, choroidal neovascular membranes, and branch and central retinal vein occlusion. The McHugh

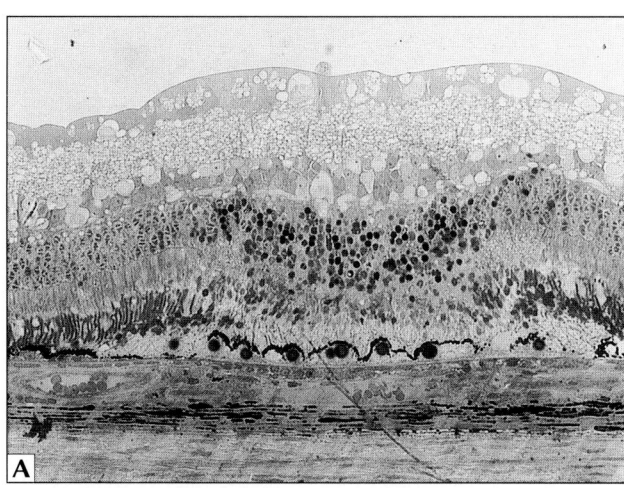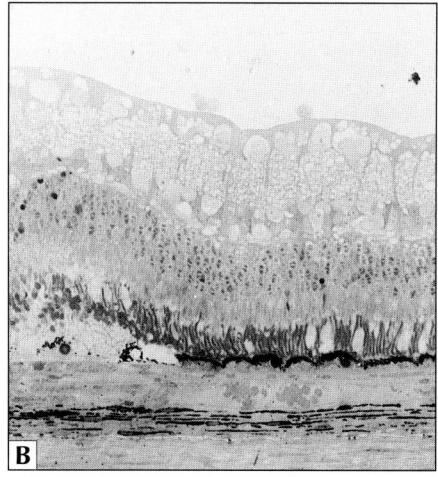
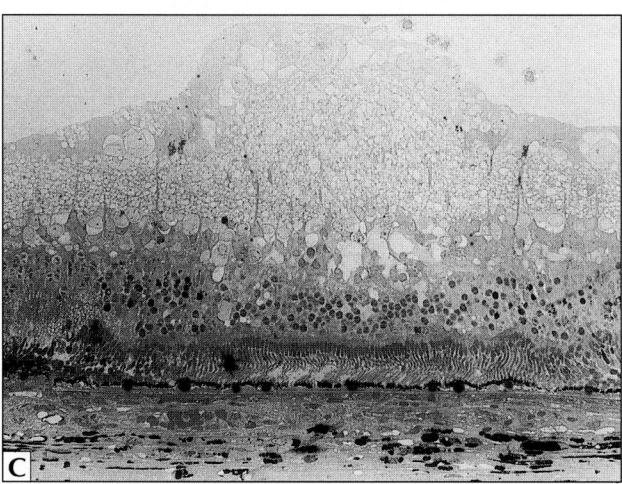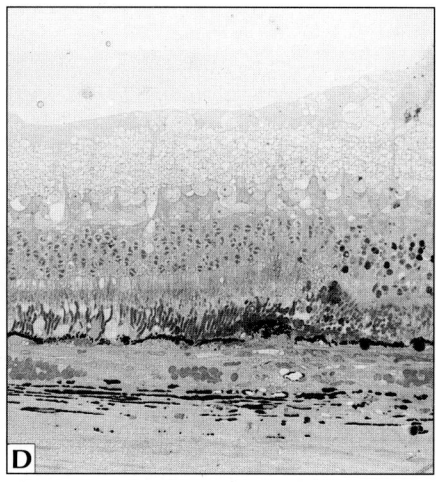

Figure 10-1 **Top,** Diode laser retinal lesion demonstrates intense coagulation necrosis of the retinal pigment epithelium and photoreceptor cells (*A*) and border between affected and unaffected retina (*B*). **Bottom,** Argon green (514.5 nm) laser retinal lesion shows damage to all layers (*C*) and border between treated and untreated retina (*D*). (*From* Brancato *et al.* [7•]; with permission.)

group encountered no side effects, such as lenticular or corneal opacities, RPE tears, or choroidal hemorrhage. RPE photocoagulation was achieved even through a layer of blood about 150 μm thick. Neovascularization had regressed 6 weeks after treatment for diabetic retinopathy, with visual acuity changes similar to those associated with other lasers. Follow-up of all patients as late as 9 months demonstrated the potential success of diode laser photocoagulation for these conditions.

The Balles group used 805-nm diode radiation at 300 to 1300 mW, 0.2 to 0.5 second, and 200 μm, and found that 4.5 times more energy, 2.5 times more power, and 1.8 times more irradiation and exposure duration were required to produce diode laser lesions that were clinically similar to those achieved with the argon laser, all consistent with the much lower absorption by the RPE of the longer wavelength. The deeper diode penetration, even greater than for krypton red light, necessitated retrobulbar anesthesia, but resulted in only four cases of subretinal hemorrhage or rupture of Bruch's membrane out of a total of over 9000 treatment exposures. There was excellent penetration through macular edema and serous retinal thickening; transmission through cataracts and hemorrhages was much greater than for shorter-wavelength lasers, with less light scattering [18]. It was also noted that because the diode radiation is invisible, there were no complaints of bright flashes. Moreover, the permanent filter blocking the diode wavelength both permits continuous viewing throughout the procedure and eliminates the clicks typically associated with movable shutters, which may startle some patients. However, the diode laser's greater beam divergence did require a greater intraocular focusing cone angle, which limited peripheral treatment.

There is experimental evidence that the diode laser can effectively produce chorioretinal adhesions, with less blood–retinal barrier destruction than with either cryotherapy or the argon laser [13,19]. Given this evidence, Haller and coworkers [20•] performed transscleral diode laser retinopexy in conjunction with scleral buckling in a series of patients with rhegmatogenous retinal detachment (Fig. 10-2). Mean power settings were 1162 mW for white patients and 342 mW for black patients, and exposure durations ranged from 1 to 9 seconds. Minor complications included a scleral thermal effect and presumed ruptures in Bruch's membrane in 30% of the patients, the latter accompanied by audible "pops." However, these problems were not encountered once the investigators used smaller, gray lesions as their endpoint. One logistic disadvantage was the longer procedure time compared with cryotherapy. Nine of 10 retinas were successfully attached at 6 months and the 10th retina redetached at 6 weeks secondary to proliferative vitreoretinopathy, but responded to reattachment. A multicenter trial is currently underway to evaluate this modality more precisely. It remains to be seen whether the average of 520 J used by the Haller team is necessary to create retinopexy, and whether such high energy will not cause some hemorrhages in a larger study group.

Glaucoma

Jacobson and coworkers [21] created diode laser peripheral iridectomies in rabbits that were similar to argon blue-green laser iridectomies. These authors speculated that the greater transmission through the iris stroma and stronger absorption by the iris pigment epithelium at 810 nm may make the diode laser preferable for this procedure, especially in dark irides. This group reported the first human iridectomies produced with the diode laser, occasionally encountering the same mild anterior lens capsule opacity sometimes seen with the argon laser, especially with longer expo-

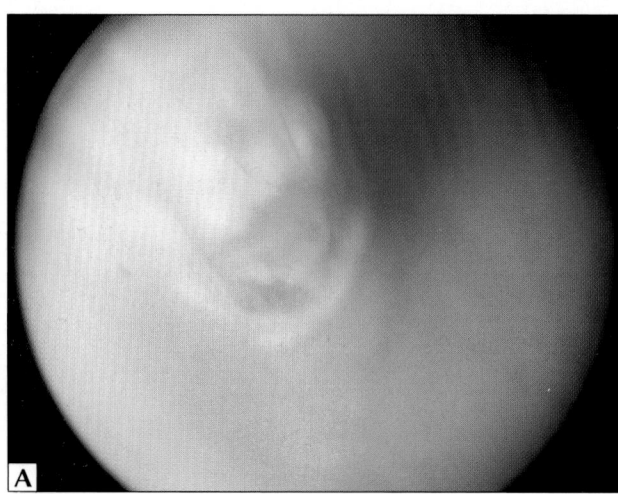

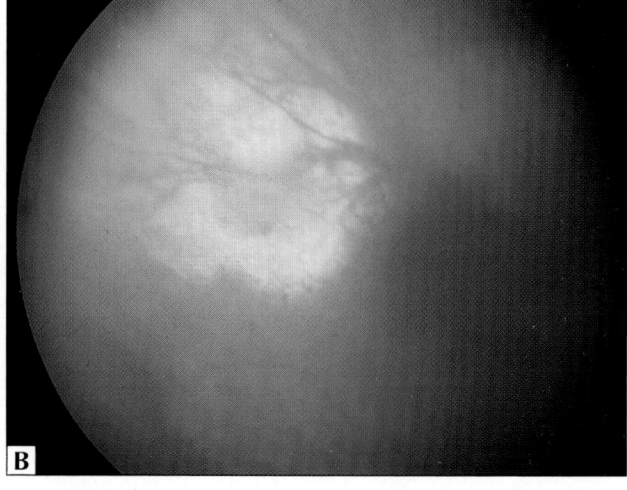

FIGURE 10-2 A, Diode laser photocoagulation lesions surrounding a retinal break 1 day after scleral buckle surgery.

B, At 6 months the lesions are pigmented and more diffuse. (*From* Haller *et al.* [20•]; with permission.)

sures and larger spot sizes [22]. In a larger clinical series, Emoto and coworkers [23•] used a two-step method of circular burns to stretch the iris (200 mW, 0.2 second, 200 µm), followed by penetrating burns (1000 mW, 0.05 second, 75 µm), with a mean total of 152 burns. Iritis developed in all patients, but responded to topical corticosteroid treatment. Other complications included pupillary distortion (70%), transient anterior lens capsule opacification (60%), intraocular pressure (IOP) rise greater than 10 mm Hg (20%), and corneal endothelial lesions (5%). Focal cataract developed in 5% of eyes but resolved within 3 months. All openings remained patent at 9 months.

McHugh and coworkers [24•] conducted a pilot clinical investigation of diode laser trabeculoplasty. They used parameters of 0.8 to 1.2 W, 0.2 second, and 100 µm, and placed 50 burns for 180 degrees, and noted that the desired exposure endpoint was a mild blanching of the pigmented portion of the trabecular meshwork. That these lesions were just above threshold was suggested by the absence of bubble formation, in contrast to that seen with the argon laser procedure. However, IOP was lowered just as much as it was with the more established laser (9.6 mm Hg at 6 months), with an even greater effect 2 to 4 weeks after the laser trabeculoplasty, possibly as a result of the deeper penetration at 810 nm. Consistent with the lighter lesions and absence of bubbles, there was no IOP spike immediately after treatment. As is sometimes seen with the argon laser, there was a mild IOP reduction in the fellow, untreated eye, suggesting that laser trabeculoplasty may cause the release of chemical mediators. These researchers also showed that the trabecular meshwork damage is histologically similar whether laser trabeculoplasty is performed with the diode or argon laser, further reflecting the procedure's independence of wavelength [25]. Indeed, in a direct clinical comparison, Brancato and coworkers [26] showed that patients undergoing diode laser trabeculoplasty retained the same lowering of IOP through 12 months as did those treated with argon laser trabeculoplasty.

Liebmann and coworkers [27] successfully created ab interno contact diode laser sclerostomies in rabbits. Schuman and coworkers [28] performed contact transscleral diode laser cyclophotocoagulation on rabbits, and found IOP lowering and ultrastructural damage similar to that achieved with the Nd:YAG laser. Work on human cadaver eyes revealed that only 75% of the energy used with the Nd:YAG laser is needed for the diode laser procedure, consistent with melanin's greater absorption of the latter's wavelength [29]. Initial clinical studies of contact diode laser cyclophotocoagulation by Gaasterland and coworkers [30] realized average IOP reductions from 36 mm Hg before laser treatment to 23 mm Hg at a 3-month follow-up, with-

out any hypotony, but with mild surface burns in 40% of patients.

ENDOLASER

As clinical experience with the diode laser has accumulated, there has been concomitant progress in refining both the laser itself and the means for delivering its output to the eye. This laser's compactness makes it particularly well suited to use with the endoprobe and indirect ophthalmoscope (Fig. 10-3). Numerous applications have been developed for endophotocoagulation since the technique was first introduced in the early 1980s. Recent uses have included treatment of a choroidal bleed in a patient following the evacuation of a subretinal clot and ablation of experimental choroidal melanomas in rabbits with high-power argon radiation [31,32]. Building on early work in animals, Smiddy [33] reported the first clinical use of diode endolaser photocoagulation, treating patients with proliferative diabetic retinopathy, proliferative vitreoretinopathy, complex retinal detachments, and retinal breaks [2•,4,34]. Exposure parameters were dictated by the specific pathology, always avoiding reaching the whitish lesions typically expected with the argon laser,

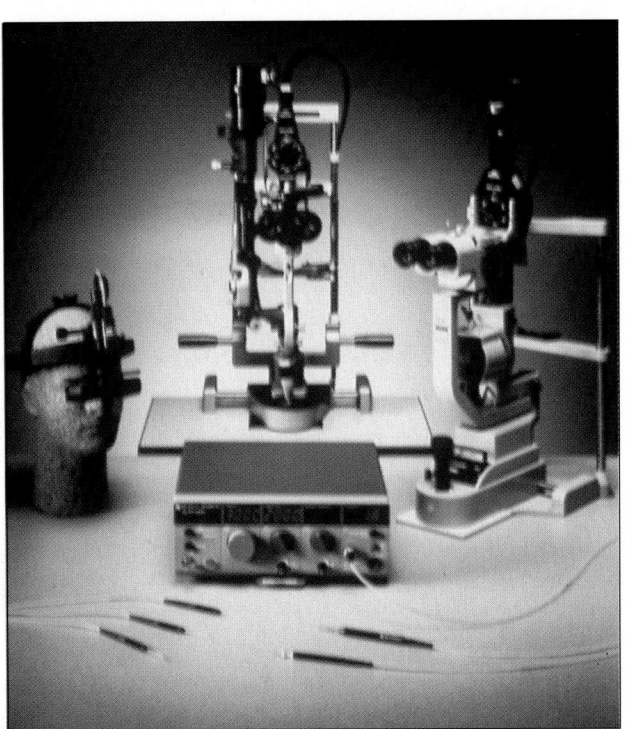

FIGURE 10-3 OcuLight SLx diode laser with the three means by which up to 2 W can be delivered to the eye: slit-lamp biomicroscope, endoprobe, and indirect ophthalmoscope. The laser console measures 10 cm X 30 cm X 30 cm, weighs 5.5 kg, and runs on either 115 or 230 V without requiring external air or water cooling. (Courtesy of Iris Medical Instruments, Mountain View, CA.)

which, with the diode laser, have been associated with iatrogenic choroidal folds [35]. As noted in other studies, treatment through small amounts of preretinal blood was facilitated by the diode's wavelength, but this had the corresponding disadvantage of preventing coagulation of bleeding stumps. Overall, it was believed that endophotocoagulation with the diode laser is as clinically efficacious as with the argon laser, but that the diode laser offers significant logistic and ergonomic advantages.

In the past few years, considerable advances have been made in probe technology, especially in conjunction with the diode laser, all aimed at maximizing the functions that can be performed by a single probe. Peyman and coworkers [36•,37] developed a couple of such 20-gauge devices, combining fiberoptic diode or argon lasers and aspiration and infusion capabilities, with one also including fiberoptic illumination. These instruments can be used to both drain subretinal fluid and photocoagulate the retinotomy site, thereby obviating repeated forays into the eye. Uram [38,39•] also constructed a 20-gauge probe that incorporated diode laser and illumination fiberoptics, but rather than an aspiration-infusion capability, his has a microendoscope with a 70-degree field of view and recording capability. When using this device, Uram was able to deliver precisely titrated laser exposures to a specific number of ciliary processes, potentially enabling more effective treatment of neovascular glaucoma. Vitreoretinal endophotocoagulation was similarly facilitated, with the probe providing a clear view even when more anterior structures would obscure the view through an operating microscope, and permitting post-treatment inspection for retinal breaks without resorting to indirect ophthalmoscopy.

LASER INDIRECT OPHTHALMOSCOPE

The laser indirect ophthalmoscope (LIO) is another instrument that has been used increasingly more during the past decade. This laser has all the advantages and disadvantages inherent in indirect ophthalmoscopy but is indispensable for selected applications. Unlike with slit-lamp delivery, the spot size is impossible to standardize because it depends on the power and position of the hand-held and headset lenses, the refractive power of the treated eye, and the presence of any intraocular gas. Macular work is not recommended given the inherent limitations in aiming. However, the field of view is greater than with other laser modalities, and in conjunction with scleral depression, this technique reduces the laser power needed for photocoagulation, probably as a result of the stretched choroid's diminished ability to dissipate heat from the RPE [40•]. The LIO is very useful in cases requiring far

peripheral treatment, such as retinal tears or peripheral neovascularization, especially those with localized lens opacities or small pupils [41]. It is essential for pneumatic retinopexy reattachment or laser treatment of retinopathy of prematurity, and has also been reported for the treatment of retinoblastoma and choroidal melanoma [42–44]. Complications include occasional choroidal hemorrhage from too intense exposures, superficial burns of the iris and cornea (which may be exacerbated by the corneal epithelial defects commonly seen after vitrectomy, especially in diabetic patients), and melted Prolene haptics (which contain copper phthalocyanine dye) [45–47].

Retinopathy of prematurity

Retinopathy of prematurity is a potentially devastating condition affecting, to some extent, about two thirds of infants with birthweight below 1251 g [48]. Cryotherapy has assumed an important role in treating retinopathy of prematurity, cutting almost in half the rate of unfavorable anatomic outcomes. Nevertheless, cryotherapy is often ineffective and has been associated with such complications as intraocular hemorrhage, retinal detachment, and scleral trauma, generally because of the pressure with which the probe is applied and the freezing process itself [49]. This pressure, along with the intravenous sedation frequently used, may also induce episodes of apnea, bradycardia, and oxygen desaturation [50].

Although the use of photocoagulation to treat retinopathy of prematurity was first proposed more than 25 years ago, it wasn't until the widespread use of the LIO that it became a viable alternative to cryotherapy. Landers and coworkers [51•] reported the first use of this technique when they used the argon laser to treat the entire area of avascular retinopathy of prema-

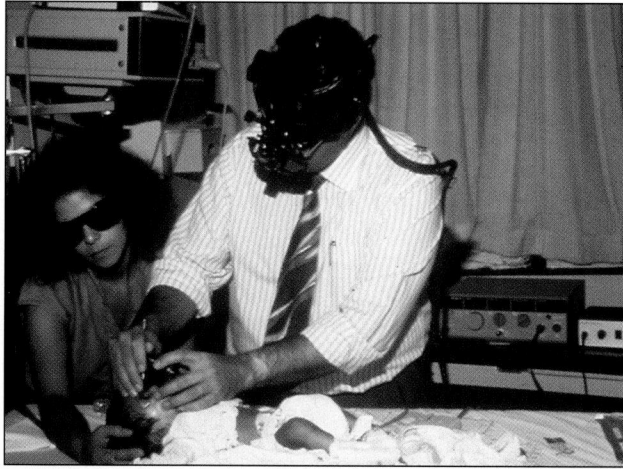

FIGURE 10-4 Diode laser indirect ophthalmoscope photocoagulation for retinopathy of prematurity. (Courtesy of Iris Medical Instruments, Mountain View, CA.)

turity. They placed 433 burns approximately 300 µm in diameter, of unspecified power, and achieved complete regression of the fibrovascular ridge and abnormal vessels at 10 weeks. Another, more extensive investigation of this therapy by Landers and coworkers [52] used an average of 696 burns of 0.5 to 0.9 W, 0.2 to 1.0 second, and 400 to 500 µm, resulting in favorable 6-month outcomes in 73% of infants with at least threshold, stage 3 "plus" disease. Whereas more recent studies have involved the use of only topical anesthesia, this group chose to use general anesthesia. Significant vitreous or preretinal blood, or a residual tunica vasculosa lentis, would particularly complicate this approach with the argon laser, whereas a small pupil or corneal irregularities would interfere with any LIO [53]. Iverson and coworkers [54] and McNamara and coworkers [55] conducted preliminary clinical trials directly comparing cryotherapy with argon LIO photocoagulation for threshold retinopathy of prematurity. Both groups concluded that photocoagulation was at least as effective as cryotherapy and that it involved less trauma to the eye.

Given its technical convenience, the diode laser has been the subject of most recent studies on photocoagulation in the treatment of retinopathy of prematurity. Fleming and coworkers [56] used the diode LIO at 180 to 200 mW, 0.3 second, and approximately 676 µm to treat infants with prethreshold, posterior retinopathy of prematurity. There were no complications, and all disease had regressed by 24 weeks. They also indicated that the criteria for treating this condition should be less stringent than those for the less aggressive anterior form of retinopathy of prematurity.

McNamara and coworkers [57•] and Hunter and Repka [58•] performed randomized trials comparing diode LIO photocoagulation and cryotherapy for the treatment of threshold retinopathy of prematurity. In the McNamara study, exposure parameters were 120 to 600 mW and 0.3 second, with an average of 959 burns placed (Fig. 10-4). Transient vitreous hemorrhages were noted in 3.6% of the laser-treated and 12.5% of the cryotherapy-treated eyes. Lid edema,

conjunctival hyperemia, and chemosis lasting 1 to 3 days were seen in all of the cryotherapy-treated eyes, whereas one laser-treated eye showed mild conjunctival hyperemia lasting only several hours. Pain was difficult to assess, but appeared to be similar to that seen in treatment with an argon laser and less than that experienced with cryotherapy. In the laser group, 25 of 28 eyes followed for 3 months and all seven of those followed for 1 year showed regression; the corresponding numbers for the cryotherapy group were 20 of 24 and all seven. Diode laser treatment thus appeared at least as efficacious as cryotherapy, and has the advantage over the argon laser of portability, permitting treatment in neonatal units that might not have access to other lasers. Moreover, as noted previously, the diode laser's wavelength would permit treatment through blood and minimize damage in infants with persistent tunica vasculosa lentis. Laser spots were placed one-half burn apart, sometimes necessitating retreatment in "skip" areas. However, it has been suggested that, as with cryotherapy, no such untreated zones need be left given the fact that photocoagulation appears at least as safe as cryotherapy [59].

Similar results were obtained by the Hunter group, despite their use of a somewhat different photocoagulation strategy. Observing that, unlike in the treatment of subretinal neovascular disease in adults, the diode laser's deeper penetration and sparing of the inner retina with its capillary endothelial precursors may be a disadvantage in treating retinopathy of prematurity, they used a clinical endpoint of creamy white lesions in an attempt to extend the laser damage to the inner retina (Fig. 10-5). In only one instance did this result in a subretinal hemorrhage consistent with a rupture of Bruch's membrane. They also noted that treatment through hazy media was easier with the diode laser than with cryotherapy. There was also much less damage to the peripheral fundus. Improvements in the delivery system decreased the beam divergence and eliminated iris clipping. Considering that all preliminary studies have supported the efficacy of photocoag-

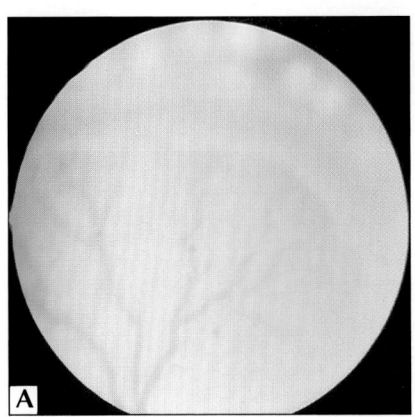 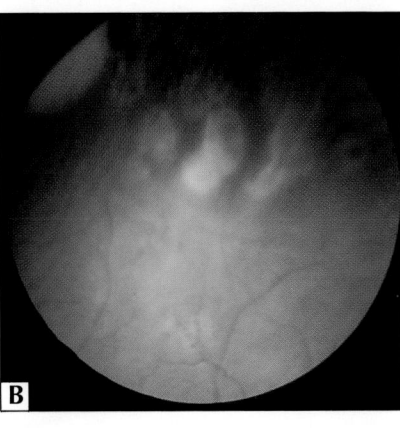

FIGURE 10-5 A, Creamy white diode laser spots, placed at 0.25- to 0.5 spot–widths apart, immediately after treatment for threshold retinopathy of prematurity. **B,** One month later, the burns have matured with minimal spreading, leaving isthmuses of intact peripheral retina, choroid, and sclera. (*From* Hunter and Repka [58•]; with permission.)

ulation and its greater tolerance in the treatment of retinopathy of prematurity, Tasman [60] has suggested that future multicenter trials concentrate on establishing the optimal threshold and parameters for laser treatment, rather than on randomized comparisons with cryotherapy.

ABLATION

The recent ophthalmic laser development with the most widespread potential applicability, and which has thus received the greatest public attention, is corneal ablation. Photorefractive keratectomy with the excimer laser at 193 nm has become a highly successful clinical procedure just 10 years after the first experimental reports, and will likely soon receive Food and Drug Administration (FDA) approval. Nevertheless, the technology and techniques are still evolving, and there have been many reports of potential alternatives or successors to the excimer laser [61–65]. Moreover, although the cornea remains the most common and suitable target for laser ablation, there is considerable interest in extending the process to intraocular structures.

Cornea

Although there are many engineering and treatment nuances among the major ophthalmic excimer lasers, the systems are much more alike than not. Significant technical hurdles had to be overcome before the excimer laser was ever used clinically, but recent enhancements and modifications have largely been variations on the same theme. Different strategies are continually being studied to optimize refractive outcome and minimize healing complications. However,

clinical considerations aside, the excimer's considerable size, cost, and energy requirement represent significant impediments to its widespread use. LaserSight, Inc. (Orlando, FL) has introduced the "mini-excimer" which, at 70 kg, weighs about one tenth as much as conventional ophthalmic excimer lasers (Fig. 10-6). It operates from a 110-V outlet, is air cooled, and uses an excimer gas mixture containing only 0.19% fluorine. Because this device can generate sufficient fluences for ablation over spot sizes of only 1.0 to 1.5 mm in diameter, it uses a computer-controlled scanning system to treat the cornea. Preliminary clinical trials for correction of myopia were conducted in China in early 1993, reportedly with good results, with phase I FDA studies scheduled for later in the year. Studies on hyperopia correction are also planned.

Although excimer laser photorefractive keratectomy for mild-to-moderate myopia is relatively predictable and successful, that for high myopia and hyperopia is much less so. An old idea that has been recently resurrected for the alteration of corneal curvature without removing any tissue is thermokeratoplasty. Seiler and coworkers [66•,67] proposed the use of the pulsed solid-state holmium-yttrium aluminum garnet (Ho:YAG) laser at 2.06 µm to create intrastromal, cone-shaped coagulations to correct hyperopia. Although still in early clinical trials, at present this is the most widely accepted means of laser therapy for hyperopia (Fig. 10-7) [68]. At least one manufacturer currently offers a single unit containing both excimer and holmium lasers (Fig. 10-8). There has also been a report of a micropulsed diode laser being used to achieve seven diopters of steepening in porcine cadaver corneas to whose surfaces indocyanine green (ICG) had been added [69].

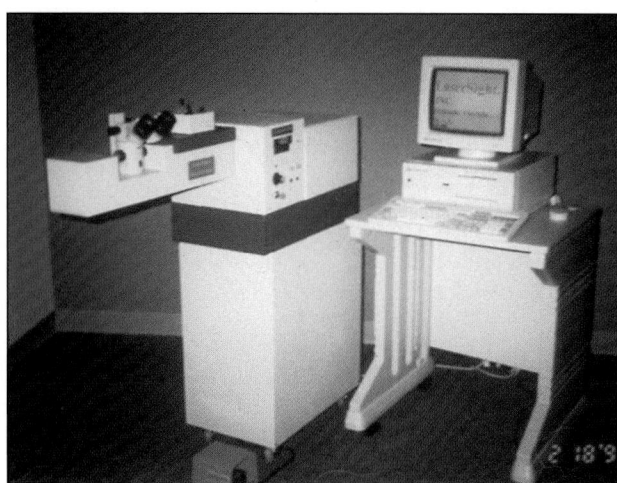

FIGURE 10-6 Compak-200 "mini-excimer." (Courtesy of LaserSight, Inc., Orlando, FL.)

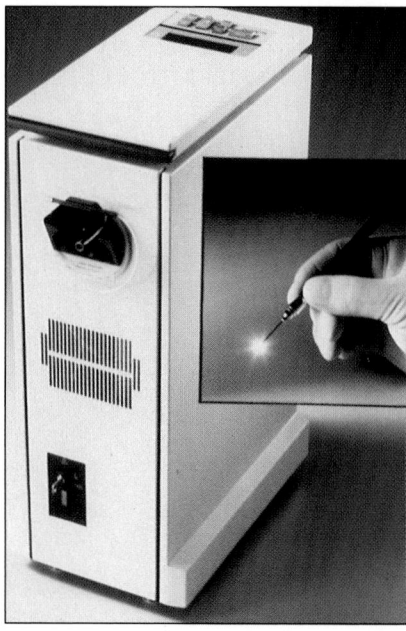

FIGURE 10-7 The gLASE 210 thulium holmium chromium-yttrium aluminum garnet laser, which produces 2.1 µm radiation at 5 Hz and up to 350 mJ, transmitted via the SUN-LITE probe. It is currently used for sclerostomies but is under early investigation for use in thermokeratoplasty treatment for hyperopia. (Courtesy of Sunrise Technologies, Fremont, CA.)

For excimer laser photorefractive keratectomy to realize its full potential, there must be disruption, if not obliteration, of what has traditionally been viewed as the inviolable Bowman's membrane. Although, in conjunction with steroids or antimetabolites, the cornea appears to heal with little or no residual scarring, the long-term implications of this procedure remain to be determined. Furthermore, studies have documented the importance of the epithelium in moderating repair and in reducing corneal haze and reversal of refractive changes after excimer ablation [70]. Some researchers have thus proposed selective intrastromal ablation without damage to the anterior layers as an alternative to excimer laser anterior ablation, although the appropriate laser remains to be determined [71].

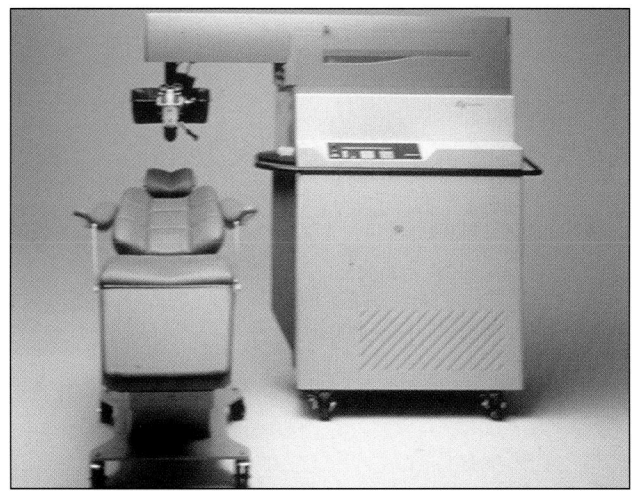

FIGURE 10-8 OmniMed laser refractive workstation, combining excimer and holmium-yttrium aluminum garnet lasers for the correction of myopia and hyperopia, respectively. The manufacturer also offers the emphasis Erodible Mask for hyperopia correction when using the excimer laser. (Courtesy of Summit Technology, Waltham, MA.)

Zysset and coworkers [72•] provided early guidance for intrastromal ablation by demonstrating that for suprathreshold Nd:YAG laser corneal lesions, the damage zone radius is proportional to the cube root of the pulse energy. Although picosecond (ps, 10^{-12}seconds) and nanosecond (ns, 10^{-9} seconds) pulses of equal energy cause approximately the same damage, because the former tend to be on the order of microjoules and the latter on the order of millijoules, in practice the use of low-energy picosecond pulses can significantly reduce collateral tissue damage. In contrast to nanosecond exposures, picosecond ones were not associated with significant shock wave propagation or cavitation bubble expansion in the primary interaction zone. However, given the low energy of individual picosecond pulses, they concluded that to achieve effective cutting or ablation, it would be necessary to use many such exposures at moderate-to-high repetition rates.

At least two companies now produce such short-pulsed lasers capable of intrastromal ablation and other applications. The Phoenix Model 2500 Ophthalmic Laser Workstation (Phoenix Laser Systems, Inc., Fremont, CA) uses a frequency-doubled, 532-nm Nd:YAG laser with 8-ns, 40- to 350-μJ pulses. It has a nominal spot size of 5 μm, with three-dimensional accuracy consistent with a 15 to 20 μm treatment area, and incorporates an eye-tracking system to eliminate effects of even subtle movements. Early attempts at intrastromal ablation (which the company terms "transepithelial stromal keratectomy") with this laser in enucleated eyes yielded vacuoles 30 to 80 μm in diameter, surrounded by compressed collagen anteriorly and edematous collagen posteriorly, without apparent endothelial damage (Fig. 10-9) [73•]. The vacuoles collapse as the fluid inside is absorbed, thereby altering the corneal curvature. Work is ongoing to determine the ablation scanning patterns necessary for correction of

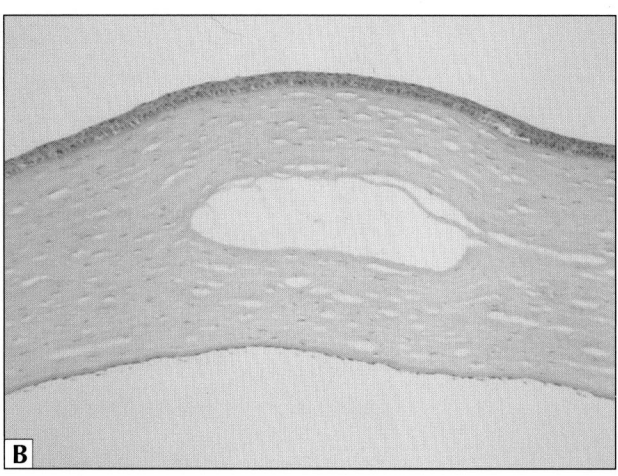

FIGURE 10-9 **A**, Slit-lamp biomicroscope and **B**, histologic views after ablation of a porcine cornea with the Phoenix Model 2500 Ophthalmic Laser Workstation. The absence of fluorescein staining reflects the intrastromal nature of the treatment. (Courtesy of Phoenix Laser Systems, Inc., Fremont, CA.)

various types of ametropia. The only procedure for which the laser has already been approved is posterior capsulotomy, but other applications in various stages of investigation, for which the laser's precision may provide unique advantages, include nuclear photofragmentation, sclerostomy, phototherapeutic keratectomy, radial keratectomy, iridectomy, and focal retinal ablation.

The neodymium-yttrium lithium fluoride (Nd:YLF) Eye Laser System (Intelligent Surgical Lasers, Inc., San Diego, CA) produces 1053-nm pulses of energy at 20 to 350 µJ, at a spot size of 7 µm or less, duration of 60 ps or less, and repetition rate of 10 to 1000 Hz (Fig. 10-10). It consists of a stable mode-locked oscillator laser operating at 80 MHz whose output is a continuous train of 1-nJ pulses, which a high-gain, Q-switched regenerative amplifier then converts to 1-mJ pulses [74]. Nd:YLF has a larger fluorescence bandwidth than does Nd:YAG, which allows pulses of shorter duration to be generated. Using an earlier Intelligent Surgical Lasers model, Frueh and coworkers [75] created intrastromal transverse excisions in rabbit corneas, which initially induced approximately 5 diopters of flattening, without intrastromal scarring. Steroids were not used, and the changes regressed by 6 weeks. Remmel and coworkers [76] demonstrated that a continuous layer of stroma could be removed in human cadaver eyes. Also using this system in human cadaver eyes, at 80 to 140 µJ, 50 ps, and 1 kHz, Niemz and coworkers [77•] scanned the laser focus in a spiral pattern to create intrastromal vacuoles of approximately 40 µm in diameter and 20 µm deep, 100 µm below Bowman's membrane, without damaging it or the epithelium. It has also been demonstrated that this process causes no acute endothelial damage [78]. However, Brown and coworkers [79•] found that ablation depth in human

and rabbit cadaver corneas was related to energy but not to programmed depth. Collagen disorganization ranged from 3 to 8 µm with 100-µJ pulses, and 10 to 20 µm at 300 µJ. The ablation effect varied with the beam path direction and plasma threshold changes within the cornea. Moreover, there was ablation of tissue anterior to the desired target, lamellar separation by plasma-gas formation without ablation, and inconsistent ablation, indicating the need for further studies and refinement of this technique. The Nd:YLF laser has also been used to create sclerectomies in human cadaver eyes, sclerostomies in rabbits, and iridotomies in patients, all with a high degree of precision [80–82]. As of mid-1993 the Intelligent Surgical Lasers had received FDA clearance only for use in performing posterior capsulotomy, but was in phase I trials for vitreolysis and phase II for cataract fragmentation. There was an open iridotomy study underway while investigational device exemptions were filed for intrastromal ablation and internal and external sclerostomy.

Taboada and coworkers [83•] described a technique they termed "intrastromal photokeratectomy," in which Q-switched Nd:YAG laser pulses at 100 ns and 500 to 2000 Hz were applied to the cornea via a contact probe. This procedure resulted in vacuoles of approximately 100 µm in diameter, localizable within 20 µm and with a transition zone between normal tissue of 0.5 µm. The track of vacuoles, which can be created in radial, wide-area, or other patterns, optically disappeared within 2 days as treated tissue dissolved into a diffusive liquid, yet the refractive effects in the rabbit and monkey eyes persisted for the 5-month duration of the study. There was no immediate or long-term damage to either the epithelium or endothelium. It remains to be seen whether intrastromal ablation with any laser can approach the precision of the

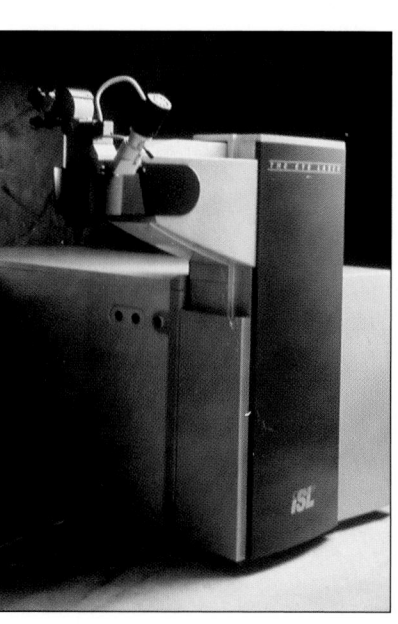

FIGURE 10-10 Neodymium-yttrium lithium fluoride Eye Laser System, with a wavelength of 1053 nm, pulse duration of 60 ps or less at a repetition rate of 10 to 1000 Hz, energy of 20 to 350 µJ, and spot size of 7 µm or less. (Courtesy of Intelligent Surgical Lasers, Inc., San Diego, CA.)

excimer laser, and whether Descemet's membrane is not more likely to push forward than Bowman's membrane backward, but potential advantages include increased patient comfort and no need to patch or instill antibiotic treatment because of retention of the epithelium, as well as lower cost and avoidance of any exposure to ultraviolet radiation.

Vitreous and retina

Although retinal photocoagulation was the first medical use of lasers, practical applications of ablation in the posterior segment have been far more elusive. The carbon dioxide (CO_2) laser at 10.6 µm has been used in animals to cut vitreous bands and drain subretinal fluid but cannot be used close to the retina, is large and inefficient, and requires an articulated arm [84,85]. Experimental vitreous membranes in rabbits were cut with the excimer laser at 308 nm, but no additional work in this area has been reported [86]. Margolis and coworkers [87•] used a solid-state, fiberoptic-coupled, 250 µs pulsed erbium-yttrium aluminum garnet (Er:YAG) laser at 2.94 µm to cut experimental vitreous membranes in rabbits at distances of 500 to 3600 µm from the retina. All attempts at cutting the membranes were successful, although 53% resulted in some form of retinal lesion—either hemorrhages or nonhemorrhagic burns. Nevertheless, the 200 to 300-µm size of the nonhemorrhagic burns was not considered a contraindication to clinical application of the technique if the membranes occurred in extramacular sites. Lin and coworkers [88] showed that the Er:YAG output creates a bubble at the tip of the fiber through which it is transmitted, which can cause thermal and mechanical tissue damage. To minimize the size and movement of this bubble, and thus the resulting damage to the retina, they suggested reducing the pulse energy to below 0.5 mJ and using a shielded tip. These steps may have their own adverse consequences—namely, requiring a higher repetition rate, and decreasing some of the advantages of laser ablation over mechanical cutting for removal of membranes tightly adherent to the retinal

surface, respectively; investigation of these issues is ongoing. Stern and coworkers [65] have suggested that use of pulses in the picosecond domain just above the ablation threshold may significantly reduce untoward thermal and mechanical effects, allowing safe cutting very near the retina.

Borirakchanyavat and coworkers [89•] attempted transection of experimental vitreous membranes by using a 250-µs pulsed Ho:YAG laser at 2.12 µm. When an optical fiber was used alone, only thin membranes could be sectioned at energy levels or repetition rates that permitted work near the retina. This problem was solved by encasing the fiber in a retinal-shielding pick, which allowed almost 75% of membranes, as close as 0.5 mm to the retina, to be completely transected. The laser directly caused one nonhemorrhagic retinal burn, whereas the pick caused two retinal injuries, including one with a small hemorrhage. Cutting precision was histologically similar to that of the CO_2 laser, but an order of magnitude less than that of the Er:YAG laser [87•]. One technical advantage of the Ho:YAG radiation is that it is much more easily transmitted by existing fiberoptics.

Selective RPE damage has been reported with the Q-switched Nd:YAG and micropulsed diode and argon lasers [90–92]. A significant impediment to the intraocular use of 193-nm excimer laser radiation is the technical difficulty in transmitting it with the necessary accuracy. Lewis and coworkers [93•] constructed a guide consisting of a fused silica lens of 1000-mm focal length and a rapidly tapered stainless steel tube whose outer diameter was that of an 18-gauge needle, with an inner diameter of 120 µm. They used this instrument to ablate bovine cadaver retinas and rabbit retinas *in vivo* after lensectomy and vitrectomy, using pulses of 0.5 to 1.2 J/cm^2 and 120 µs, at 30 to 100 Hz. Once a low pressure stream of air was used to displace the thin layer of adherent fluid from the area to be treated, they were able to achieve retinal ablation with the precision typically associated with the cornea (Fig. 10-11). Possible applications include ablation of epiretinal mem-

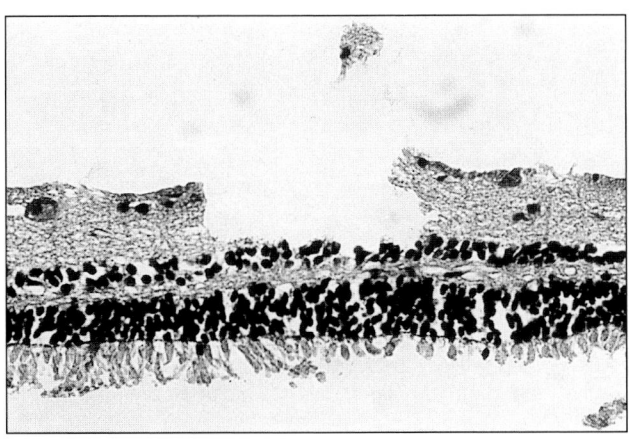

FIGURE 10-11 Forty-µm-deep ablation to the inner nuclear layer in a bovine retina, created with the argon fluoride excimer laser at 1.2 J/cm^2/pulse. (*From* Lewis *et al.*[93•]; with permission.)

branes, as even a slight amount of underlying fluid would protect the retina, and the creation of precise retinotomies and retinectomies.

MISCELLANEOUS APPLICATIONS

Liposomes

Zeimer and coworkers [94•,95] and Khoobehi and coworkers [96–98,99•] have conducted a series of studies on the intravenous injection of liposomes containing drugs or dye. Low-level irradiation with argon blue-green or dye yellow light is used to achieve heat-induced localized release in the retinal vasculature of those substances from the miniature phospholipid containers with a transition temperature of 41°C. Potential applications include measurement of blood flow and selective angiography. Work on the latter has shown that with a spot size of 1.5 to 2.0 mm centered on the optic disc and energy densities of 0.5 to 3.4 J/cm², it is possible to obtain multiple angiograms up to 3 hours after dye injection (Fig. 10-12) [99•]. Possible advantages of this technique include reduction of choroidal fluorescence, which permits optimal viewing of the retinal microcirculation, and clear separation of arterial and venous fluorescence. Selective angiography of a suspected leaking vessel could be documented by specifically targeting it with the laser. Blood flow might be monitored during and after laser treatment for tumors and angiomas. Before any clinical use, however, more extensive tissue damage studies are needed, as are data on the potential toxicity of the liposomes and carboxyfluorescein dye.

Scleral buckling

Scleral buckling is the standard procedure for the treatment of rhegmatogenous retinal detachment, but is not without its complications. Alternate treatments such as pneumatic retinopexy also have side effects and generally have more limited applicability. In a search for a method that would avoid episcleral sutures and large exoplants, Ren and coworkers [100•] used the Ho:YAG laser on human cadaver eyes to induce tissue shrinkage and create a buckling effect (Fig. 10-13). Five 250-µs pulses were applied via a fiberoptic probe held approximately 5 mm from the sclera to achieve a fluence of 11.3 ± 1.2 J/cm², which affected only the outer two thirds of the sclera; there was no damage to the remaining sclera or the underlying retina. Although their system was successful, they speculated that a continuous-wave laser tunable over the 1.8 to 2.4-µm range would permit more controllable treatment, adjustable to the various absorption characteristics of pathologic sclera. They also suggested the possibility of combining this technique with laser retinopexy, the early clinical results of which were promising [20•].

Tissue welding

The use of lasers to join tissue without the need for sutures has been an attractive but elusive goal, and remains the subject of periodic studies. Burstein and coworkers [101•] used the continuous-wave hydrogen

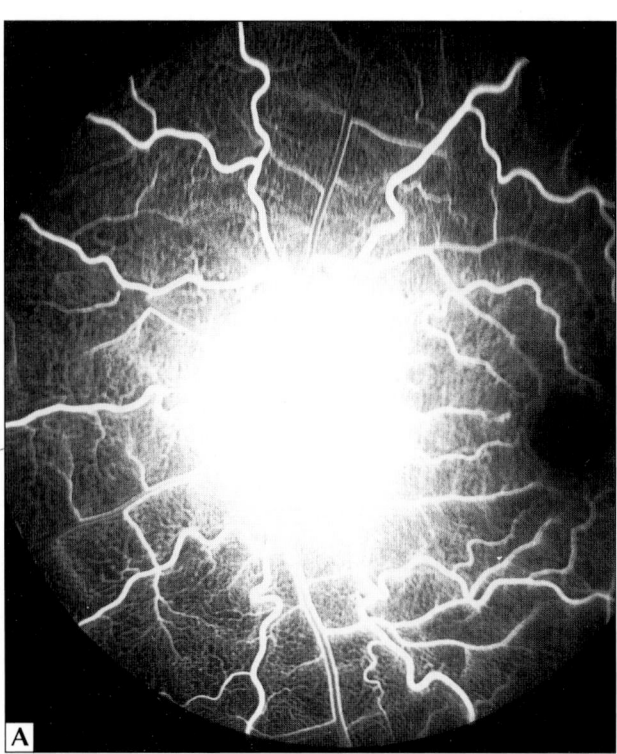

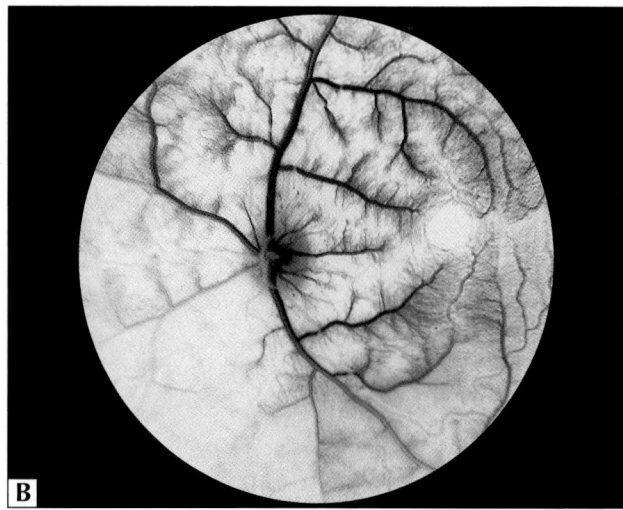

FIGURE 10-12 **A**, Selective angiogram in a squirrel monkey taken 1.4 seconds after beginning a 1.5-second exposure with argon blue-green light (visible as the bright area). Also visible is the passage of dye through the arteries and capillaries and its early entrance into the inferior temporal vein. **B**, At 0.6 seconds after completion of the laser exposure, dye has exited the arteries and that in the capillaries has begun to enter the veins. (*From* Khoobehi *et al.* [99•]; with permission.)

fluoride laser to seal corneal incisions in porcine cadaver eyes. The welding spot size of approximately 0.2 mm in diameter was moved across the incision at a rate of 1 mm per minute. The fundamental mode, with a wavelength of 2579 nm and power of 30 mW, produced a weld approximately 100 μm deep, which failed at 14 mm Hg, whereas the overtone at 1340 nm and 320 mW created a weld 300 μm deep that withstood pressures of up to 34 mm Hg. Scleral welding was found to be less successful. Considerably greater resistance was noted by Khadem and coworkers [102•] in human cadaver eyes in which corneal incisions had been sealed with a fibrinogen mixture containing a photosensitive singlet oxygen generator activated by an argon blue-green laser to cross-link a protein solder with stromal collagen. Wolf and coworkers [103•] used the diode laser to convert ICG–enhanced fibrinogen to fibrin in rabbit retinas, and speculated that this procedure may provide a quick chorioretinal adhesion, thereby assisting in the treatment of retinal breaks and retinotomies.

FUTURE DEVELOPMENTS

Ophthalmologists were the first physicians to develop clinical applications for lasers, a trend that continues today. Whereas in the past decade photodisruption, and, increasingly, ablation, have joined photocoagulation as established procedures, there is good reason to believe that the field of ophthalmic lasers is far from mature. New instruments and techniques are continually being developed, and few go untested for potential ophthalmic use.

The diode laser is revolutionary more for economic and ergonomic reasons than because it provides some fundamentally new laser–tissue interaction. Its low cost and easy portability will permit treatment in remote areas, including many third-world nations. Just as

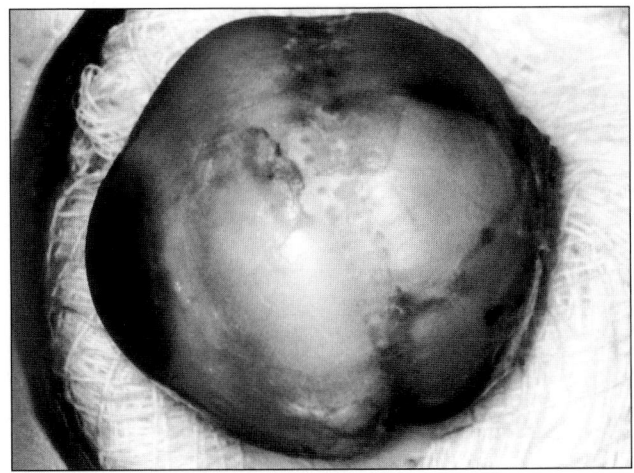

Figure 10-13 Human cadaver eye with scleral buckle created by three circumferential rows of holmium-yttrium aluminum garnet spots. (*From* Ren *et al.* [100•]; with permission.)

GaAlAs diode technology has been improved in the past several years so that sufficient power is now available for many applications, the future holds the promise that, with new materials, useful diode output will be achieved at visible wavelengths, perhaps supplanting the much bulkier and less efficient argon, krypton, and dye lasers. At present, diodes are beginning to replace flashlamps and other lasers as pumping sources for visible wavelengths [104]. If sufficient energy can be generated by Q-switched diode lasers, they might be used in place of Nd:YAG laser photodisruption.

Work on laser modification of corneal curvature is proceeding so rapidly that, even before the excimer laser has received FDA approval, potential replacements are being studied. Although tremendous engineering efforts have resulted in a substantially reliable instrument, the excimer remains a very large and expensive device. There is also concern about exposure to fluorine gas. The mini-excimer may prove to be a viable alternative, but is just beginning to undergo clinical investigation. Other improvments in the excimer itself might include the addition of real-time eye tracking and tissue-depth monitoring; possible approaches to the latter include femtosecond (10^{-15}s) laser optical ranging and optical coherence domain reflectometry [105,106].

Early worries about possible mutagenesis appear to have subsided (except for radiation at around 248 nm, which has not been used clinically), and, despite the achievement of infrared laser ablation, researchers have not been able to duplicate the precision realized by the argon fluoride excimer laser. As such, several investigators are studying solid-state, ultraviolet alternatives to the excimer laser. Researchers from the Bascom Palmer Eye Institute are collaborating with LaserSight, Inc. on the use of the Nd:YAG fifth harmonic at 213 nm (achieved with a combination of cesium-dihydrogen-arsenate and barium borate crystals) for possible ablation [107•,108]. Because, unlike with the excimer laser, sufficient energy for ablation can only be achieved with a small spot size, tissue removal is effected by scanning a 0.5 to 1.0-mm beam across the cornea in a precise pattern to achieve the desired profile [109•]. Preliminary results in cadaver and rabbit eyes revealed ablations similar to those of the argon fluoride excimer laser, with damage zones less than 1-μm wide and no step-like transition zones [110,111]. Although commercial availability is at least several years away, another goal of this group is the development of a laser capable of generating several harmonics at various pulse durations, potentially also permitting photocoagulation and photodisruption [112•]. Researchers at Tufts University and Schwartz Electro-Optics (Concord, MA) are investigating ablation with the solid-state titanium-sapphire laser, using barium borate crystals to frequency-quadruple its 10-ns, 10-Hz output to 205 to 225 nm [113]. Although it is very inefficient, the free electron laser is capable of generating a wide range of infrared wavelengths and allows independent variation of wavelength, energy, and pulse duration. Very preliminary studies have shown achievement of corneal ablation, but it remains to be seen whether the use of the free electron laser is preferable to that of the solid-state infrared lasers [114,115]. Novatec Laser Systems, Inc. (San Diego, CA) indicates that its LightBlade laser is capable of corneal surface, intrastromal, and intraocular ablation, and includes an eye-tracking system, but clinical trials of the as-yet-unspecified "deep ultraviolet solid state" device have yet to begin as of late 1993.

Whereas laser removal of primary cataracts remains a popular misconception, reality may be catching up with myth. Photophacofragmentation is the process of using pulsed laser energy to soften a cataractous lens to facilitate aspiration at the time of surgery; studies involving the use of the Nd:YAG laser for this process have been reported [116,117]. Early work with the excimer laser has given way to the study of the very-short-pulsed Nd:YLF and frequency-doubled Nd:YAG and mid-infrared lasers for the dissolution of cataracts [118,119]. One possibility is the aspiration of lens remnants through a very small incision, through which some polymer capable of reconstituting the lens, perhaps restoring accomodation, could be injected [120].

REFERENCES AND RECOMMENDED READING

Recently published papers of particular interest have been highlighted as:
• Of interest
•• Of outstanding interest

1. Birngruber R, Hillenkamp F, Gabel VP: Theoretical investigations of laser thermal retinal injury. *Health Phys* 1985, 48:781–796.

2.• Puliafito CA, Deutsch TF, Boll J, *et al.*: Semiconductor laser endophotocoagulation of the retina. *Arch Ophthalmol* 1987, 105:424–427.

First report of therapeutically useful diode laser lesions. Burns in rabbit retinas were similar to those created with the argon laser, but with histologic damage limited to the outer retina.

3. Brancato R, Pratesi R: Applications of diode lasers in ophthalmology. *Lasers Ophthalmol* 1987, 1:119–129.

4. Smiddy WE, Hernandez E: Histopathologic results of retinal diode laser photocoagulation in rabbit eyes. *Arch Ophthalmol* 1992, 110:693–698.

5. Brancato R, Pratesi R, Leoni G, *et al.*: Retinal photocoagulation with diode laser operating from a slit lamp microscope. *Lasers Light Ophthalmol* 1988, 2:73–78.

6. Brancato R, Pratesi R, Leoni G, *et al.*: Semiconductor diode laser photocoagulation of human malignant melanoma. *Am J Ophthalmol* 1989, 107:295–296.

7.• Brancato R, Pratesi R, Leoni G, *et al.*: Histopathology of diode and argon laser lesions in rabbit retina: a comparative study. *Invest Ophthalmol Vis Sci* 1989, 30:1504–1510.

Detailed histologic comparison of retinal lesions produced with argon and diode lasers. The diode laser caused zones of coagulation necrosis and vacuolation in the RPE, whereas sensory retina damage was confined to photoreceptor cells and nuclei of the inner nuclear layer.

8. McHugh JDA, Marshall J, Capon M, *et al.*: Transpupillary photocoagulation in the eyes of rabbit and human using a diode laser. *Lasers Light Ophthalmol* 1988, 2:125–143.

9. Wallow IHL, Sponsel WE, Stevens TS: Clinicopathologic correlation of diode laser burns in monkeys. *Arch Ophthalmol* 1991, 109:648–653.

10. Jennings T, Fuller T, Vukich JA, *et al.*: Transscleral contact retinal photocoagulation with an 810-nm semiconductor diode laser. *Ophthalmic Surg* 1990, 21:492–496.

11. Peyman GA, Naguib KS, Gaasterland D: Transscleral application of a semiconductor diode laser. *Lasers Surg Med* 1990, 10:569–575.

12. Fankhauser F, Kwasniewska S, Henchoz P-D, *et al.*: Versatility of the cw-Nd:YAG and diode lasers in ocular surgery. *Ophthalmic Surg* 1993, 24:225–231.

13. Menchini U, Trabucchi G, Brancato R, *et al.*: Can the diode laser (810 nm) effectively produce chorioretinal adhesion? *Retina* 1992, 12:S80–S86.

14. Chong LP, Kohen L, Kelsoe W, *et al.*: Selective RPE damage by micro-pulse diode laser photocoagulation [Abstract]. *Invest Ophthalmol Vis Sci* 1992, 33(suppl):722.

15. Trokel S, Wapner F, Schubert H: Contact transscleral retinal photocoagulation using a micropulsed diode laser [Abstract]. *Invest Ophthalmol Vis Sci* 1992, 33(suppl):1311.

16.• McHugh JDA, Marshall J, ffytche TJ, *et al.*: Initial clinical experience using a diode laser in the treatment of retinal vascular disease. *Eye* 1989, 3:516–527.

Early clinical trial of diode laser photocoagulation of retinal vascular diseases. Follow-up at 9 months demonstrated the potential success of this method.

17.• Balles MW, Puliafito CA, D'Amico DJ, *et al.*: Semiconductor diode laser photocoagulation in retinal vascular disease. *Ophthalmology* 1990, 97:1553–1561.

Early clinical trial of diode laser photocoagulation of retinal vascular diseases. Compared with argon laser lesions, those produced with the diode laser required more energy and power, consistent with the lower absorption by the RPE of the diode's longer wavelength. Although this requirement necessitated retrobulbar anesthesia, subretinal hemorrhages occurred in only 0.04% of exposures. Transmission through cataracts, hemorrhages, macular edema, and serous retinal thickening was greater than with the argon laser. Patients preferred the lack of bright flashes or filter clicks.

18. Balles MW, Puliafito CA: Semiconductor diode lasers: a new laser light source in ophthalmology. *Int Ophthalmol Clin* 1990, 30:77–83.

19. Sato Y, Berkowitz BA, Wilson CA, *et al.*: Blood-retinal barrier breakdown caused by diode vs argon laser endophotocoagulation. *Arch Ophthalmol* 1992, 110:277–281.

20.• Haller JA, Lim JI, Goldberg MF: Pilot trial of transscleral diode laser retinopexy in retinal detachment surgery. *Arch Ophthalmol* 1993, 111:952–956.

Transscleral diode laser retinopexy in conjunction with scleral buckling for rhegmatogenous retinal detachment. Attachments were successful, but three of 10 patients experienced ruptures of Bruch's membrane accompanied by "pops." An average total energy of 520 J per eye was used.

21. Jacobson JJ, Schuman JS, El Koumy H, *et al.*: Diode laser peripheral iridectomy. *Int Ophthalmol Clin* 1990, 30:120–122.

22. Schuman JS, Puliafito CA, Jacobson JJ: Semiconductor diode laser peripheral iridotomy. *Arch Ophthalmol* 1990, 108:1207–1208.

23.• Emoto I, Okisaka S, Nakajima A: Diode laser iridotomy in rabbit and human eyes. *Am J Ophthalmol* 1992, 113:321–327.

Clinical trial of diode laser iridotomy. Iritis developed in all patients but responded to topical steroid treatment. Also complicating some cases were pupillary distortion, IOP rise, corneal endothelial lesions, and transient anterior lens capsule opacification. All openings remained patent at 9 months.

24.• McHugh D, Marshall J, ffytche TJ, *et al.*: Diode laser trabeculoplasty (DLT) for primary open-angle glaucoma and ocular hypertension. *Br J Ophthalmol* 1990, 74:743–747.

Pilot trial of diode laser trabeculoplasty. The desired exposure endpoint was a mild blanching of the pigmented trabecular meshwork, which was achieved without bubble formation. IOP reduction was similar to that produced with the argon laser, without the usual initial spike.

25. McHugh D, Marshall J, ffytche TJ, *et al.*: Ultrastructural changes of human trabecular meshwork after photocoagulation with a diode laser. *Invest Ophthalmol Vis Sci* 1992, 33:2664–2671.

26. Brancato R, Carassa R, Trabucchi G: Diode laser compared with argon laser for trabeculoplasty. *Am J Ophthalmol* 1991, 112:50–55.

27. Liebmann JM, Katz NR, McCormick SA, *et al.*: Ab interno contact diode laser sclerostomy: a rabbit model [Abstract]. *Invest Ophthalmol Vis Sci* 1993, 34(suppl):1070.

28. Schuman JS, Jacobson JJ, Puliafito CA, *et al.*: Experimental use of semiconductor diode laser in contact transscleral cyclophotocoagulation in rabbits. *Arch Ophthalmol* 1990, 108:1152–1157.

29. Schuman JS, Noecker RJ, Puliafito CA, *et al.*: Energy levels and probe placement in contact transscleral semiconductor diode laser cyclophotocoagulation in human cadaver eyes. *Arch Ophthalmol* 1991, 109:1534–1538.

30. Gaasterland DE, Abrams DA, Belcher CD, *et al.*: A multicenter study of contact diode laser transscleral cyclophotocoagulation in glaucoma patients. *Invest Ophthalmol Vis Sci* 1992, 33(suppl):1019.

31. Thomas MA, Halperin LS: Subretinal endolaser treatment of a choroidal bleeding site. *Am J Ophthalmol* 1990, 109:742–744.

32. Jaffe GJ, Mieler WF, Burke JM, *et al.*: Photoablation of ocular melanoma with a high-powered argon endolaser. *Arch Ophthalmol* 1989, 107:113–118.

33. Smiddy WE: Diode laser photocoagulation. *Arch Ophthalmol* 1992, 110:1172–1174.

34. Duker JS, Federman JL, Schubert H, *et al.*: Semiconductor diode laser endophotocoagulation. *Ophthalmic Surg* 1989, 20:717–719.

35. Diskin J, Maguire AM, Margherio RR: Choroidal folds induced with diode endolaser. *Arch Ophthalmol* 1992, 110:754.

36.• Peyman GA, Lee KJ: Multifunction endolaser probe. *Am J Ophthalmol* 1992, 114:103–104.

The authors report development of a 20-gauge intraocular probe combining a diode laser, fiberoptic illumination, and aspiration and infusion capabilities.

37. Peyman GA, D'Amico DJ, Alturki WA: An endolaser probe with aspiration capability. *Arch Ophthalmol* 1992, 110:718.

38. Uram M: Ophthalmic laser microendoscope ciliary process ablation in the management of neovascular glaucoma. *Ophthalmology* 1992, 99:1823–1828.

39.• Uram M: Ophthalmic laser microendoscope endophotocoagulation. *Ophthalmology* 1992, 99:1829–1832.

Describes design of a 20-gauge intraocular probe incorporating a diode laser, illumination, and a microendoscope with recording capability.

40.• Friberg TR: Principles of photocoagulation using binocular indirect ophthalmoscope laser delivery systems. *Int Ophthalmol Clin* 1990, 30:89–94.

Review of LIO theory.

41. Friberg TR: Clinical experience with a binocular indirect ophthalmoscope laser delivery system. *Retina* 1987, 7:28–31.

42. Friberg TR, Eller AW: Pneumatic repair of primary and secondary retinal detachments using a binocular indirect ophthalmoscope laser delivery system. *Ophthalmology* 1988, 95:187–193.

43. Augsburger JJ, Faulkner CB: Indirect ophthalmoscope argon laser treatment of retinoblastoma. *Ophthalmic Surg* 1992, 23:591–593.

44. Augsburger JJ, Muller D, Kleineidam M: Planned combined I-125 plaque irradiation and indirect ophthalmoscope laser therapy for choroidal malignant melanoma. *Ophthalmic Surg* 1993, 24:76–81.

45. Irvine WD, Smiddy WE, Nicholson DH: Corneal and iris burns with the laser indirect ophthalmoscope. *Am J Ophthalmol* 1990, 110:311–313.

46. Rubinfeld RS, Pilkerton AR, Zimmerman LE: A corneal complication of indirect ophthalmic laser delivery systems. *Am J Ophthalmol* 1990, 110:206–208.

47. Morley MG, Frederick AR: Melted haptic as a complication of the indirect ophthalmic laser delivery system. *Am J Ophthalmol* 1992, 113:584–586.

48. Palmer EA, Flynn JT, Hardy RJ, *et al.*: Incidence and early course of retinopathy of prematurity. *Ophthalmology* 1991, 98:1628–1640.

49. Cryotherapy for Retinopathy of Prematurity Cooperative Group: Multicenter trial of cryotherapy for retinopathy of prematurity: one-year outcome—structure and function. *Arch Ophthalmol* 1990, 108:1408–1416.

50. Cryotherapy for Retinopathy of Prematurity Cooperative Group: Multicenter trial of cryotherapy for retinopathy of prematurity: preliminary results. *Arch Ophthalmol* 1988, 106:471–479.

51.• Landers MB, Semple HC, Ruben JB, *et al.*: Argon laser photocoagulation for advanced retinopathy of prematurity. *Am J Ophthalmol* 1990, 110:429–431.
First report of diode LIO to treat entire area of avascular retinopathy of prematurity.

52. Landers MB, Toth CA, Semple HC, *et al.*: Treatment of retinopathy of prematurity with argon laser photocoagulation. *Arch Ophthalmol* 1991, 110:44–47.

53. Schechter RJ: Laser treatment of retinopathy of prematurity. *Arch Ophthalmol* 1993, 111:730–731.

54. Iverson DA, Trese MT, Orgel IK, *et al.*: Laser photocoagulation for threshold retinopathy of prematurity. *Arch Ophthalmol* 1991, 109:1342–1343.

55. McNamara JA, Tasman W, Brown GC, *et al.*: Laser photocoagulation for stage 3+ retinopathy of prematurity. *Ophthalmology* 1991, 98:576–580.

56. Fleming TN, Runge PE, Charles ST: Diode laser photocoagulation for prethreshold, posterior retinopathy of prematurity. *Am J Ophthalmol* 1992, 114:589–592.

57.• McNamara JA, Tasman W, Vander JF, *et al.*: Diode laser photocoagulation for retinopathy of prematurity: preliminary results. *Arch Ophthalmol* 1992, 110:1714–1716.
Randomized trial comparing diode LIO and cryotherapy for treatment of retinopathy of prematurity. The laser method was at least as efficacious as cryotherapy, and involved less vitreous hemorrhage and conjunctival hyperemia, with no lid edema or chemosis.

58.• Hunter DG, Repka MX: Diode laser photocoagulation for threshold retinopathy of prematurity: a randomized study. *Ophthalmology* 1993, 100:238–244.
Randomized trial comparing diode LIO and cryotherapy for treatment of retinopathy of prematurity. Although these researchers used an endpoint of creamy white lesions, they encountered only one case of subretinal hemorrhage. They suggested that LIO may prove to be the treatment of choice for retinopathy of prematurity.

59. Drack AV, Burke JP, Pulido JS, *et al.*: Transient punctate lenticular opacities as a complication of argon laser pho-

toablation in an infant with retinopathy of prematurity. *Am J Ophthalmol* 1992, 114:583–584.

60. Tasman W: Threshold retinopathy of prematurity revisited. *Arch Ophthalmol* 1992, 110:623–624.

61. Loertscher H, Mandelbaum S, Parrish RK, *et al.*: Preliminary report on corneal incisions created by a hydrogen fluoride laser. *Am J Ophthalmol* 1986, 102:217–221.

62. Stern D, Puliafito CA, Dobi ET, *et al.*: Infrared laser surgery of the cornea: studies with a Raman-shifted neodymium:YAG laser at 2.8 and 2.92 μm. *Ophthalmology* 1988, 95:1434–1441.

63. Peyman GA, Badaro RM, Khoobehi B: Corneal ablation in rabbits using an infrared (2.9-μm) erbium:YAG laser. *Ophthalmology* 1989, 96:1160–1170.

64. Bende T, Jean B, Matallana M, *et al.*: Wet areal ablation with the erbium:YAG laser (2.94 μm): first results. *Lasers Light Ophthalmol* 1992, 5:39–44.

65. Stern D, Schoenlein RW, Puliafito CA, *et al.*: Corneal ablation by nanosecond, picosecond, and femtosecond lasers at 532 and 625 nm. *Arch Ophthalmol* 1989, 107:587–592.

66.• Seiler T, Matallana M, Bende T: Laser thermokeratoplasty by means of a pulsed holmium:YAG laser for hyperopic correction. *Refract Corneal Surg* 1990 6:335–339.
Initial report of Ho:YAG laser thermokeratoplasty used to steepen corneal curvature and reduce myopia.

67. Seiler T: Ho:YAG laser thermokeratoplasty for hyperopia. *Ophthalmol Clin North Am* 1992, 5:773–780.

68. Moreira H, Campos M, Sawusch MR, *et al.*: Holmium laser thermokeratoplasty. *Ophthalmology* 1993, 100:752–761.

69. Wapner F, Eaton A, Schubert H, *et al.*: Micropulsed diode laser dye-enhanced thermokeratoplasty. *Invest Ophthalmol Vis Sci* 1992, 33(suppl):769.

70. Tuft SJ, Zabel RW, Marshall J: Corneal repair following keratectomy: a comparison between conventional surgery and laser photoablation. *Invest Ophthalmol Vis Sci* 1989, 10:1769–1777.

71. Troutman RC, Véronneau-Troutman S, Jakobiec FA, *et al.*: A new laser for collagen wounding and strabismus surgery: a preliminary report. *Trans Am Ophthalmol Soc* 1986, 84:117–132.

72.• Zysset B, Fujimoto JG, Puliafito CA, *et al.*: Picosecond optical breakdown: tissue effects and reduction of collateral damage. *Lasers Surg Med* 1989, 9:193–204.
Picosecond pulses, which tend to be on the order of microjoules, cause significantly less damage than do nanosecond pulses on the order of millijoules. High repetition microjoule pulses are necessary for effective tissue cutting.

73.• Rowsey JJ, Bowyer BL, Margo CE, *et al.*: Intrastromal ablation of corneal tissue using a frequency doubled Nd:YAG laser. *Invest Ophthalmol Vis Sci* 1993, 34(suppl):1247.
Initial use of the frequency-doubled Nd:YAG laser with 8-ns, 40- to 350-μJ pulses to create intrastromal ablation in enucleated eyes. As the resulting vacuoles collapsed, corneal curvature was altered.

74. Bado P, Bouvier M, Coe JS: Nd:YLF mode-locked oscillator and regenerative amplifier. *Opt Lett* 1987, 12:319–321.

75. Frueh BE, Bille JF, Brown SI: Intrastromal relaxing incisions with a picosecond infrared laser. *Lasers Light Ophthalmol* 1992, 4:165–168.

76. Remmel RM, Dardenne CM, Bille JF: Intrastromal tissue removal using an infrared picosecond Nd:YLF ophthalmic laser operating at 1053 nm. *Lasers Light Ophthalmol* 1992, 4:169–173.

77.• Niemz MH, Hoppeler TP, Juhasz T, *et al.*: Intrastromal ablation for refractive corneal surgery using picosecond infrared laser pulses. *Lasers Light Ophthalmol* 1993, 5:149–155.

Report of the use of the Nd:YLF laser at 1053 nm, 50-ps pulses at 80 to 140 µJ and 1 kHz, to produce intrastromal ablation in human cadaver eyes.

78. Nissen M, Speaker MG, Davidian ME, *et al.*: Acute effects of intrastromal ablation with the Nd:YLF picosecond laser on the endothelium of rabbit eyes. *Invest Ophthalmol Vis Sci* 1993, 34(suppl):1246.

79.• Brown DB, O'Brien WJ, Schultz RO: Nd:YLF picosecond laser capabilities and ultrastructure effects in corneal ablations. *Invest Ophthalmol Vis Sci* 1993, 34(suppl):1246.

Report of difficulties with Nd:YLF intrastromal ablation, including collagen disorganization of up to 20 µm and unpredictability of ablation depth and effect.

80. Cooper HM, Schuman JS, Puliafito CA, *et al.*: Picosecond neodymium:yttrium lithium fluoride laser sclerectomy. *Am J Ophthalmol* 1993, 115:221–224.

81. Park SB, Kim JC, Aquavella JV: Nd:YLF laser sclerostomy. *Ophthalmic Surg* 1993, 24:118–120.

82. Frangie JP, Park SB, Aquavella JV: Peripheral iridotomy using Nd:YLF laser. *Ophthalmic Surg* 1992, 23:220–221.

83.• Taboada J, Poirier RH, Yee RW, *et al.*: Intrastromal photorefractive keratectomy with a new optically coupled laser probe. *Refract Corneal Surg* 1992, 8:399–402.

The authors used Nd:YAG 100-ns pulses at 500 to 2000 Hz to create 100-µm intrastromal vacuoles in animal eyes, localizable to within 20 µm and with a transition zone between normal tissue of 0.5 µm.

84. Meyers SM, Bonner RF, Rodrigues MM, *et al.*: Phototransection of vitreal membranes with the carbon dioxide laser in rabbits. *Ophthalmology* 1983, 90:563–568.

85. Engel JM, Blair NP, Harris D, *et al.*: Use of the carbon dioxide laser in the drainage of subretinal fluid. *Arch Ophthalmol* 1989, 107:731–734.

86. Pellin MJ, Williams GA, Young CE, *et al.*: Endoexcimer laser intraocular ablative photodecomposition. *Am J Ophthalmol* 1985, 99:483–484.

87.• Margolis TI, Farnath DA, Destro M: Erbium-YAG laser surgery on experimental vitreous membranes. *Arch Ophthalmol* 1989, 107:424–428.

The authors cut experimental vitreous membranes with the Er:YAG laser as close as 500 µm to the retina, but experienced some form of retinal lesion in 53% of cases.

88. Lin CP, Stern D, Puliafito CA: High-speed photography of Er:YAG laser ablation in fluid. *Invest Ophthalmol Vis Sci* 1990, 31:2546–2550.

89.• Borirakchanyavat S, Puliafito CA, Kliman GH, *et al.*: Holmium-YAG laser surgery on experimental vitreous membranes. *Arch Ophthalmol* 1991, 109:1605–1609.

Report of the use of the Ho:YAG laser to cut experimental vitreous membranes. Encasing the optical fiber in a retinal shielding pick improved cutting efficiency and allowed treatment within 500 µm of the retina. There were few retinal lesions, but cutting precision was similar to that achieved with the CO_2 laser and an order of magnitude less than that with the Er:YAG laser.

90. Huie TY, Chang CJ, Tso MOM: Localized surgical debridement of RPE by Q-switched neodymium: YAG laser [Abstract]. *Invest Ophthalmol Vis Sci* 1993, 34(suppl):959.

91. Chong LP, Kohen L: A retinal laser which damages only the RPE: ultrastructural study [Abstract]. *Invest Ophthalmol Vis Sci* 1993, 34(suppl):960.

92. Roider J, Michaud N, Flotte T, *et al.*: Selective RPE photocoagulation by 1 µsec laser pulses [Abstract]. *Invest Ophthalmol Vis Sci* 1993, 34(suppl):960.

93.• Lewis A, Palanker D, Hemo I, *et al.*: Microsurgery of the retina with a needle-guided 193-nm excimer laser. *Invest Ophthalmol Vis Sci* 1992, 33:2377–2381.

The authors constructed a guide for 193-nm retinal ablation with an excimer laser. Treatment of animal eyes showed precision similar to that of corneal ablation with this laser.

94.• Zeimer RC, Khoobehi B, Niesman MR, *et al.*: A potential method for local drug and dye delivery in the ocular vasculature. *Invest Ophthalmol Vis Sci* 1988, 29:1179–1183.

Initial report of laser-induced local release in the retina of dye and drugs from liposomes.

95. Zeimer RC, Guran T, Shahidi M, *et al.*: Visualization of the retinal microvasculature by targeted dye delivery. *Invest Ophthalmol Vis Sci* 1989, 30:1459–1465.

96. Khoobehi B, Niesman MR, Peyman GA, *et al.*: Repetitive, selective angiography of individual vessels of the retina. *Retina* 1989, 9:87–96.

97. Khoobehi B, Peyman GA, Niesman MR, *et al.*: Measurement of retinal blood velocity and flow rate in primates using a liposome-dye system. *Ophthalmology* 1989, 96:905–912.

98. Khoobehi B, Char CA, Peyman GA: Assessment of laser-induced release of drugs from liposomes: an in vitro study. *Lasers Surg Med* 1990, 10:60–65.

99.• Khoobehi B, Peyman GA, Vo K: Laser-triggered repetitive fluorescein angiography. *Ophthalmology* 1992, 99:72–79.

Use of a 1.5 to 2.0-mm argon laser spot centered on the optic disc, with energy densities of 0.5 to 3.4 J/cm^2, permitted sufficient dye release from liposomes to obtain angiograms up to 3 hours after injection in animals.

100.• Ren Q, Simon G, Parel J-M, *et al.*: Laser scleral buckling for retinal reattachment. *Am J Ophthalmol* 1993, 115:758–762.

Circumferential rows of Ho:YAG laser spots create a buckling effect in cadaver eyes, without damaging the underlying retina.

101.• Burstein NL, Williams JM, Nowicki MJ, *et al.*:Corneal welding using hydrogen fluoride lasers. *Arch Ophthalmol* 1992, 110:12–13.

Hydrogen fluoride laser burns enabled incisions in cadaver corneas to withstand pressures of up to 34 mm Hg.

102.• Khadem JJ, Truong TV, Ernest JT: Laser activated tissue glue. *Invest Ophthalmol Vis Sci* 1993, 34(suppl):1247.

Incisions in cadaver corneas sealed with a fibrinogen mixture that contained a photosensitive singlet oxygen generator activated by an argon blue-green laser to cross-link a protein solder with stromal collagen withstood pressures as high as 154 mm Hg.

103.• Wolf MD, Arrindell L, Han DP: Retinectomies treated by diode laser activated indocyanine green dye-enhanced fibrinogen glue. *Invest Ophthalmol Vis Sci* 1992, 33(suppl):1316.

A diode laser converted ICG–enhanced fibrinogen to fibrin in rabbit retinas.

104. Pratesi R, Brancato R, Trabucchi G: Miniature laser for retinal photocoagulation: the self-doubling 532 nm neodymium-yttrium aluminum borate (NYAB) microlaser. *Invest Ophthalmol Vis Sci* 1992, 33(suppl):1317.

105. Stern D, Lin W-Z, Puliafito CA, *et al.*: Femtosecond optical ranging of corneal incision depth. *Invest Ophthalmol Vis Sci* 1989, 30:99–104.

106. Huang D, Wang J, Lin CP, *et al.*: Micron-resolution ranging of cornea anterior chamber by optical reflectometry. *Lasers Surg Med* 1991, 11:419–425.

107.• Ren Q, Gailitis RP, Thompson K, *et al.*: Corneal refractive surgery using an ultra-violet (213 nm) solid state laser. *Proc Ophthalmic Tech* 1991, 1423:129–139.

Description of principles of corneal ablation with the frequency-quintupled Nd:YAG laser.

108. Gailitis RP, Ren Q, Thompson KP, *et al.*: Solid state UV laser ablation (213 nm) of the cornea and synthetic epikeratoplasty material. *Invest Ophthalmol Vis Sci* 1991, 32(suppl):996.

109.• Manns F, Ren Q, Parel J-M, *et al.*: Investigation of an algorithm for photo-refractive keratectomy using a scanning beam delivery system. *Invest Ophthalmol Vis Sci* 1993, 34(suppl):800.

Wide-area corneal ablation may be achieved by using computer-assisted scanning of a 0.5- to 1.0-mm laser beam.

110. Ren Q, Simon G, Parel J-M, *et al.*: Investigation of laser-harmonic (213 nm) solid state laser for photo-refractive keratectomy (PRK). *Invest Ophthalmol Vis Sci* 1993, 34(suppl):1245.

111. Culbertson W, Simon G, Ren Q, *et al.*: 213 nm solid state laser photo-refractive keratectomy: in vivo studies. *Invest Ophthalmol Vis Sci* 1993, 34(suppl):1245.

112.• Lin JT: A multiwavelength solid state laser for ophthalmic applications. *Proc Ophthalmic Tech II* 1992, 1644:266–275.

Discussion of a possible all-in-one ophthalmic laser, incorporating multiple Nd:YAG harmonics and pulse durations to achieve ablation, photocoagulation, and photodisruption.

113. Feld JR, Lin CP, Woods WJ, *et al.*: Cornea ablation studies at wavelengths between 205 and 225 nm using a tunable solid state laser. *Invest Ophthalmol Vis Sci* 1992, 33(suppl):1105.

114. Bende T, Jean B, Matallana M, *et al.*: Photoablation with the free electron laser between 2.8 and 6.2 microns wavelength. *Invest Ophthalmol Vis Sci* 1993, 34(suppl):1246.

115. Logan RA, O'Day DM, Haglund RF, *et al.*: Preliminary observations on the effects of the free electron laser on corneal tissue. *Invest Ophthalmol Vis Sci* 1993, 34(suppl):1246.

116. Zelman J: Photophaco fragmentation. *J Cataract Refract Surg* 1987, 13:287–289.

117. Chambless WS: Neodymium:YAG laser phacofracture: an aid to phacoemulsification. *J Cataract Refract Surg* 1988, 14:180–181.

118. Nanevicz TM, Prince MR, Gawande AA, *et al.*: Excimer laser ablation of the lens. *Arch Ophthalmol* 1986, 104:1825–1829.

119. Gailitis RP, Patterson SW, Samuels MA, *et al.*: Comparison of laser phacovaporization using the Er-YAG and the Er-YSGG laser. *Arch Ophthalmol* 1993, 111:697–700.

120. Haefliger E, Parel J-M, Fantes F, *et al.*: Accommodation of an endocapsular silicone lens (phaco-ersatz) in the non-human primate. *Ophthalmology* 1987, 94:471–477.

SELECT BIBLIOGRAPHY

Krauss JM: Contemporary ophthalmic lasers. In *New Frontiers in Medical Device Technology*. Edited by Rosen A and Rosen H. New York: John Wiley & Sons; 1994.

Krauss JM, Puliafito CA, Steinert RF: Photocoagulation. In *Principles and Practice of Ophthalmology: Basic Sciences*. Edited by Albert DM, Jakobiec FA. Philadelphia: WB Saunders; 1994:1346–1360.

Krauss JM, Puliafito CA, Steinert RF: Photoablation. In *Principles and Practice of Ophthalmology: Basic Sciences*. Edited by Albert DM, Jakobiec FA. Philadelphia: WB Saunders; 1994:1384–1408.

Berlin MS, ed.: *Ophthalmology Clinics of North America: Lasers in Ophthalmology: An Update*. Philadelphia: WB Saunders; 1993.

Noyori K, Shimizu K, Trokel S: *Ophthalmic Laser Therapy*. Tokyo: Igaku-Shoin; 1992.

Steinert RF, Puliafito CA, Krauss JM: Photodisruption. In *Principles and Practice of Ophthalmology: Basic Sciences*. Edited by Albert DM, Jakobiec FA. Philadelphia: WB Saunders; 1994:1360–1383.

Weingeist TA, Sneed SR: *Laser Surgery in Ophthalmology: Practical Applications*. East Norwalk, CT: Appleton & Lange; 1992.

CHAPTER *11*

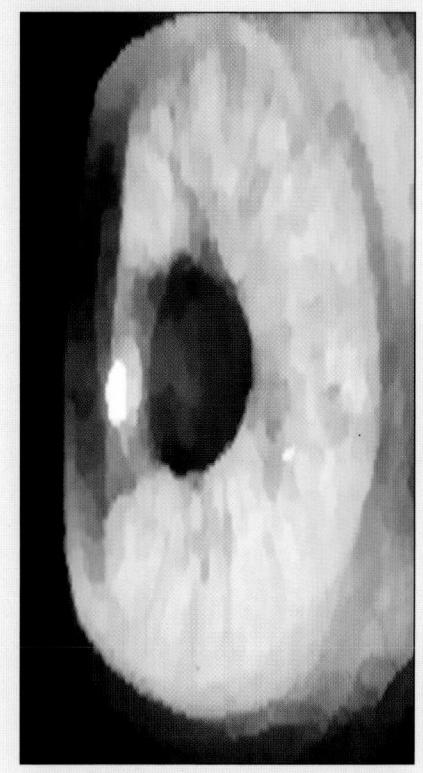

INDOCYANINE GREEN DYE–ENHANCED DIODE LASER PHOTOCOAGULATION OF SUBFOVEAL CHOROIDAL NEOVASCULARIZATION

ALLEN C. HO
DAVID R. GUYER

Exudative Age-Related Macular Degeneration

Age-related macular degeneration is the leading cause of severe visual loss in elderly persons living in developed countries [1]. Exudative age-related macular degeneration, the form associated with choroidal neovascularization, develops in relatively few patients with the disease; however, it accounts for most of the cases of legal blindness associated with this condition. In particular, subfoveal choroidal neovascularization associated with age-related macular degeneration is known to have a poor natural history [2,3].

The Macular Photocoagulation Study Group has published a series of reports since 1982 that have provided guidelines for the performance of laser photocoagulation of extrafoveal, juxtafoveal, and subfoveal choroidal neovascularization associated with age-related macular degeneration [4–7]. Although these landmark studies have demonstrated the beneficial results of receiving laser photocoagulation for choroidal neovascularization as compared with the natural course of the disease, ophthalmologists are still vexed by several problems, including the relentless progression of the disease, a relatively high recurrence rate of choroidal neovascularization after laser photocoagulation, the lack of an effective therapy for occult choroidal neovascularization (choroidal neovascularization that is not well defined by fluorescein angiography), and the coincident loss of central visual acuity associated with subfoveal laser photocoagulation.

Management of Subfoveal Choroidal Neovascularization

The Macular Photocoagulation Study Group reported that, on average, patients with well-defined subfoveal choroidal neovascularization lost three lines of vision after the performance of laser photocoagulation [7]. With time, however, this group of patients experienced less severe visual loss, loss of contrast sensitivity, and loss of reading speed when compared with patients exposed to the natural course of the disease [7]. Certain subgroups in the Macular Photocoagulation Study Group's subfoveal photocoagulation study, however, did not experience the initial drop in visual acuity after foveal laser photocoagulation (S Fine, Personal communication). Because of the immediate loss of central visual acuity associated with foveal ablation in the treatment of subfoveal

choroidal neovascularization, others have attempted foveal-preserving techniques through the use of laser photocoagulation, surgical excision, and antiangiogenic pharmacotherapy.

In a controlled clinical trial that evaluated 160 eyes, Coscas and coworkers [8] reported that "perifoveal" laser photocoagulation may be effective in preserving vision and providing more effective low vision rehabilitation of eyes with subfoveal choroidal neovascularization compared with eyes exposed to the natural course of the disease. In 1992, Tornambe and coworkers [9] published results of a nonrandomized, uncontrolled study of 40 eyes that were treated with foveal-sparing scatter macular laser photocoagulation for subfoveal choroidal neovascularization. These two studies challenged the tenet that complete laser obliteration of choroidal neovascularization is necessary for a favorable outcome. It may be that laser photocoagulation induces a release of local inhibitors of choroidal neovascularization [10,11]. By avoiding laser photocoagulation of the fovea, these investigators attempted to reduce the amount of initial visual acuity loss associated with subfoveal ablation for choroidal neovascularization. These two studies were limited by their length of patient follow-up and one study was nonrandomized and uncontrolled. Nevertheless, these reports described intriguing alternatives to the performance of direct foveal ablation.

The surgical approach to the excision of subretinal hemorrhagic complications of choroidal neovascularization was introduced in 1988 by De Juan and Machemer [12]. In 1992, Lambert and coworkers [13] described the most encouraging results for surgical excision of subfoveal choroidal neovascularization associated with age-related macular degeneration. Seventy percent of their patients with 20/200 vision or worse demonstrated modest visual improvement at a 6-month follow-up. In the same year, Thomas and coworkers [14], as well as Berger and Kaplan [15], reported visual improvement in patients who had surgical excision of choroidal neovascularization associated with the presumed ocular histoplasmosis syndrome, but less favorable results with choroidal neovascularization associated with age-related macular degeneration. These authors could not recommend widespread application of this foveal-preserving microsurgical technique until better case selection and longer-term follow-up was generated. Our initial experience with indocyanine green (ICG)–guided surgical excision of occult subfoveal choroidal neovascularization associated with age-related macular degeneration has demonstrated that this procedure can afford visual stabilization for these patients; however, only rarely does it achieve visual improvement [16]. A multicenter controlled clinical study is in progress to address these issues.

In 1991, Fung and coworkers [17] reported their initial experience with the use of an antiangiogenic pharmacotherapeutic agent, interferon alfa, to cause regression of choroidal neovascularization associated with age-related macular degeneration. Because interferon alfa had shown efficacy in promoting the regression of hemangiomas of infancy, as well as in causing the regression of iris neovascularization in an experimental eye model, it was thought to have potential in causing the regression of choroidal neovascularization associated with age-related macular degeneration [18,19]. The drug is subcutaneously administered and its most common clinical side effects include influenza-like illness, fatigue, and decreased blood counts. Preliminary reports from uncontrolled studies have both supported and raised doubts about the ability of interferon alfa to cause regression of choroidal neovascularization [20]. A multicenter, randomized, controlled clinical study is underway to evaluate the safety and efficacy, if any, of this drug.

Because of the problems associated with these techniques in the management of choroidal neovascularization, we have explored the use of ICG dye–enhanced diode laser photocoagulation in the treatment of choroidal neovascularization associated with age-related macular degeneration. ICG is a dye

approved by the Food and Drug Administration that has a fortuitously similar peak absorption spectra (805 nm) to the peak emission spectra of the semiconductor diode laser (Fig. 11-1). Theoretically, this technique may be used to destroy selectively subfoveal choroidal neovascularization with relative sparing of the neighboring retina (Fig. 11-2). Due to the infrared wavelengths associated with ICG peak absorption and diode laser peak emission, this technique may also be better able to penetrate through turbid fluid, blood, pigment, and pigment epithelial detachments (PEDs) associated with occult choroidal neovascularization. The goals of dye–enhanced diode laser photocoagulation are to close selectively and entirely the choroidal neovascularization complex and to minimize damage to the overlying retina, thereby decreasing the amount of immediate visual acuity loss associated with subfoveal laser photocoagulation treatment.

INDOCYANINE GREEN VIDEOANGIOGRAPHY

To understand the potential benefits and limitations of ICG dye–enhanced laser photocoagulation, it is important to review the physiologic characteristics and distribution of ICG dye, as well as its diagnostic imaging capabilities.

Indocyanine green dye characteristics and distribution

Indocyanine green dye is a tricarbocyanine dye that has been used as a research tool in ophthalmic angiog-

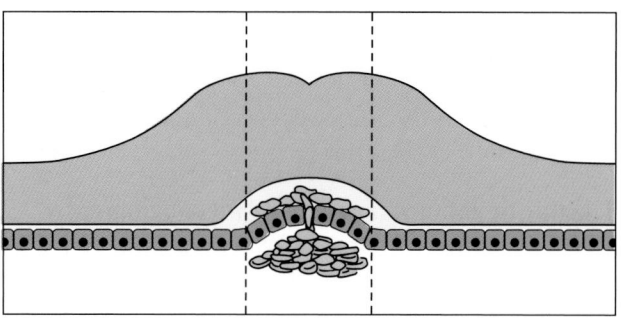

FIGURE 11-2 Theoretical concept of indocyanine green (ICG) dye–enhanced diode laser photocoagulation. ICG dye retention within choroidal neovascularization permits ICG dye–enhanced diode laser photocoagulation with selective destruction of choroidal neovascularization.

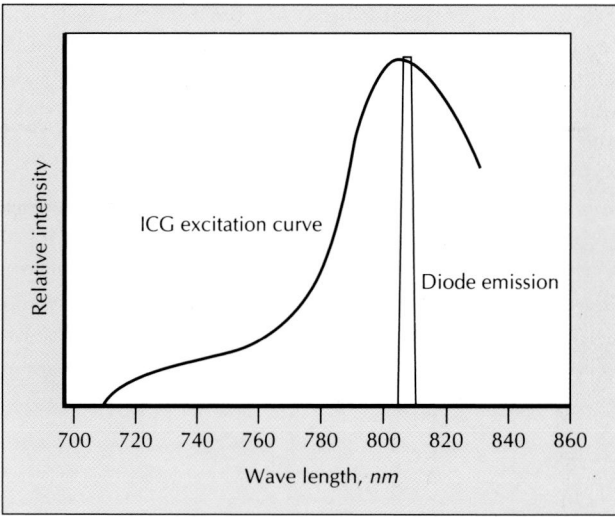

FIGURE 11-1 The peak emission of the diode laser corresponds with near peak absorption of indocyanine green dye.

raphy since 1970 (Fig. 11-3) [21]. With improvement in digital systems, scanning laser ophthalmoscopes, and infrared cameras, ICG videoangiography has become useful in the delineation of some cases of occult choroidal neovascularization [22–25]. ICG is highly bound to serum proteins such as albumin and the lipoproteins (98%), and is considered to be an essentially nondiffusible dye within the normal retinal vasculature (Fig. 11-4) [26]. In the choroidal circulation, ICG leaks less from the choriocapillaris and demonstrates selective retention in and around most choroidal neovascularization, with less leakage than sodium fluorescein [23–25,27]. Recently, Green and coworkers have correlated ICG videoangiographic hyperfluorescence with histopathologic demonstration of choroidal neovascularization (Green and coworkers, Personal communication).

Indocyanine green dye is a relatively safe angiographic dye, but it is contraindicated in patients who have a known allergy to iodine-based dyes or an underlying liver insufficiency. Nausea and vomiting are uncommon side effects during ICG angiography, and, in one series of 700 ICG angiograms, no side effects were reported [28]. One report described a similar safety and adverse reaction profile for ICG and fluorescein angiography [29]. The dye is excreted via the hepatobiliary system [30].

We have recently identified ICG leakage into the retina in some cases of occult choroidal neovascularization. Therefore, diagnostic ICG videoangiography should be performed before any therapeutic consideration with ICG dye. Approximately 11% of eyes with occult choroidal neovascularization will leak ICG dye into cystoid spaces within the retina (average postinjection time, 20 minutes), presumably from a choroidal neovascular source. This leakage is a probable contraindication to the use of dye–enhanced laser photocoagulation (Fig. 11-5)[31].

Diagnostic indocyanine green videoangiography

Recently, several groups have reported results from the use of digital ICG videoangiography as an adjunctive technique to fluorescein angiography in the detection and delineation of occult choroidal neovascularization [23–25]. In particular, Yannuzzi and coworkers [23] have reported that this technique appears to be useful for the detection of occult choroidal neovascularization, neovascularization associated with PEDs, and recurrent choroidal neovascularization. Overall 39% of 129 eyes with occult choroidal neovascularization identified by fluorescein angiography were converted to eyes with well-delineated choroidal neovascularization based on information added by ICG videoangiography. Enhanced imaging was due, in part, to the fact that ICG can better penetrate through overlying blood or serosanguinous fluid because of its infrared absorption and emission characteristics.

Patients with PED were often noted to have diffuse pooling of fluorescein dye beneath the PED. Because ICG dye is more tightly bound to serum proteins, there was less leakage of dye beneath the PED and often a focal area of hyperfluorescence corresponding to presumed choroidal neovascularization (Figs. 11-6 and 11-7).

Similarly, ICG angiography is useful in the detection of occult recurrent choroidal neovascularization after previous laser photocoagulation. In one study, ICG videoangiography confirmed the presence of recurrence in 15 (94%) of 16 eyes [30]. In seven (44%) of the patients, ICG videoangiography converted occult recurrent choroidal neovascularization to well-delineated areas of ICG hyperfluorescence. Furthermore, in seven of these eyes, ICG videoangiography provided the only evidence for recurrent disease. With ICG videoangiography, prior laser photocoagulation scars are relatively hypofluorescent. Because there is less leakage of ICG dye from the surrounding choriocapillaris, there is improved resolution of recurrent choroidal neovascularization as a result of improved contrast.

Although preliminary pilot studies are encouraging for ICG–guided laser photocoagulation of primary occult and recurrent occult choroidal neovascularization secondary to age-related macular degeneration, further prospective randomized studies are necessary

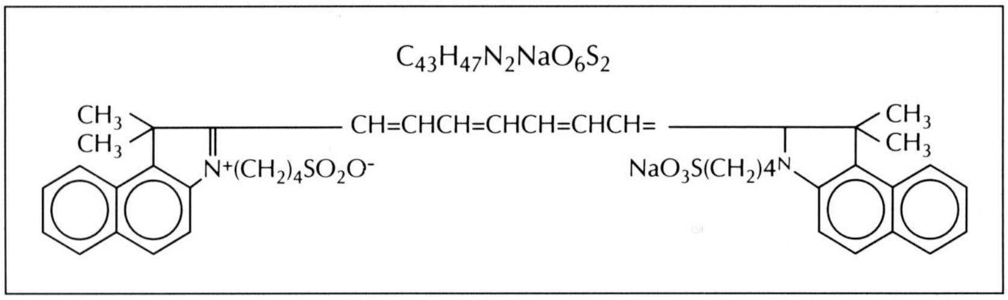

$$C_{43}H_{47}N_2NaO_6S_2$$

FIGURE 11-3 Indocyanine green is a tricarbocyanine dye.

to confirm these findings [32–34]. Until that time, the clinical, fluorescein angiographic, and laser photocoagulation standards of the Macular Photocoagulation Study Group should be followed.

We believe that ICG videoangiography will serve as an important adjunctive technique to fluorescein angiography in the delineation of occult choroidal neovascularization. At this time, fluorescein angiography is still superior in delineating well-defined choroidal neovascularization, and we use this imaging modality to define areas of choroidal neovascularization for ICG dye–enhanced diode laser photocoagulation. The resolution of lacy-fine capillaries at the borders of areas of classic choroidal neovascularization is often better with

fluorescein angiography than with ICG videoangiography. Nevertheless, because ICG is selectively retained in and around areas of choroidal neovascularization, we have sought to exploit this property with dye–enhanced diode laser photocoagulation.

INDOCYANINE GREEN DYE–ENHANCED DIODE LASER PHOTOCOAGULATION

Randomized, prospective controlled clinical trials of ICG dye–enhanced laser photocoagulation are still pending. Several preliminary pilot studies (Guyer and coworkers, Reichel and coworkers, Olk and coworkers) are in

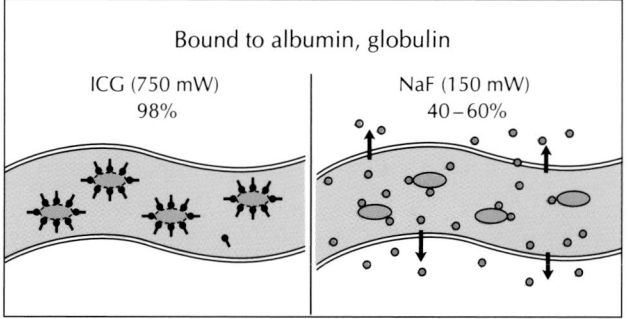

FIGURE 11-4 Indocyanine green is 98% bound to serum proteins, whereas sodium fluorescein is only 40% to 60% bound to serum proteins.

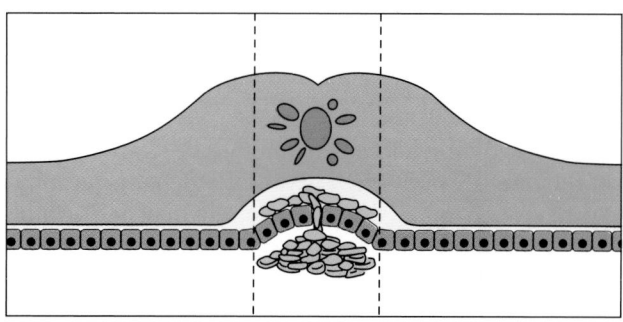

FIGURE 11-5 Indocyanine green (ICG) dye leakage within cystoid retinal spaces is a potential relative contraindication to ICG dye–enhanced diode laser photocoagulation. Diode laser photocoagulation could cause dye-enhanced destruction of the neurosensory retina.

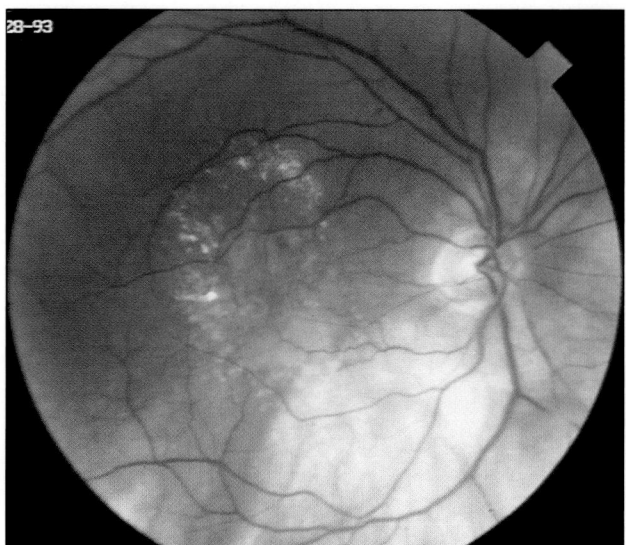

FIGURE 11-6 Exudative macular degeneration. Red-free photograph of a retinal pigment epithelial detachment with lipid exudation.

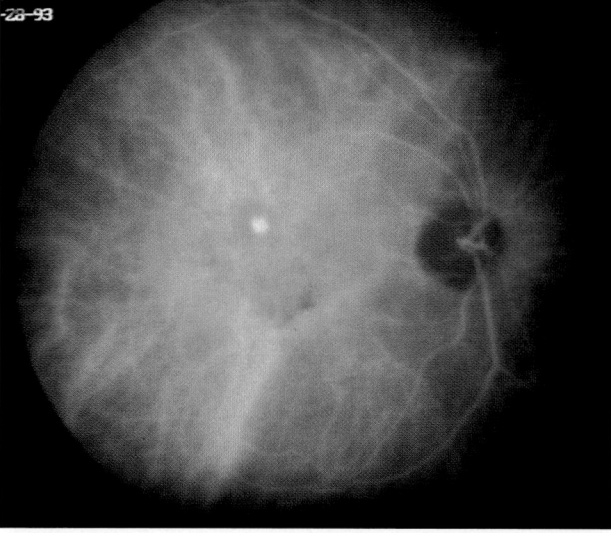

FIGURE 11-7 Diagnostic indocyanine green angiography demonstrating a focal area of hyperfluorescence of presumed choroidal neovascularization beneath the retinal pigment epithelial detachment (See Fig. 11-6).

progress and appear to be somewhat promising. We describe our current protocol and experience with this technique.

Patient selection

For patients with subfoveal choroidal neovascularization, ICG dye–enhanced diode laser photocoagulation may cause closure of the choroidal neovascularization with relative sparing of the adjacent neurosensory retina. Choroidal neovascularization that is obscured by blood or fluid is better imaged with ICG videoangiography, and the diode laser is thought to penetrate more effectively through these fluids. In addition, ICG videoangiography may permit delineation of focal choroidal neovascularization associated with retinal PED. Dye–enhanced diode laser photocoagulation theoretically allows for better energy penetration to these lesions.

Imaging protocol

Diagnostic fluorescein angiography is used and may be simultaneously performed with ICG videoangiography. We have had no adverse reactions when performing both simultaneously. Fluorescein angiography is performed in the usual fashion by using Kodak tri-X film and an injection of sodium fluorescein, 10%, into a peripheral arm vein. Our experience has been with the dye–enhanced diode laser photocoagulation of well-defined areas of subfoveal choroidal neovascularization (by fluorescein angiography). Reischel and coworkers have used ICG guidance as well (Reischel and coworkers, Personal communication).

Diagnostic ICG videoangiography should be performed before any therapeutic consideration of dye–enhanced laser photocoagulation. If ICG dye leakage is noted to be present within the retina, then dye–enhanced laser photocoagulation is not performed. We perform a standard imaging protocol as described in detail by Yannuzzi and coworkers [23], and images are displayed on a high-resolution, 1024-line monitor. Hard-copy print from the system is obtained from a digital continuous printer. Because of a lack of dye within the retinal vasculature during late ICG studies, hyperfluorescent areas of ICG dye are warped and traced onto red-free fundus photographs or additional ICG dye is injected into an antecubital vein to delineate the retinal vasculature and its relationship to the choroidal neovascularization [35]. With the Topcon Imaging System (TopconAmerica Corporation, Paramus, NJ), we have found that the late studies, (30 to 40 minutes), are particularly helpful in delineating choroidal neovascularization. Diagnostic ICG videoangiography is performed with ICG dye, 25 mg diluted in 3 mL of sterile aqueous solvent. After appropriate detection and delineation of choroidal neovascularization by ICG and fluorescein angiography, and after noting a lack of intraretinal ICG dye leakage, we consider a therapeutic application of ICG dye–enhanced diode laser photocoagulation. In particular, eyes that demonstrate subfoveal choroidal neovascularization and good initial visual acuity (20/100 or better) may benefit from this technique. Informed consent is obtained from each patient.

Therapeutic dye–enhanced laser photocoagulation

During therapeutic dye–enhanced diode laser photocoagulation of choroidal neovascularization, we use 5 mg of ICG dye per kilogram of body weight injected

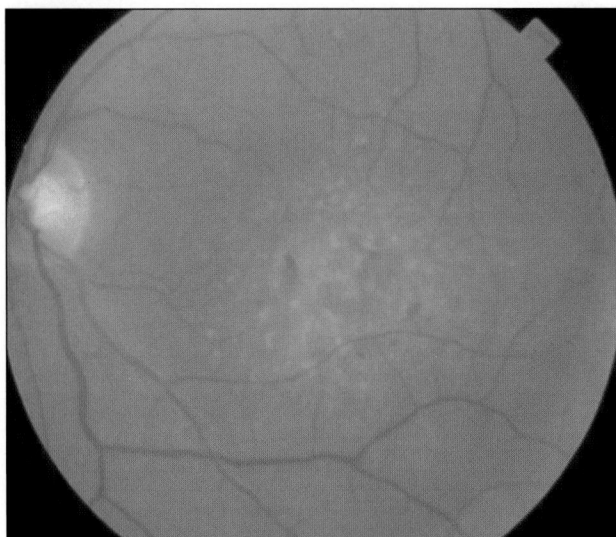

FIGURE 11-8 Confluent soft drusen with intraretinal hemorrhage temporal to the fovea. Fluorescein angiogram demonstrated well-delineated subfoveal choroidal neovascularization.

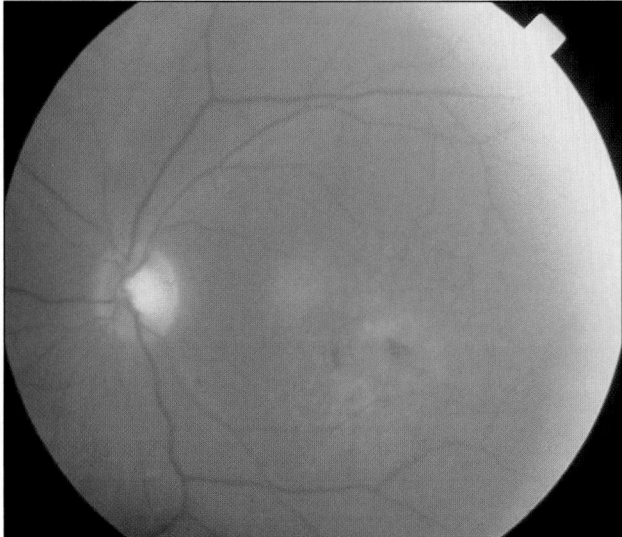

FIGURE 11-9 Immediately after treatment with indocyanine green dye–enhanced diode laser photocoagulation of the subfoveal choroidal neovascularization. Note the light grey treatment endpoint at the fovea.

via an anticubital vein, followed immediately by a 5.0-mL flush of sterile saline. It should be noted that the appropriate dosage of ICG dye injection is unknown. Recently, we have used as little as 0.5 to 1 mg/kg of body weight. The dye injection is performed while the patient is seated at a slit-lamp instrument adapted with a diode laser (Oculight SLx, Iris Medical Instruments, Mountain View, CA). Typically, we use a laser spot size of 200 μm and a duration of 0.5 to 1.0 second. Power considerations are important because the endpoint of treatment is a mild gray burn. We specifically try to avoid a white burn, which might indicate associated neurosensory retinal photocoagulation. The starting power is 150 mW, and we increase the power by 50-mW increments until we achieve the desired threshold lesion.

A threshold lesion is first created outside the area of interest without ICG dye, the goal being a mild gray-brown reaction underneath the retina. The power setting is noted and then the power is halved as a starting energy for the foveal ICG dye–enhanced reaction. Confluent areas are applied to the area of choroidal neovascularization as determined by the initial diagnostic fluorescein angiogram.

We attempt to cover the entire area of presumed choroidal neovascularization, including the foveal avascular zone if involved (Figs. 11-8 and 11-9). The treatment endpoint is a mild gray-brown reaction. We commence the laser treatment within 2 to 5 minutes after the bolus of therapeutic ICG dye is administered by the peripheral vein. With this technique, we were able to obliterate choroidal neovascularization in eight of 10 eyes (80%) (Figs. 11-10 and 11-11). The median

number of treatments needed to obtain angiographic closure of areas of choroidal neovascularization was 1.5 (range, 1–3). The median power used was 475 mW (range, 250–900 mW). Median exposure time was 0.25 ms (range, 0.2–0.5 ms). In this study, the median refractive preoperative vision was 20/130 (range 20/40 to count fingers). The median follow-up period was 12 weeks (range, 5 to 21 weeks). Median refracted final visual acuity was 20/200 (range, 20/100 to 20/200). Four of the 10 eyes (40%) had improved or unchanged vision after treatment.

SUMMARY

Although randomized prospective controlled clinical trials led by the Macula Photocoagulation Study Group have improved our ability to treat subfoveal choroidal neovascularization associated with age-related macular degeneration, the ability to treat this disease with preservation of visual acuity is largely unsatisfactory. As a result, a variety of alternative techniques, including surgical excision of choroidal neovascular membranes and the use of antiangiogenic pharmacologic therapeutic agents and new foveal-sparing laser techniques, including perifoveal laser photocoagulation and ICG dye–enhanced laser photocoagulation, have begun to emerge. It is important to emphasize that these alternative techniques are still investigational. Prospective, randomized, controlled clinical studies as well as histopathologic correlations are required to determine what role, if any, ICG dye–enhanced diode laser photocoagulation will play in the treatment of choroidal neovascularization.

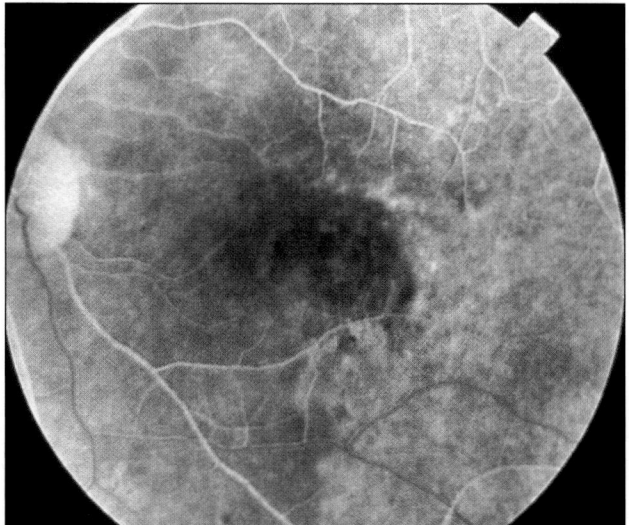

FIGURE 11-10 Arterial-phase fluorescein angiogram with patchy choroidal filling 2 weeks after subfoveal indocyanine green dye–enhanced diode laser photocoagulation.

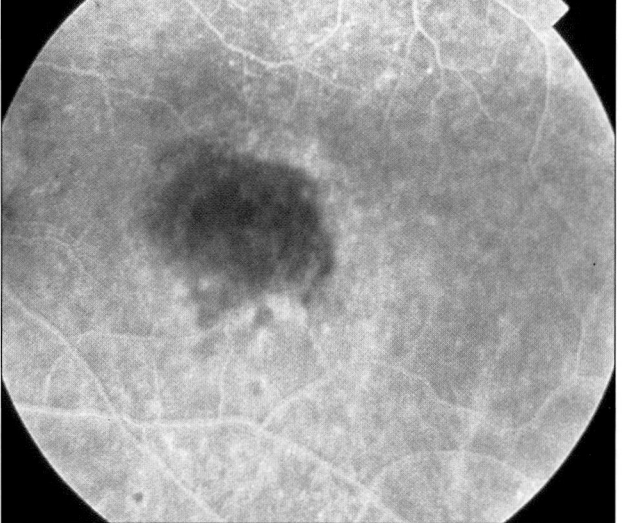

FIGURE 11-11 Recirculation-phase fluorescein angiogram demonstrating closure of the subfoveal choroidal neovascular membrane with indocyanine green dye–enhanced diode laser photocoagulation.

REFERENCES AND RECOMMENDED READING

Recently published papers of particular interest have been highlighted as:
• Of interest
•• Of outstanding interest

1. Ferris FL, Fine SL, Hyman L: Age-related macular degeneration and blindness due to neovascular maculopathy. *Arch Ophthalmol* 1984, 102:1640–1642.

2. Bressler SB, Bressler NM, Fine SI, *et al.*: Natural course of choroidal neovascular membranes within the foveal avascular zone in senile macular degeneration. *Am J Ophthalmol* 1982, 93:157–163.

3. Guyer DR, Fine SL, Maguire MG, *et al.*: Subfoveal choroidal neovascular membranes in age-related macular degeneration: visual prognosis in eyes with relatively good visual acuity. *Arch Ophthalmol* 1986, 104:702–705.

4. Macular Photocoagulation Study Group: Argon laser photocoagulation for senile macular degeneration: result of a randomized clinical trial. *Arch Opthlalmol* 1982, 100:912–918.

5. Macular Photocoagulation Study Group: Argon laser photocoagulation for neovascular maculopathy: five-year results from randomized clinical trials. *Arch Ophthalmol* 1991, 109:1109–1114.

6. Macular Photocoagulation Study Group: Krypton laser photocoagulation for neovascular lesions in age-related macular degeneration: results of a randomized clinical trial. *Arch Ophthalmol* 1990, 108:816–824.

7••. Macular Photocoagulation Study Group: Laser photocoagulation of subfoveal neovascular lesions in age-related macular degeneration: results of a randomized clinical trial. *Arch Ophthalmol* 1991, 109:1220–1231.

8. Coscas G, Soubrane G, Ramahefasolo C, *et al.*: Perifoveal laser treatment for subfoveal choroidal new vessels in age-related macular degeneration: results of a randomized clinical trial. *Arch Ophthalmol* 1991, 109:1253–1265.

9. Tornambe PE, Poliner LS, Hovey LJ, *et al.*: Scatter macular photocoagulation for subfoveal neovascular membranes in age-related macular degeneration: a pilot study. *Retina* 1992, 12:305–314.

10. Glaser BM, Campochiaro PA, Davis JL, *et al.*: Retinal pigment epithelial cells release inhibitors of neovascularization. *Ophthalmology* 1987, 94:780–784.

11. Miller H, Miller B, Ryan SJ: The role of retinal pigment epithelium in the involution of subretinal neovascularization. *Invest Ophthalmol Vis Sci* 1986, 27:1644–1652.

12. De Juan E Jr, Machemer R: Vitreous surgery for hemorrhagic and fibrous complications of age-related macular degeneration. *Am J Ophthalmol* 1988, 105:25–29.

13. Lambert HM, Capone A Jr, Aaberg TM, *et al.*: Surgical excision of subfoveal neovascular membranes in age-related macular degeneration. *Am J Ophthalmol* 1992, 113:257–262.

14. Thomas MA, Grand GM, Williams DF, *et al.*: Surgical management of subfoveal choroidal neovascularization. *Ophthalmology* 1992, 99:952–968.

15. Berger AS, Kaplan HJ: Clinical experience with the surgical removal of subfoveal neovascular membranes. *Ophthalmology* 1992, 99:969–976.

16. Ho AC, Fisher YL, Sorenson JA, *et al.*: IC6 guided subretinal surgery for occult choroidal neovascularization [Abstract]. *Invest Ophthalmol* 1994, 35:1712.

17. Fung WE: Interferon alpha 2a for treatment of age-related macular degeneration. *Am J Ophthalmol* 1991, 112:349–350.

18. White CW, Sonheimer HM, Crouch EC, *et al.*: Treatment of pulmonary hemangiomatosis with recombinant interferon alpha-2a. *N Engl J Med* 1989, 320:1197–1200.

19. Miller JW, Steinson WG, Folkman J: Regression of experimental iris neovascularization with systemic alpha-interferon. *Ophthalmology* 1993, 100:9–14.

20. Guyer DR, Adamis AP, Gragoudas ES, *et al.*: Systemic antiangiogenic therapy for choroidal neovascularization: what is the role of interferon alfa? *Arch Ophthalmol* 1992, 110:1383–1384.

21. Kogure K, David NJ, Yamanouchi U, *et al.*: Infrared absorption angiography of the fundus circulation. *Arch Ophthalmol* 1970, 83:209–214.

22. Guyer DR, Puliafito CA, Mones JN, *et al.*: Digital indocyanine-green angiography in chorioretinal disorders. *Ophthalmology* 1992, 99:287–291.

23. Yannuzzi LA, Slakter JS, Sorenson JA, *et al.*: Indocyanine green videoangiography of choroidal neovascularization. *Retina* 1992, 12:191–223.

24. Scheider A, Kaboth A, Neuhauser L: Detection of subretinal neovascular membranes with indocyanine green and an infrared scanning laser ophthalmoscope. *Am J Ophthalmol* 1992, 113:45–51.

25. Destro M, Puliafito CA: Indocyanine green videoangiography of choroidal neovascularization. *Ophthalmology* 1989, 96:846–853.

26. Riva CE, Ben-Sira I, Feke GT: Flow and diffusion of indocyanine green and fluorescein dyes in the fovea centralis. *Exp Eye Res* 1977, 24:15–23.

27. Hayashi K, Hasegawa Y, Tokoro T, *et al.*: Value of indocyanine green angiography in the diagnosis of occult choroidal neovascular membrane. *Jpn J Clin Ophthalmol* 1988, 42:827–829.

28. Bischoff PM, Flower RW: Ten years experience with choroidal angiography using indocyanine green dye: a new routine examination or an epilogue? *Doc Ophthalmol* 1985, 60:235–291.

29. Hope-Ross M, Yannuzzi LA, Guyer DR, *et al.*: Indocyanine green angiography complications. *Ophthalmology* 1994, 101:529–533.

30. Cherrick GR, Stein SW, Leevy CM, Davidson CS: Indocyanine green: observations on its physical properties, plasma decay, and hepatic extraction. *J Clin Invest* 1960, 39:592–600.

31. Ho AC, Yannuzzi LA, Guyer DR, *et al.*: Intraretinal leakage of indocyanine green dye. *Ophthalmology* 1994, 101:534–541.

32. Sorenson JA, Yannuzzi LA, Slakter JS, *et al.*: A pilot study of indocyanine green videoangiography guided diagnosis and treatment of recurrent choroidal neovascularization. *Arch Ophthalmol* 1994, in press.

33. Slakter JS, Yannuzzi LA, Sorenson JA, *et al.*: A pilot study of digital indocyanine green videoangiography guided laser photocoagulation of occult choroidal neovascularization in age-related macular degeneration. *Arch Ophthalmol* 1994, in press.

34. Regillo CD, Benson WE, Maguire JI, Annesley WH Jr: Indocyanine green angiography and occult choroidal neovascularization. *Ophthalmology* 1994, 101:280–288.

35. Brucker AJ, Brant A, Nyberg W: Landmark injection for localization of choroidal lesions using indocyanine green angiography. *Retina* 1993, 13:169–171.

36. Balles MW, Puliafito CP, Kliman GH, *et al.*: Indocyanine green dye enhanced diode laser photocoagulation of subretinal neovascular membranes [Abstract]. *Invest Ophthalmol* 1990, 31:282.

Select Bibliography

Balles MW, Puliafito CP, Kliman GH, *et al.*: Indocyanine green dye enhanced diode laser photocoagulation of subretinal neovascular membranes [Abstract]. *Invest Ophthalmol* 1990, 31:282.

Macular Photocoagulation Study Group: Laser photocoagulation of subfoveal neovascular lesions in age-related macular degeneration: results of a randomized clinical trial. *Arch Ophthalmol* 1991, 109:1220–1231.

Puliafito CA, Destro M, To K, *et al.*: Dye-enhanced photocoagulation of choroidal neovascularization (Association for Research in Vision and Ophthalmology abstracts). *Invest Ophthal Vis Sci* 1988, 29(suppl):414.

Regillo CD, Benson WB, Maguire JI, *et al.*: Indocyanine green angiography and occult choroidal neovascularization: diagnostic and therapeutic yield. *Ophthalmology* 1994, 101:280–288.

Slakter JS, Yannuzzi LA, Sorenson JA, *et al.*: A pilot study of digital indocyanine green videoangiography guided laser photocoagulation of occult choroidal neovascularization in age-related macular degeneration. *Arch Ophthalmol* 1994, in press.

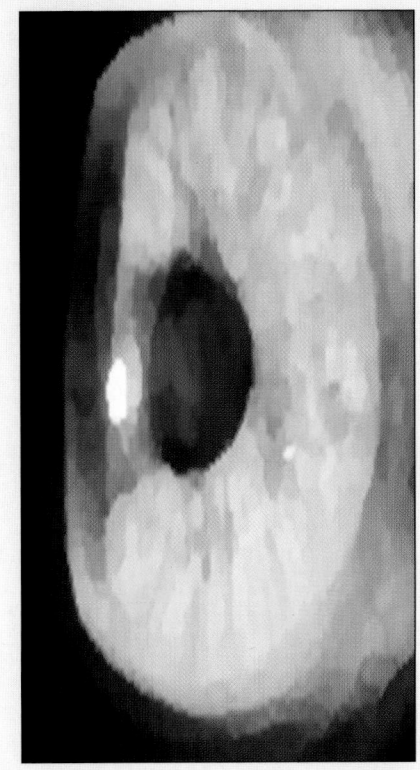

CHAPTER 12

THE FUTURE OF LASER PHOTOCOAGULATION IN RETINAL DISEASES

ROSARIO BRANCATO
FRANCESCO BANDELLO
GIUSEPPE TRABUCCHI

Although several clinical trials have demonstrated the efficacy of lasers in the treatment of many retinal vascular diseases, research has been directed in recent years toward the setting up of new laser sources. The clinical trials that have been carried out have demonstrated that the efficacy of these new laser instruments (double-frequency neodymium-yttrium aluminum garnet [Nd:YAG] laser, diode laser) is similar to that of traditional gas ion lasers; furthermore, these new instruments are less expensive and cumbersome to operate, making retinal photocoagulation available for a greater number of patients. Nevertheless, some disadvantages have also been noted, thus making it impossible to consider these new instruments as components of the ideal laser system. Preliminary experiments carried out with frequency-doubled microlasers emitting in the visible (532 nm) spectrum have resulted in the probability that in the near future an ideal tunable microlaser will be available for use in retinal photocoagulation.

Two important events have marked the development of laser applications in the treatment of retinal diseases over the past few years: 1)new-wave lasers have confirmed both their efficacy and their limitations in several clinical trials conducted with patients affected by retinal diseases and, 2)the development of newer instruments has been proposed. Experimental studies have shown that these lasers have useful features that make it probable that they will be used in clinical practice in the near future.

NEW-WAVE LASERS FOR RETINAL PHOTOCOAGULATION

Together with other colleagues in Europe, we started to use lasers in clinical practice in the early 1970s. During the ensuing years we found laser treatment of retinal diseases to be efficient and useful. The Diabetic Retinopathy Study and the Early Treatment Diabetic Retinopathy Study demonstrated the benefits obtained by argon laser photocoagulation in reducing the risk for severe visual loss in patients with proliferative diabetic retinopathy and in those affected by diabetic macular edema (Fig. 12-1) [1,2]. The Macular Photocoagulation Study showed that argon laser photocoagulation can reduce the risk for severe visual loss caused by subretinal new vessels in patients affected by age-related macular degeneration and ocular histoplasmosis [3–6]. Several controlled clinical trials have demonstrated the efficacy of both krypton laser photocoagulation in preventing visual loss in patients with ocular histoplasmosis, and of argon laser photocoagulation in preventing visual loss in patients with occlusive retinal vein diseases [6–9].

Although these important results have substantially modified the therapy for many retinal vascular diseases, further research over the past 5 years has greatly enhanced the development of new laser systems in the hope that they may offer advantages or improvements in treatment over the established gas ion laser technology. In particular, laser research is working toward finding an effective and safe laser source with the following major important technical features: high electrical and optical efficiency, the need for an ordinary electrical power supply, and no need of water cooling. With these characteristics, the laser sources should be more compact and have lower purchase and maintenance costs. These requirements are important because it must eventually be possible for these lasers to be used to attend to the needs of developing countries also. The features of the new laser systems, developed over the past 5 years, meet these requirements and offer distinct advantages over traditional gas ion lasers (Fig. 12-2).

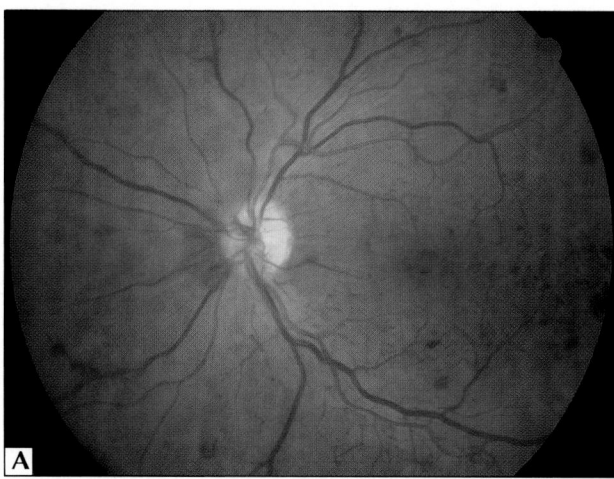

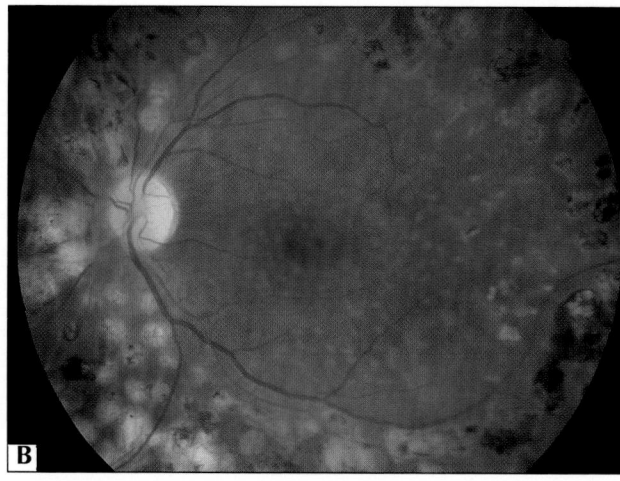

FIGURE 12-1 A, The figure shows a case of proliferative diabetic retinopathy with new vessels at the disk and elsewhere.

B, Argon green laser photocoagulation of the whole ischemic retina allowed a complete regression of proliferative lesions.

FREQUENCY-DOUBLED NEODYMIUM-YTTRIUM ALUMINUM GARNET LASER

Francis L'Esperance was the first to attempt to replace the ion lasers with a solid-state laser in 1971 [10]. This laser used a flash lamp as its pump source and a Nd:YAG rod combined with a frequency-doubling crystal, instead of the ionic gas tube, as its cavity. The resulting laser was far less cumbersome and emitted at 1064 nm and 532 nm. Studies carried out with infrared radiation (1064 nm) demonstrated that photocoagulative treatment of the retina frequently involved undesired side effects, such as choroidal hemorrhages and rupture of Bruch's membrane [11]. These side effects are probably caused by the use of high energy levels, necessary because of the low levels of infrared radiation absorbed by the melanin. In our experience, the use of these high energy levels also exposes the patient to the risk of damage to the lens. Because of these complications, radiation emitted in 1064-nm wavelengths is infrequently used for retinal photocoagulation. By filtering the infrared radiation and using only the visible component (532 nm), it is possible to produce radiation in which the effects on the tissue are very similar to those seen after use of the monochromatic argon green wavelength (514 nm) [12,13]. The first prototypes of the double-frequency Nd:YAG laser, which emitted a monochromatic green radiation only, were produced in the late 1980s. The limitations of these systems were a tendency to overheat and low electrical and optical efficiency.

It has only been over the last few years that the technical improvements in frequency-doubling crystal technology have made possible the development of frequency-doubled Nd:YAG lasers in which these limitations are significantly reduced. The results of the first clinical study involving the use of the frequency-doubled Nd:YAG laser were published in 1991 [14]. In this study, two groups of 10 eyes in patients affected by proliferative diabetic retinopathy were randomly treated with argon green and frequency-doubled Nd:YAG lasers. Regression of new vessels and evolution of visual acuity were similar in the two treatment groups after a mean follow-up time of 6 months.

The technical advantages of the arc lamp-pumped frequency-doubled Nd:YAG laser over the argon laser are the same as those that solid-state lasers have over ionic gas ones and can be summarized as follows: longer operating life, lower maintenance costs, greater reliability, reduced expense, smaller size, and greater portability. In addition, the frequency-doubled Nd:YAG laser does not require water cooling and operates on normal 220-V monophasic alternate current (Fig. 12-2B). Although, as already noted, the frequency-doubled Nd:YAG lasers commercially available are more efficient from an electrical and optical point of view, and have the advantage of an efficient air-cooling system, some technical drawbacks still exist—*ie*, a short delay between activation of the foot switch and appearance of the laser beam, and some problems in coupling the laser with the slit lamp.

SEMICONDUCTOR DIODE LASER

The medical applications of the diode laser, developed in 1962, were limited by its relatively low power output. Later advances in semiconductor technology led to the development of gallium-aluminum-arsenide laser diodes, which can emit continuous-wave, mono-

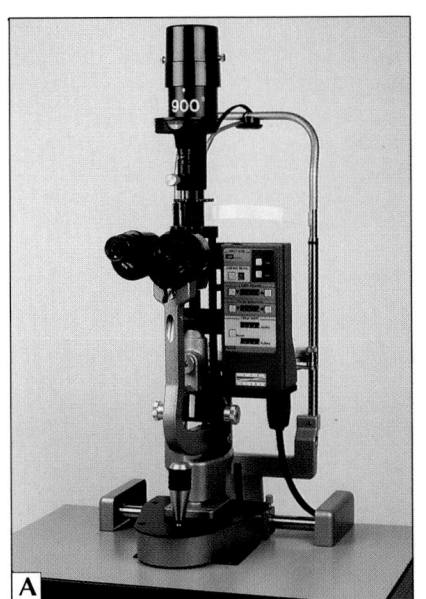 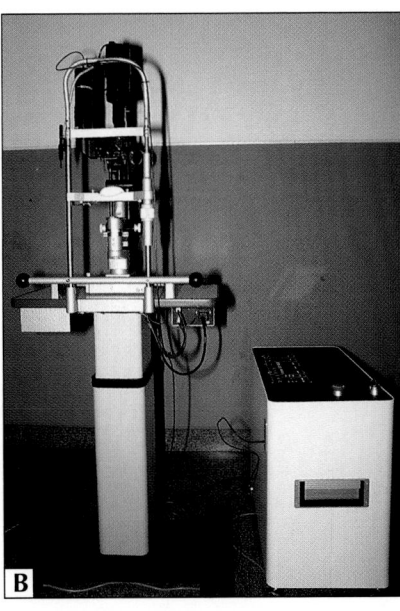

FIGURE 12-2 The figures show two commercially available examples of new laser systems: **A**, a diode laser and **B**, a double-frequency neodymium-yttrium aluminum garnet laser. The size is very small in comparison with that of traditional gas ion lasers.

chromatic, coherent laser light in excess of 1 W (Fig. 12-3). The light emitted by currently available diodes is in the near infrared range with wavelengths ranging from 780 to 840 nm. The diode laser was first used on the eye between 1987 and 1989; these first treatments were carried out by using endophotocoagulation and transpupillary delivery systems (15••,16,17,18•,19). These studies demonstrated that photocoagulative effects on both rabbit and human eyes were similar to those produced by conventional lasers from a histologic point of view, although the diode laser produced deeper photocoagulation than did the argon laser [18•,19].

After these first applications, two reports appeared in the literature by McHugh and coworkers [20] and Balles and coworkers [21••] describing the results obtained when using the transpupillary diode laser in the treatment of retinal vasculopathies. These articles described the results obtained when using the diode laser on 33 and 30 eyes, respectively, of patients affected by proliferative diabetic retinopathy, choroidal neovascular membrane (CNV) associated with age-related macular degeneration, branch retinal vein occlusion (BRVO), central retinal vein occlusion (CRVO), clinically significant diabetic macular edema, and Coats' disease. No treatment-associated complications and only minimal patient discomfort were reported. In Balles's caselist, patients treated with both diode and argon green lasers required 4.5±1.8 times greater mean laser energy with the diode compared with the argon laser to create ophthalmoscopically similar lesions; furthermore, patients complained of moderate-to-marked pain in 10 of 23 (43%) treatments that were initiated with the patient receiving topical anesthesia.

Noyori and coworkers [22] reported other successful treatments in 1990 with the use of the diode laser in patients affected by various retinal vascular diseases. In this study as well, some clinical side effects, such as pain during treatment and large areas of post-treatment chorioretinal atrophy, were reported. The limits of the narrow power range available to produce satisfactory retinal lesions were also emphasized. The results of diode laser treatment in nine eyes with parafoveal CNVs because of age-related macular degeneration or angioid streaks were recently reported by Ulbig and coworkers [23]. The authors reported results similar to those generally with the use of the argon laser.

None of the studies so far mentioned were designed with the aim of comparing, from a clinical standpoint, the therapeutic effects of the diode laser with those obtained through use of the conventional ion lasers. The first study carried out with this goal was published in 1990 and described the results of a comparative study in which the diode and argon green lasers were randomly selected to perform panretinal photocoagulation in two groups of patients affected by proliferative diabetic retinopathy [24]. At a 6-month follow-up, the percentage of cases with regression of retinal neovascularization was similar in the two groups. The sample size in this study was then increased to 44 eyes and the mean follow-up period extended to more than 2 years [25•]. In this last trial, the percentage of new vessel regression was 100% in diode-treated eyes and 91% in argon green–treated eyes. Three major problems emerged in the application of diode laser treatments: 1)the intensity of burns was difficult to judge by appearance alone; 2)satisfactory thermal retinal lesions could be produced from only a very narrow power range; and 3)thermal effect was strongly influenced by the pigmentation of the treated areas of the retina [26]. There was a strong possibility, therefore, of producing an unintentional variation in retinal irradiation. The study hypothesized that both the overdosage (energy dependent) and the deeper effects of infrared radiation (wavelength dependent) may play a role in causing the large areas of chorioretinal atrophy typical in diode laser–treated eyes (Fig. 12-4).

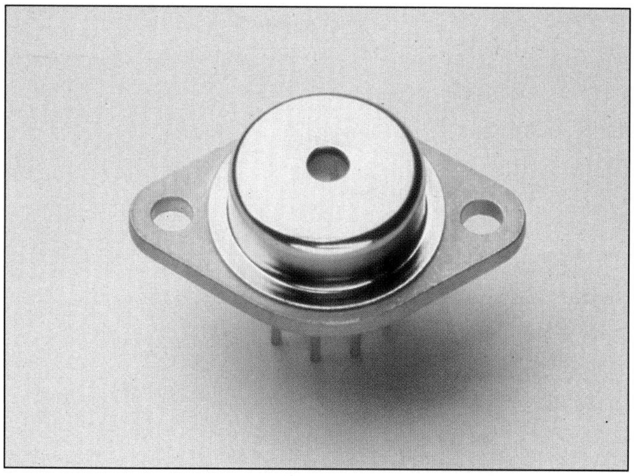

FIGURE 12-3 Self-doubling crystal neodymium-yttrium aluminum borate. The diode is very small.

The use of the diode laser in the treatment of patients affected by macular degeneration with subretinal neovascular membrane who had received intravenous injections 20 minutes before laser application with indocyanine green (ICG) (5 mg/kg) has also been proposed [21••]. ICG accumulates in and around the subretinal neovascular nets after having been cleared from the surrounding circulation and acts as a chromophore for selective absorption of 805-nm laser light, potentially enhancing thermal damage to neovascular membranes. As reported by Balles and coworkers [21••], in three cases of neovascular membranes closure was achieved by using an ophthalmoscopic treatment goal of a mild grey-white color change in the lesion, rather than the intense retinal whitening typically used. Although this was one of the most interesting applications of the diode laser for retinal photocoagulation in retinal vascular diseases, no further reports have been published on the use of this technique.

Excellent results have also been reported with the use of the diode laser in transpupillary prophylaxis for retinal detachment and in vitreoretinal surgery [27,28]. Use of the diode laser as an endophotocoagulator has spread so rapidly that it is now more widely used in the operating room than is the argon laser because of its compact size and reliability. More recently, a report was published on the use of the diode laser in the field of retinal detachment surgery to produce a transscleral retinopexy [29]. The objective was to use this laser in place of transscleral cryopexy. This goal is possible to achieve because the scleral tissue is transparent to all radiation wavelengths ranging from 800 to 1064 nm.

In 1989 we reported the results of transscleral chorioretinal photocoagulation in humans in which continuous-wave Nd:YAG laser radiation was brought into contact with the sclera through a fiberoptic [30]. Its greater affinity with melanin certainly makes the diode laser wavelength (810 nm) more suitable for this type of application. The pilot study in which 10 patients underwent contact transscleral retinopexy produced brilliant results in the production of an adhesive effect [29]. The clinical advantages are smaller rupture of the blood–retinal barrier in comparison with that induced by transscleral cryopexy; the ability to treat through the sclera and through the buckling elements; and the possibility to use the aiming beam to better identify the areas of the retina to be treated. Diode-laser transscleral retinopexy is more time consuming, however, and requires more treatment spots than does cryopexy because only a few large retinal spots are customarily created in cryotherapy. Furthermore, the retinal photocoagulated areas created by the diode laser are less evident for the surgeon than are the large retinal whitenings created by cryotherapy.

Further very interesting clinical possibilities arise from the fact that this laser source can be coupled with an indirect ophthalmoscope, which makes it possible to carry out transpupillary retinal photocoagulation in children affected by threshold stage 3+ retinopathy of prematurity. The results reported by McNamara and coworkers [31•] of a study of 32 infants showed that this laser treatment is just as effective as is transscleral cryopexy. There are many clinical advantages in using the diode laser for this type of treatment. Many infants who reach threshold retinopathy of prematurity are in tenuous health, making transfer to another facility hazardous. In addition, neonatologists prefer to have the infant treated in the intensive care nursery. The advantage of the portable diode laser with indirect ophthalmoscope delivery is that it can be transported to the

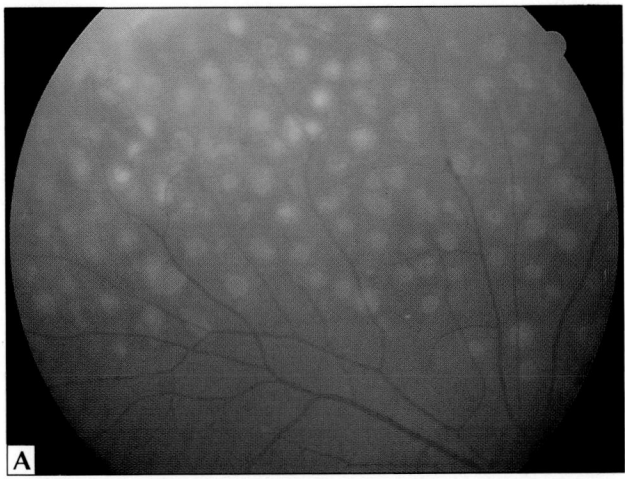
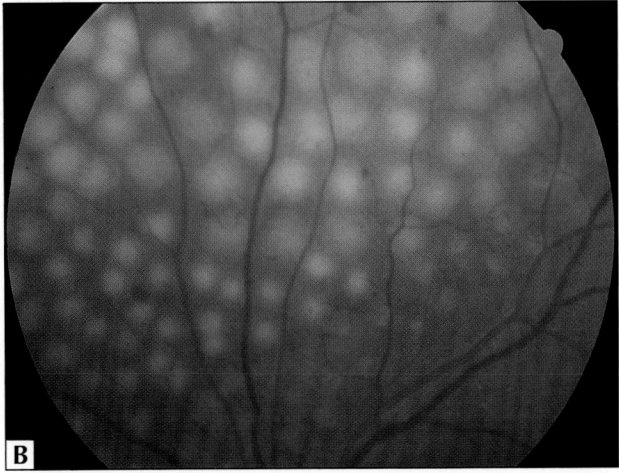

FIGURE 12-4 A, When the diode laser is used to perform a panretinal photocoagulation, the spots must be gray and noncontiguous. B, Panretinal photocoagulation, carried out by argon green laser, must consist of white contiguous spots.

infant rather than vice versa. The inflammation produced by transscleral cryopexy is very severe, resulting in lid edema, conjunctival hyperemia, and chemosis. The parents are usually upset by the swelling and redness of their children's eyes. Diode transpupillary photocoagulation does not produce these alterations.

The data reported since 1987 indicate that our originally reported projections on the future use of the diode laser for ophthalmologic purposes were correct [15••]. In retinal photocoagulation, in particular, the therapeutic effects of the diode laser appear to be similar to those of ion lasers. The most important clinical advantages of the diode laser include decreased light scatter at longer wavelengths and low level of light absorption in nuclear sclerotic cataracts, mild intravitreal hemorrhage, and intraretinal hemorrhage. However, on the basis of our experience, we believe that the infrared radiation of the diode laser cannot really substitute for the visible wavelengths. We believe that (apart from the transscleral procedure) the best results in retinal photocoagulation are obtained with green light.

On the other hand, we consider the technologic characteristics of diode laser systems to be very important—*ie*, their compact size, portability, and ordinary electrical power requirements (Fig. 12-5). These features go a long way toward satisfying the economic and widespread distribution criteria mentioned earlier. The current goal is to develop a laser source with the technical advantages of the diode laser but that emits visible green radiation.

A NEW LASER FOR RETINAL PHOTOCOAGULATION: MICROLASER

In 1987, we suggested using the coherent light emitting diode, also known as the *semiconductor diode laser*,

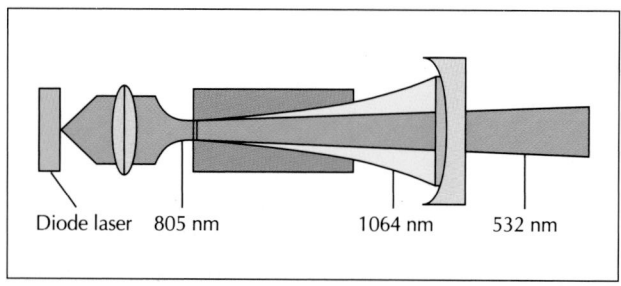

instead of flash lamps to pump the laser and thus to obtain a very compact laser for ophthalmologic applications [15••]. The use of frequency-doubled microlasers emitting in the visible (532 nm) and in the infrared (1064 nm) spectra has already been reported [32,33]. Preliminary experiments have been carried out with the aid of laboratory prototypes of these lasers emitting in the green light spectrum. Because of the power–energy limitations in the green line (100 to 150 mW), retinal photocoagulation was produced only in rabbit eyes. The advent of high-quality autoduplicating crystals (neodymium-yttrium aluminum borate, neodymium-potassium tiranyl phosphate, and so forth) and of the higher power resources of the new-generation diode lasers make it probable that a microlaser will be developed in the near future that will be able to emit effective radiation in the green spectrum (Fig. 12-5). Optical parameters oscillators are also very interesting nonlinear devices that generate light that can be tuned from ultraviolet to infrared. Microlaser pumping of optical parameters oscillators represents a very promising approach toward the establishment of an extremely compact solid-state source of coherent radiation that is continuously tunable from 300 to 3000 nm [34].

Bearing in mind that microlasers generating radiation in the whole visible spectrum will soon be available, we believe that these new-wave lasers can be considered a further step toward the development of the ideal compact laser system to be used in performing retinal photocoagulation.

ACKNOWLEDGMENT

The authors are grateful to Piergiorgio Gobbi, PhD, for his kind assistance in reviewing the manuscript.

FIGURE 12-5 Self-doubling system that makes possible the monochromatic-green emission of the microlaser.

Diode laser   805 nm   1064 nm   532 nm

REFERENCES AND RECOMMENDED READING

Recently published papers of particular interest have been highlighted as:
- Of interest
- • Of outstanding interest

1. The Diabetic Retinopathy Study Research Group: Photocoagulation treatment of proliferative diabetic retinopathy: the second report of diabetic retinopathy study findings. *Ophthalmology* 1978, 85:82–106.

2. Early Treatment Diabetic Retinopathy Study Research Group: Photocoagulation for diabetic macular edema: early treatment diabetic retinopathy study report number 1. *Arch Ophthalmol* 1985, 103:1796–1806.

3. Macular Photocoagulation Study Group: Argon laser photocoagulation for senile macular degeneration: results of a randomized clinical trial. *Arch Ophthalmol* 1982, 100:912–918.

4. Macular Photocoagulation Study Group: Argon laser photocoagulation for neovascular maculopathy: three year results from randomized clinical trials. *Arch Ophthalmol* 1986, 104:694–701.

5. Macular Photocoagulation Study Group: Argon laser photocoagulation for ocular histoplasmosis: results of a randomized clinical trial. *Arch Ophthalmol* 1983, 101:1347–1357.

6. Macular Photocoagulation Study Group: Krypton laser photocoagulation for neovascular lesions of ocular histoplasmosis: results of a randomized clinical trial. *Arch Ophthalmol* 1987, 105:1499–1507.

7. Branch Vein Occlusion Study Group: Argon laser scatter photocoagulation for prevention of neovascularization and vitreous hemorrhage in branch vein occlusion. *Arch Ophthalmol* 1986, 104:34–41.

8. Branch Vein Occlusion Study Group: Argon laser scatter photocoagulation for macular edema in branch vein occlusion. *Am J Ophthalmol* 1984, 98:271–282.

9. Magargal LE, Brown GC, Augsburger JJ, *et al.*: Efficacy of panretinal photocoagulation in preventing neovascular glaucoma following ischemic central retinal vein obstruction. *Ophthalmology* 1982, 89:780–783.

10. L'Esperance FA Jr: Clinical photocoagulation with the frequency-doubled neodymium yttrium-aluminum-garnet laser. *Am J Ophthalmol* 1971, 71:631–638.

11. van der Zypen E, Fankhauser F, Kwasniewska S, *et al.*: Transpupillary irradiation of the rabbit retina with the cw-Nd:YAG laser. *Invest Ophthalmol Vis Sci* 1990, 31:29–40.

12. Mosier MA, Champion J, Liaw LH, *et al.*: Retinal effects of the frequency-doubled YAG laser (532 nm). *Invest Ophthalmol Vis Sci* 1987, 28:1288–1305.

13. Jalkh AE, Pflibsen K, Pomerantzeff O, *et al.*: A new solid-state, frequency-doubled neodymium-YAG photocoagulation system. *Arch Ophthalmol* 1988,106:847–849.

14. Brancato R, Bandello F, Trabucchi G, *et al.*: Frequency-doubled Nd:YAG laser versus argon-green laser photocoagulation in proliferative diabetic retinopathy. *Lasers Light Ophthalmol* 1991, 2:97–102.

15.•• Brancato R, Pratesi R: Applications of diode lasers in ophthalmology. *Lasers Light Ophthalmol* 1987, 1:119–129.

In this article the different applications of the diode laser in ophthalmic therapy were first proposed.

16. Puliafito CA, Deutsch TF, Boll J, *et al.*: Semiconductor laser endophotocoagulation of the retina. *Arch Ophthalmol* 1987, 105:424–427.

17. Brancato R, Pratesi R, Leoni G, *et al.*: Retinal photocoagulation with diode laser operating from a slit lamp microscope. *Lasers Light Ophthalmol* 1988, 2:7378.

18.• Brancato R, Pratesi R, Leoni G, *et al.*: Histopathology of diode and argon laser lesions in rabbit retina. *Invest Ophthalmol Vis Sci* 1989, 30:1504–1510.

One of the first studies evaluating the tissue effect of diode laser radiation on rabbit chorioretina.

19. McHugh JDA, Marshall J, Capon M, *et al.*: Transpupillary retinal photocoagulation in the eyes of rabbit and human using diode laser. *Lasers Light Ophthalmol* 1988, 2:125–143.

20. McHugh JDA, Marshall J, ffytche TJ, *et al.*: Initial clinical experience using a diode laser in the treatment of retinal vascular disease. *Eye* 1989, 3:516–527.

21.•• Balles MW, Puliafito CA, D'Amico DJ, *et al.*: Semiconductor diode laser photocoagulation in retinal vascular disease. *Ophthalmology* 1990, 97:1553–1561.

In addition to being one of the first papers to describe the clinical applications of the diode laser in *Ophthalmology*, it also reports on three cases of dye-enhanced diode laser photocoagulation of neovascular membranes in age-related macular degeneration.

22. Noyori K, Noyori S, Ryutaro O: Clinical trial of diode laser photocoagulation: a preliminary report. *Lasers Light Ophthalmol* 1990, 2:81–87.

23. Ulbig MW, McHugh DA, Hamilton AM: Photocoagulation of choroidal neovascular membranes with a diode laser. *Br J Ophthalmol* 1993, 77:218–221.

24. Brancato R, Bandello F, Trabucchi G, *et al.*: Argon and diode laser photocoagulation in proliferative diabetic retinopathy: a preliminary report. *Lasers Light Ophthalmol* 1990, 3:233–237.

25.• Bandello F, Brancato R, Trabucchi G, *et al.*: Diode versus argon-green laser panretinal photocoagulation in proliferative diabetic retinopathy: a randomized study in 44 eyes with a long follow-up time. *Graefe's Arch Clin Exp Ophthalmol* 1993, 221:491–494.

This is the first and only clinical trial carried out to compare the effects of the diode and argon green laser on proliferative diabetic retinopathy.

26. Brancato R, Bandello F, Trabucchi G: Does wavelength matter when photocoagulating eyes with macular degeneration or diabetic retinopathy [Letter]? *Arch Ophthalmol* 1994, 112:156–157.

27. Menchini U, Trabucchi G, Brancato R, *et al*.: Is the diode laser (810nm) effective to produce chorioretinal adhesion? *Retina* 1992, 12:580–586.

28. Duker JS, Federman JL, Schubert H, *et al*.: Semiconductor diode laser endophotocoagulation. *Ophthalmic Surg* 1989, 10:717–719.

29. Haller JA, Lim JI, Goldberg MF: Pilot trial of transscleral diode laser retinopexy in retinal detachment surgery. *Arch Ophthalmol* 1993, 111:952–956.

30. Brancato R, Leoni G, Trabucchi G, *et al*.: Contact transscleral irradiation of human chorioretina with cw Nd:YAG laser. *Ophthalmic Res* 1989, 21:1–7.

31.• McNamara AJ, Tasman W, Vander JF, *et al*.: Diode laser photocoagulation for retinopathy of prematurity. *Arch Ophthalmol* 1993, 110:1714–1716.

The results of a randomized study carried out in eyes affected by retinopathy of prematurity are described, and the advantages of diode laser treatment over traditional cryotherapy are emphasized.

32. Pratesi R, Brancato R, Trabucchi G: Miniature laser for retinal photocoagulation: the self-doubling 532nm Neodymium-Yttrium Alluminum Borate (NYAB) microlaser. *Invest Ophthalmol Vis Sci* 1992, 33(suppl):3126.

33. Gobbi PG, Brancato R, Agnesi A, *et al*.:New compact laser source at 532nm for chorioretinal photocoagulation, based on all-solid state technology. *Invest Ophthalmol Vis Sci* 1993, 34(suppl):1226.

34. Brancato R, Pratesi R, *et al*.: Miniature lasers: new potentials for ophthalmology [Editorial]. *Ital J Ophthalmol* 1991, 4:257.

SELECT BIBLIOGRAPHY

Brancato R, Bandello F: Chorioretinal photocoagulation by different laser sources. *Methods in Neurosciences* 1991, 7:111–121.

Brancato R, Menchini U: *Microchirurgia Laser in Oftalmologia*. Milano: Ghedini Ed; 1989.

L'Esperance FA Jr: *Ophthalmic Lasers*. St. Louis: The CV Mosby Company; 1989.

Noyori K, Shimizu K, Trokel S: *Ophthalmic Laser Therapy*. Tokyo-New York: Igaku-Shoin; 1992.

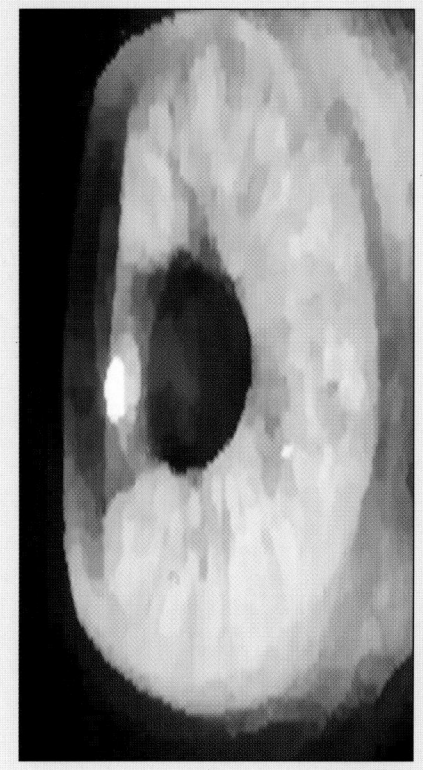

CHAPTER 13

PHOTODYNAMIC THERAPY FOR OCULAR TUMORS AND NEOVASCULARIZATION

ROBERT HAIMOVICI
JOAN W. MILLER
EVANGELOS S. GRAGOUDAS

Photodynamic therapy (PDT) combines the application of low-intensity light with a photosensitizing agent to produce tissue effects. Early investigations in animal models and early pilot studies of human ocular tumors have yielded mixed results with earlier-generation photosensitizers. More recently, PDT with newer photosensitizing agents has shown more encouraging results. These newer photosensitizing agents have increased absorption at longer wavelengths and produce diminished skin photosensitivity. The improved efficacy of PDT demonstrated in recent experimental studies suggests that PDT shows promise as a primary treatment modality for ocular neovascularization and tumors.

PHOTODYNAMIC THERAPY FOR HUMAN MALIGNANCIES

The foundation for modern PDT consists of a large body of observations and investigations into the nature of photodynamic reactions that has spanned most of this century [1••,2]. The modern era of clinical PDT (then termed *photoradiation therapy*) began in the 1970s when reports were made of long-term cures after light radiation treatment of animal tumors 24 to 48 hours after intravenous hematoporphyrin administration [3,4]. In the following years, numerous clinical studies were performed that evaluated patients with malignancies at various sites, including the bladder, lung, head and neck, brain, blood, uterus, and gastrointestinal tract. Most reports concluded that superficial and minimally invasive disease responds best to PDT. The treatment of large tumors generally required higher light or photosensitizer doses to produce a complete response and

were associated with an increased rate of complications. These earlier studies often lacked standardized inclusion criteria, treatment protocols and endpoints, definition of response rates, and lengths of follow-up, making interpretation of the results difficult. Improved photosensitizers, advances in photosensitizer delivery and light dosimetry, and the adoption of increasingly rigorous study designs should allow clinicians and regulatory agencies to evaluate the efficacy of PDT in comparison with other more established forms of therapy.

Mechanism of action

Photodynamic therapy requires the administration of a photosensitizing dye, usually intravenously, which localizes to the target tissues. Light irradiation of these tissues elevates the photosensitizer from its electronic ground state to a higher level (excited) triplet state. The excited photosensitizer quickly returns to the ground state, and, in the process, transfers energy to molecular oxygen. This energy transfer leads to the formation of singlet oxygen (type II mechanism), which reacts with proteins, nucleic acids, and lipid membranes [5]. When the excited photosensitizer transfers energy to other compounds, superoxide, hydroxyl, and other free radicals may be formed. (type I mechanism) [6]. Cellular injury mediated by singlet oxygen is the predominant mechanism of tissue injury involved with PDT and requires adequate levels of oxygen in the target tissues. Photodynamic tissue effects are not dependent on increasing the temperature of the target tissues and thus differ from conventional thermal photocoagulation or dye-enhanced thermal photocoagulation.

The factors governing the effectiveness of a given photosensitizer are multifactorial and depend in part on its photophysical, and physicochemical properties.

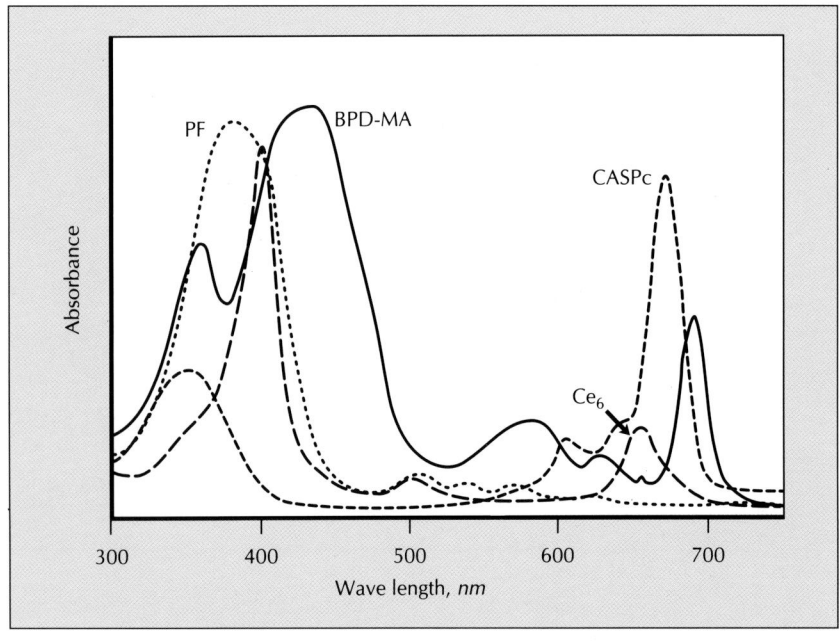

FIGURE 13-1 Absorption spectra of selected photosensitizers that have been used in photodynamic therapy. PF—photofrin; BPD- MA—benzoporphyrin derivative monoacid ring A; Ce6—chlorin e6; CASPc—chloroaluminum sulfonated phthalocyanine. (*From* Liu and Anderson [1••]; with permission.)

The absorption spectrum of the photosensitizer dictates the wavelengths of the radiation beam that may be suitable for PDT. Generally, the wavelength(s) selected coincide with an absorption maximum of the photosensitizer. The absorption spectrum of several photosensitizers that have been used in ophthalmology are superimposed in Figure 13-1. Other important considerations include the metabolism, ph, and route of administration of the photosensitizer. A key consideration in PDT for tumors is the ability of the photosensitizer to localize preferentially in malignant tissues, which leads to tissue damage within these tumors and less collateral damage to surrounding tissues [7]. Neoplastic tissues and neovascularization have increased numbers of low-density lipoprotein receptors [8]. When porphyrin photosensitizers are pre-incorporated into liposomes or precomplexed with lipoproteins, their delivery to neoplastic tissues is increased [9,10]. When the concentration of the photosensitizer in normal tissues is high, unwanted phototoxicity to normal structures may occur.

There is evidence that the subcellular mechanism of damage to neoplastic cells differs with the photosensitizer studied [11]. Some photosensitizers cause damage primarily to the plasma membrane and mitochondria and others cause nuclear or lysosomal damage. Despite evidence for direct damage to tumor cells under some circumstances, most data suggest that occlusion of tumor vasculature is an important mechanism leading to tumor cell death. PDT-induced damage to endothelial cells results in platelet adhesion and degranulation, leading to stasis and aggregation of blood cells and vascular occlusion. Tumor cell necrosis results from the subsequent tissue ischemia [12].

Many light sources can be used for PDT, including broad-band light from incandescent or arc lamps, or monochromatic light from tunable argon-pumped dye lasers, or diode lasers. Broad light bands may enhance the photodynamic effect if they excite secondary absorption peaks of the photosensitizer. Slit-lamp delivery allows for spatial confinement and is particularly suited to intraocular applications [13••,14]. PDT is typically performed with low irradiances such as 150 to 200 mW/cm^2, at which setting photochemical mechanisms predominate over thermal ones. A practical difficulty of performing PDT via the slit lamp with irradiances is maintaining proper alignment of the beam for prolonged periods. For example, when using 692 nm light and a 1250-µm-spot size diameter, 150 J/cm^2 delivered at 150 mW/cm^2 requires a treatment time of 16 minutes and 36 seconds, whereas the same energy delivered at 300 mW/cm^2 can be performed in half the time, or 8 minutes and 18 seconds. The mild hyperthermia that may be produced with higher irradiances may act synergistically with PDT to potentiate cell killing [15]. In experimental animal models, significant

thermal effects as demonstrated by collagen degradation were not observed with irradiances of up to 1800 mW/cm^2 [16].

PHOTOSENSITIZERS IN OPHTHALMOLOGY

Several major classes of photosensitizers have been used *in vitro* and in animal models for the study of mechanisms of photodynamic injury and to develop an optimal agent for PDT for human malignancies (Table 13-1). Among these agents, the tetrapyrroles, phthalocyanines, benzophenoxazines, and xanthenes have been used for ocular applications. Porphyrin derivatives such as hematoporphyrin derivative (HPD) and porfimer sodium (Photofrin) are the most widely studied photodynamic agents. HPD is a complex mixture of porphyrins that is synthesized from hematoporphyrin [17]. PDT with HPD is generally performed with a 630-nm wavelength light to increase tissue penetration and decrease absorption by other tissue chromophores. Drawbacks of this agent are its small absorption peak at longer wavelengths (Fig. 13-1) and the prolonged skin photosensitivity lasting 1 month or more after therapy. Porfimer sodium is a partially purified component of HPD that is more potent and produces less skin toxicity than does HPD [18]. Porfimer sodium has been approved for human use in Canada for the treatment of superficial bladder cancer and applications to health regulatory agencies have been submitted in Japan and in several European countries.

The chlorins, bacteriochlorins, and benzoporphyrin derivatives are newer porphyrin derivatives with favorable properties that have recently been used for PDT (Table 13-1). Chlorin derivatives such as monoaspartyl chlorin e$_6$ are effective photosensitizers in animal tumor models [19]. Bacteriochlorin a is a chlorin derivative that has an absorption maximum at 760 nm

TABLE 13-1	THERAPEUTIC PHOTOSENSITIZERS USED FOR THE TREATMENT OF OCULAR TUMORS AND NEOVASCULARIZATION

Xanthene derivatives
  Rose bengal
Tetrapyrrole derivatives
  Hematoporphyrin derivative
  Photofrin (porfimer sodium)/dihematoporphyrin ether
  Benzoporphyrin derivative
Chlorins and bacteriochlorins
  Chlorin e6
  Bacteriochlorin a
Phthalocyanines
  Chloroaluminum sulfonated phthalocyanine

and a higher molar absorption coefficient compared with HPD [20]. Benzoporphyrin derivative (BPD) is another modified porphyrin that has an absorption maximum of about 690 nm and is phototoxic *in vivo*. BPD is rapidly inactivated or cleared from the body with no significant phototoxicity after 24 hours [21]. Its safety and efficacy after intravenous administration is currently being evaluated in human clinical trials [22]. Compared with HPD, these newer-generation photosensitizers share important characteristics, such as higher absorption peaks at longer wavelengths and diminished phototoxicity.

Phthalocyanines are another class of photosensitizers with a strong absorption band at 675 nm [23,24]. Central metals such as zinc and aluminum are incorporated into their structure to increase the triplet state and singlet oxygen yields. Their solubility and cellular localization is at least partially determined by the number and charge of their side chains. The phthalocyanines are cleared more rapidly and produce substantially less skin toxicity than HPD, PFII, or dihematoporphyrin ether (DHE) [24]. Their safety for use in humans has not yet been determined. Xanthene derivatives also have photosensitizing properties [25,26]. Rose bengal is a halogenated fluorescein derivative with increased singlet oxygen yields and photosensitizing ability that has been used to produce photochemically mediated vascular damage of ocular vessels [27–29,30••].

OCULAR TUMORS AND NEOVASCULARIZATION

Accumulating knowledge regarding the mechanism of photochemically mediated injury suggests that it may offer improved selectivity compared with conventional thermal photocoagulation for selected ocular disorders. The initial distribution of photoactive dyes in vascular structures after intravenous administration and the high transmission of the ocular media (cornea, lens, and vitreous) may allow destruction of vascular structures in the eye, with reduced collateral damage to adjacent tissues. The enhanced binding to new vessels (including those associated with neoplastic tissues) exhibited by porphyrin photosensitizers may increase this selectivity. To investigate this possibility, a variety of experimental and human studies have been performed using PDT for the treatment of ocular tumors and neovascularization.

Ocular melanoma

Iris and ciliary body melanoma

There have been several case reports describing PDT for the treatment of human iris and ciliary body melanoma. In 1984, Tse and coworkers [31•] treated two ciliary body melanomas and one iris melanoma with HPD and transcorneal red light (xenon arc lamp or argon pumped dye laser at 630 nm), with low irradiances (18–200 mW/cm^2) and high fluences (1400 J/cm^2 and 2566 J/cm^2). There was incomplete necrosis of both tumors as shown by histopathologic examination, but the tumor treated with the higher fluence showed an increased depth of necrosis. The iris melanoma received 1080 J/cm^2 and showed complete clinical response. One year later, few residual tumor cells at the peripheral iris were seen histopathologically. Sery and coworkers [32] treated a patient with diffuse multinodular iris melanoma with HPD given at 2.5 mg/kg and 632-nm red light from an argon-pumped dye laser delivered by a fiberoptic probe and found no response.

A combined photodynamic and photothermal approach for the treatment of iris melanoma has also been reported. Chambers and coworkers [33] treated a patient with iris melanoma with DHE, 2.5 mg/kg, and 647 nm and 676 nm of red light (76 J/cm^2, 31,850 mW/cm^2). The tumor was subsequently re-treated with 544 nm green light and similar treatment parameters, with noticeable surface whitening. A transient iritis developed and the tumor regressed from 1 to 6 months after treatment, with no evidence of recurrence after 13 months. In 1992, Davidorf and Davidorf [18] treated four patients with iris melanoma with either HPD or DHE. Their first patient was treated with HPD, 2.5 mg/kg, and 630 nm of red light at 1.72×10^6 J/cm^2 and developed severe refractory iritis requiring enucleation. A histopathologic evaluation of the eye revealed subtotal tumor necrosis. The other three patients were given DHE and were treated with a combination of krypton red and argon green laser light delivered through a slit lamp until there was a whitening of the tumor surface. All three patients had complete clinical regression of the tumor.

Some complications noted with PDT for human iris and ciliary body melanomas such as iris neovascularization and neovascular glaucoma are also seen with other treatment modalities [31•,34]. Severe uveitis is associated with high fluences and photosensitizer doses and may be the result of sudden and extensive necrosis of neoplastic tissues [18,35•]. This complication might theoretically be minimized by the treatment of large tumors in multiple sessions.

These pilot human studies have been inconclusive with regard to the efficacy of PDT and indicate the need for an improved understanding of light dosimetry and other factors limiting photodynamic injury. Accordingly, investigators at our institution and others have pursued PDT research using experimental models. The simplest tumor model is the Greene hamster melanoma model in which Greene hamster melanoma cells are grown in culture and are injected into the anterior chamber of rabbits [36–41]. Tumor nodules rapidly proliferate, filling the anterior chamber, and, if untreated, eventually lead to ocular perforation. The photosensitizer is injected intravenously via an ear vein and the anterior segment tumors are treated with laser light at the absorption maximum of the photosensitizer using an optical fiber or with the slit lamp. The optimal time interval from injection of the photosensitizer to light irradiation may depend on the photosensitizer chosen and is a current area of investigation. Immediately after light irradiation, there may be no discernible change in the appearance of the tumor, or surface hemorrhages, vascular occlusion or narrowing, and surface edema and exudate may be noted. Anterior chamber inflammation and a slight increase in the size of the tumors (caused by edema) may be seen in the days following treatment. Anterior segment fluorescein angiography as early as 20 minutes after treatment shows profound hypofluorescence, indicating occlusion of surface tumor vessels [39].

Studies using the Greene hamster model and HPD or DHE have in most cases shown only partial tumor necrosis by histopathologic examination—results similar to those reported in humans [36]. Complete necrosis has been reported in small tumors of up to 4 mm in height with HPD, 2.5 mg/kg, and a fluence of 102 J/cm^2 or greater (irradiance: 71 mW/cm^2) [38,40]. When using this model, high doses of HPD (7.5–10

mg/kg) or energy levels of more than 180 J/cm^2 caused unacceptable ocular toxicity, including corneal and conjunctival edema, and intraocular hemorrhage and inflammation [38]. Histopathologic study of eyes after experimental anterior chamber melanoma with HPD phototherapy suggests that occlusion of tumor vessels is the predominant mechanism responsible for tumor necrosis [41]. Direct PDT effects on tumors have also been reported [41].

In our laboratory, this anterior chamber model has been used to study the feasibility of PDT with newer-generation photosensitizers such as chloraluminum sulfonated phthalocyanine (CASPc) or benzoporphyrin derivative monoacid (BPD-MA) [35•,42,43]. Panagopoulos and coworkers [35•] performed PDT 24 hours after the intravenous administration of CASPc, 5 mg/kg, using 675 nm red light at nonthermal power densities (63–216 mW/cm^2) (Fig. 13-2). Tumors treated with light or dye alone showed continued growth. Four eyes treated with 3 to 10 J/cm^2 (10–48 mW/cm^2) after intravenous CASPc administration experienced tumor regrowth after initial growth arrest. Eyes that received 20 J/cm^2 or greater had permanent growth arrest, which was confirmed histopathologically. Those that received the highest light doses (57–60 J/cm^2) or

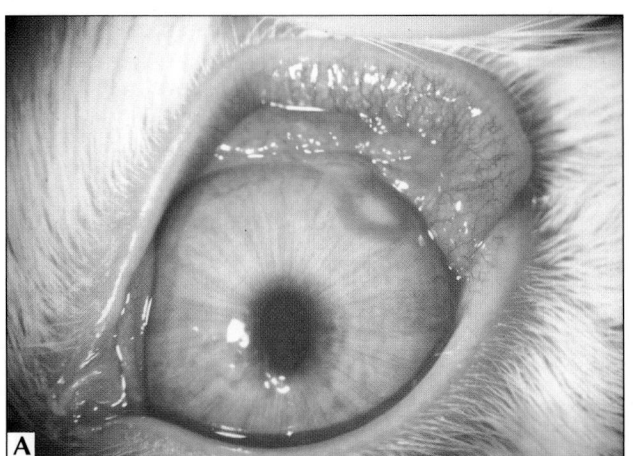

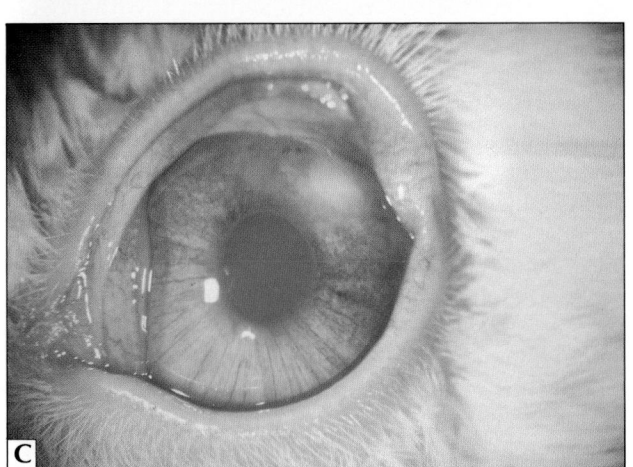

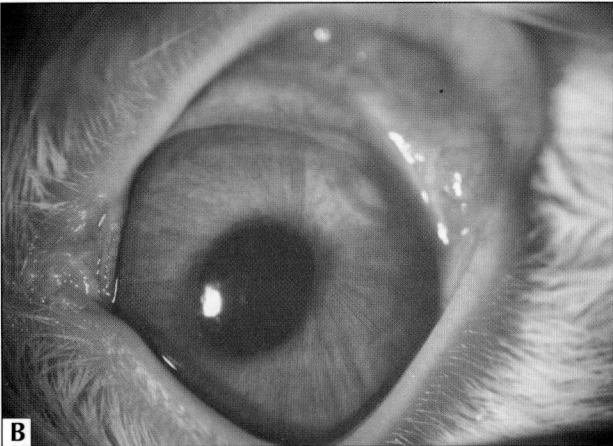

FIGURE 13-2 Experimentally implanted Greene hamster melanoma treated with chloroaluminum sulfonated phthalocyanine and 675 nm red light. **A,** Pretreatment anterior segment photograph shows iris tumor nodules. **B,** Immediately after treatment, the tumor is unchanged but is surrounded by iris pallor. **C,** Four days after treatment, there is pallor and necrosis of the tumor. (*From* Panagopoulos *et al.* [35]; with permission.)

very high doses of CASPc (16–30 mg/kg) showed permanent growth arrest but developed corneal edema, hyphema, and severe anterior segment inflammation.

Others used the same model to perform PDT using BPD-MA precomplexed with low-density lipoprotein (Schmidt and coworkers, Unpublished data). This mode of delivery has been shown in animal models to increase dye accumulation in experimental tumors [10]. After irradiation with 692 nm of red light using energies of 100 J/cm^2 (150 mW/cm^2), necrosis of anterior chamber tumors was seen histopathologically. PDT using newer photosensitizers such as CASPc and BPD appears to be effective in the treatment of Greene hamster melanoma tumors (Schmidt and coworkers, Unpublished data). However, the Greene hamster melanoma models have several limitations. Physical damage to adjacent structures such as the cornea and lens, which has been observed with this model, may be related in part to the abnormal location of these tumors as well as to the effects of PDT. Tumor cells that are not visible at the time of PDT remain untreated and continue to grow and preclude long-term follow-up of affected eyes. The Greene hamster models have also been criticized as a melanoma model because their lack of pigmentation may make these tumors more susceptible to PDT-mediated injury. Newer models with pigmented melanoma cells may address this criticism.

Choroidal melanoma
Clinical studies
The treatment of choroidal melanoma with PDT has been described in a few clinical reports. Tse and coworkers [31•] treated three patients with choroidal melanoma with HPD, 3 to 5 mg/kg, and transcorneal red light delivered via a xenon arc lamp or an argon pumped dye laser (630 nm). Two patients treated with 64 or 850 J/cm^2 showed no histologic evidence of tumor necrosis. The third patient received a higher fluence (2160 J/cm^2) but there was only limited tumor necrosis to a depth of 2 to 3 mm. Bruce [44,45] treated 24 patients with choroidal melanoma between 1982 and 1985 with HPD, 2.5 mg/kg, followed 72 hours later by trancorneal and transcleral exposure to 630 nm red light (200–6800 J/cm^2) from an argon pumped dye laser. Skin sensitivity, chemosis, iritis, and reduced visual acuity occurred in all 24 patients. Improvement in visual acuity occurred only in patients with tumors greater than 4 mm from the macula. Postoperative conjunctival chemosis and iritis were treated with topical steroids and cycloplegic drops, with resolution occurring within 6 weeks. Less common complications were cataract, vitritis, choroidal detachment, and exudative retinal detachment. Patients with small- and medium-sized tumors responded best, but no definitive statement was made regarding the numbers of patients cured [44]. An interim report by the same author had previously stated that complete regression

was seen in eight of the 11 patients with small tumors (<500 mm^3), whereas large tumors remained stable for 3 to 4 months, but all tumors regrew [44,45]. Histopathologic specimens from 10 eyes treated with PDT and subsequently enucleated for tumor recurrence or lack of initial response were reported to show extrascleral extension in three patients and viable and necrotic tumor, inflammation, and chorioretinal scarring in all 10 patients (Bruce RA, Personal communication).

Murphree and coworkers [46•] treated seven patients with choroidal melanoma with HPD, 2.5 mg/kg, and transcorneal and transcleral red light, and reported only one complete response in a patient with an amelanotic melanoma who was treated twice. More recently, Favilla and coworkers [47••] treated 19 patients with choroidal melanoma with HPD, 5 to 7.5 mg/kg, and transpupillary (and transcleral in three patients) 620 to 630 nm red light (Fig. 13-3). All tumors were less than 10 mm in height and all but one were less than 7 mm in height. Complete response was recorded in six patients who had light or moderately pigmented tumors. No regression was seen in eight patients, five of whom had darkly pigmented tumors.

In general, these studies indicate that small melanomas or those that are nonpigmented or lightly pigmented may respond favorably to PDT, whereas large melanomas are not responsive. Increased light absorption by chromophores such as melanocytes or blood may contribute to the incomplete eradication of large tumors [32]. Other possible factors include the choice of photosensitizer, low or inhomogenous oxygen concentrations within the tumor, or inadequate distribution or quenching of the photosensitizer. The results of these studies indicate that PDT for choroidal melanomas has not yet proved to be as effective as have existing methods of treatment such as charged-particle and plaque radiotherapy [48].

Experimental studies
Investigators in our laboratory and elsewhere have treated experimental choroidal melanoma with newer-generation photosensitizers [43,49,50,51••]. In these experiments, tumor cells such as the Greene hamster melanoma are injected into the suprachoroidal space, and growth is monitored by indirect ophthalmoscopy, fundus photography, and, in some cases, echography, and color Doppler imaging [50]. Tumors are then treated with laser light delivered via the slit lamp. In a joint effort between the Wellman Laboratories at Massachusetts General Hospital and the Laser Research Laboratory at the Massachusetts Eye and Ear Infirmary, Schmidt and coworkers [43] treated experimental subchoroidal Greene hamster melanoma with BPD-MA, 2 mg/kg, precomplexed with lipoprotein and 692 nm of red light. Complete necrosis of tumors was confirmed by histopathologic examination after treatment with

100 J/cm². Complications included transient vitritis and a self-limited exudative retinal detachment in 50% of treated eyes, which largely resolved within 48 hours. As described previously, the Greene hamster melanoma model, whether in the anterior or posterior segment, may be easier to treat with PDT because of its lack of pigmentation. To overcome this problem, Hu and coworkers [52] in our laboratory have established a pigmented choroidal melanoma model in the rabbit and have used it to evaluate the effect of PDT on the destruction of choroidal melanoma. Tumor-bearing rabbits were injected with CASPc, 5mg/kg, and 24 hours later, tumors were irradiated with 675 nm of red light from an argon pumped dye laser. Complete tumor arrest was accomplished with light doses of 35 to 60 J/cm² [49]. These experimental studies suggest that PDT with newer photosensitizing agents and modified treatment strategies holds promise for the treatment of human choroidal melanoma.

Retinoblastoma

Clinical studies

There are few reports of patients with retinoblastoma who have been treated with PDT. Murphree and coworkers [46•] treated six patients with recurrent retinoblastoma with HPD and subthermal threshold 630 nm red light. Despite initial regression, there was resumption of tumor growth in all six patients. Ohnishi and coworkers [53] performed PDT with HPD, 2.5 and 5 mg/kg, and the argon laser (488–514.5 nm) in five children with retinoblastoma. Four of the five eyes had had previous ionizing radiation treatment. In the case treated initially with PDT using HPD, 5 mg/kg (300 mW/cm², 270 J/cm²), angionecrosis, thrombus formation, and tumor cell death were seen to a depth of about 6 mm. Choroidal hemorrhage developed in one patient during PDT and was stopped by thermal photocoagulation. Tractional retinal detachment occurred in another child and was attributed to excessive ionizing radiation. Using an approach similar to that of Ohnishi, Murphree [54] successfully treated two patients with recurrent retinoblastoma with HPD followed by continuous-wave argon green laser photocoagulation. The lack of pigmentation in retinoblastoma should facilitate tissue penetration and increase the efficacy of PDT. However, this treatment approach is likely to be ineffective in eyes with vitreous seeding because the absence of tumor vasculature in these areas would preclude photosensitizer

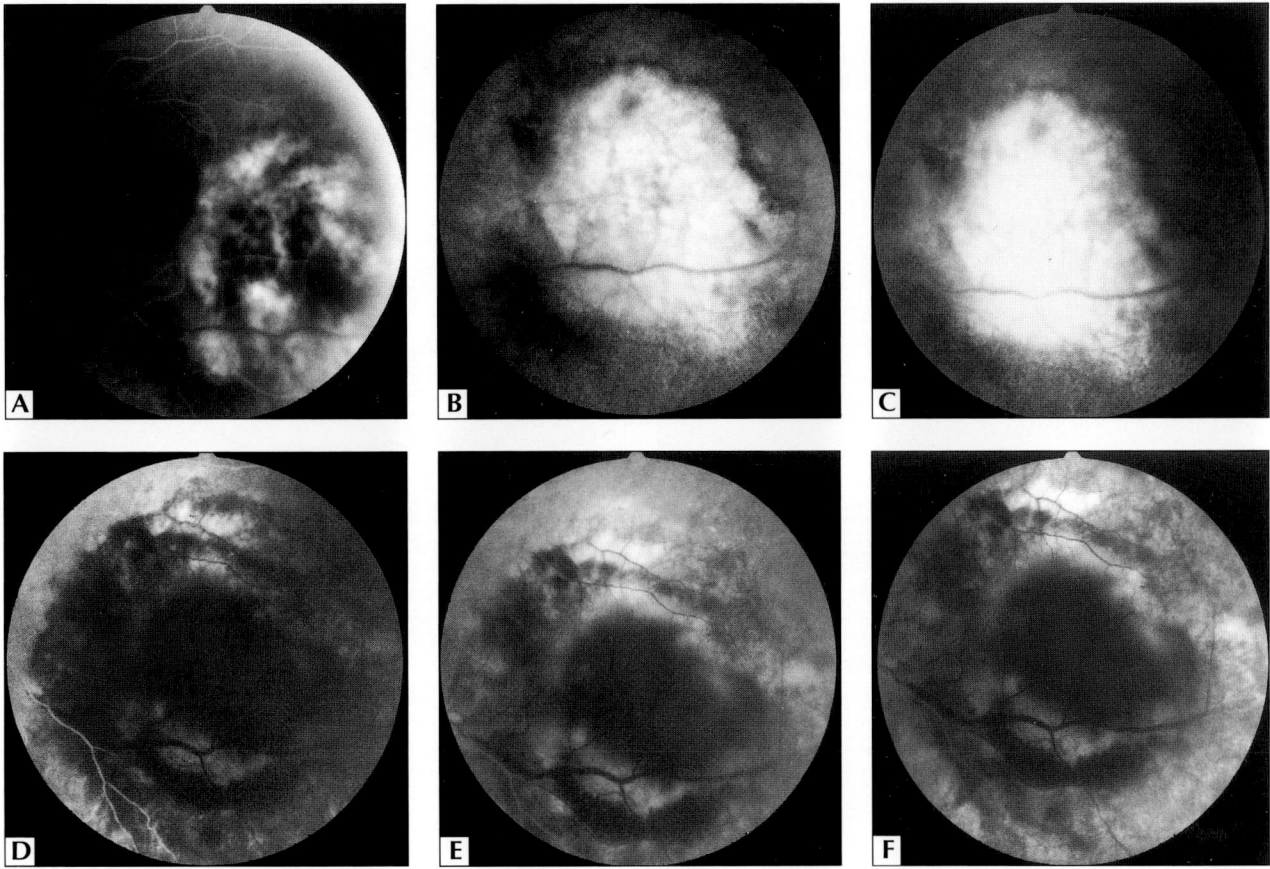

FIGURE 13-3 A, Early, **B**, Middle, **C**, Late frames of fluorescein angiography of choroidal melanoma. **D**, Early, **E**, Middle, **F**, Late frames after photodynamic therapy with hemato-porphyrin derivative; there is decreased leakage of fluorescein from surface vessels. (*From* Favilla *et al.* [47••]; with permission.)

uptake [55•]. It is difficult to draw any conclusions based on the limited treatment experience with this modality. In animal models, necrosis of experimental retinoblastoma-like tumors can be produced after PDT, but high photosensitizer doses may be associated with complications such as retinal edema, detachment, and choroidal hemorrhage [55–58]. Pending further reports, the treatment of human retinoblastoma with PDT remains investigational.

Ocular neovascularization

The rationale for using PDT to occlude pathologic neovascularization arose from observations first recognized in treating tumors. Porphyrin photosensitizing dyes preferentially localize to neovascular tissue in tumors and elsewhere and tumor damage from PDT occurs secondary to vascular occlusion. The mechanism of vascular thrombosis in the eye is similar to that previously described for ocular tumors and its rate is also directly related to light intensity, photosensitizer doses, and oxygen concentration [27–29]. The potential for PDT to produce selective closure of ocular neovascularization with decreased collateral damage to other structures has been investigated in several experimental studies.

Iris neovascularization

We are not aware of any published reports of the use of PDT for human iris neovascularization, although there have been reports using animal models. Experimental iris neovascularization may be produced in primates by photothermal occlusion of major retinal veins [59]. Using this model, Packer and coworkers [60] treated iris neovascularization with HPD, 3 mg/kg, and 675 nm red light (200 mW/cm^2, 540 J/cm^2). Twenty-four hours after PDT there was marked reduction in fluorescein staining as seen by iris angiography, but a substantial inflammatory anterior chamber reaction. Iris neovascularization later recurred in one eye, which was then re-treated. Using a similar model, Miller and coworkers [30••] in this laboratory treated experimental iris neovascularization with intravenous CASPc, 0.5 to 1.0 mg/kg, and 675 nm red laser light (200 mW, 34–102 J/cm^2) and found thrombotic occlusion of iris neovascularization as early as 1 hour after treatment (Fig. 13-4). Leaky iris vessels reappeared by day 7 in one treated eye, without evidence for recanalization of PDT-treated vessels. Minimal anterior chamber reaction and a transient rise in intraocular pressure occurred after treatment. The treatment of clinical iris

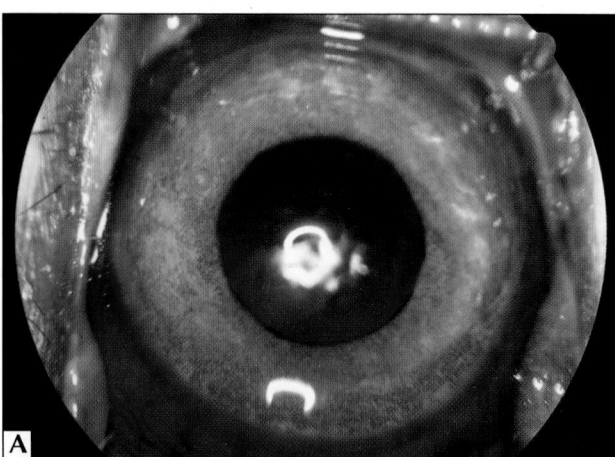

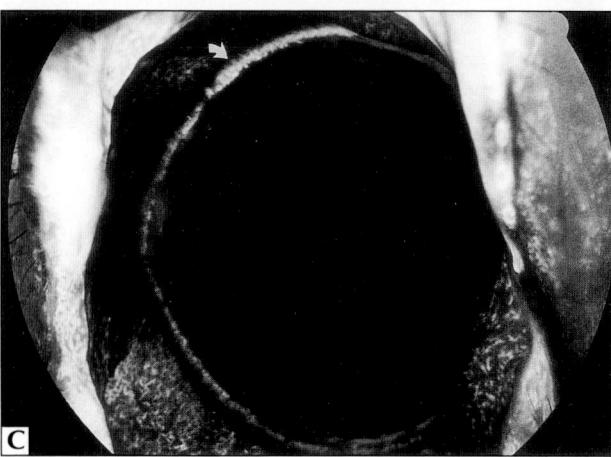

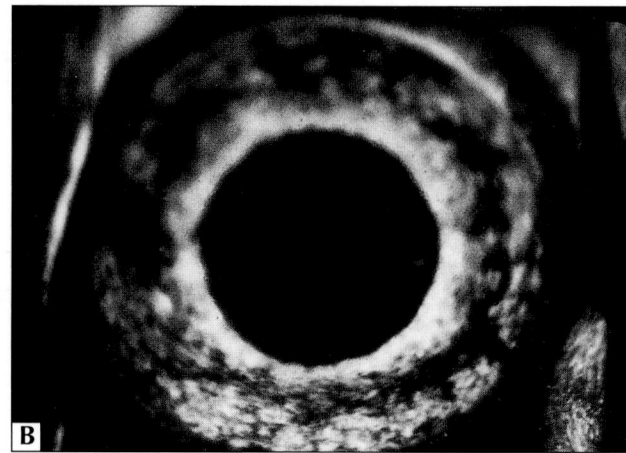

FIGURE 13-4 Photodynamic therapy for experimental iris neovascularization. **A,** Florid iris neovascularization is seen on iris photograph. **B,** New iris vessels leak on fluorescein angiogram. **C,** After treatment, there is marked hypoperfusion of iris vasculature by fluorescein angiography. (*From* Miller and coworkers [30••]; with permission.)

neovascularization with PDT may have a role as adjunctive therapy in combination with standard retinal ablation.

Choroidal neovascularization

There have been several attempts to study the feasibility of PDT for the treatment of choroidal neovascularization. Experimental choroidal neovascularization can be produced in monkeys with high-power argon laser photocoagulation [61•]. These membranes arise at the site of photocoagulation-induced breaks in Bruch's membrane, grow over a period of weeks, and then spontaneously involute. Thomas and Langhofer [62] treated one eye of a cynomolgus monkey with experimental choroidal neovascularization with DHE, 8 mg/kg, and argon green laser light. A single 1.6-J/cm² burn (200 μm, 0.1 second, 100 mW) 12 hours after DHE led to histologic evidence of occlusion of the neovascular complex but without occlusion of the choriocapillaris. An identical lesion treated without DHE did not show occlusion of the neovascular membrane. In a recent study using the same model, Miller and Miller [13••] irradiated experimental choroidal neovascular membranes after the injection of rose bengal, 40 mg/kg, with 1.5 to 7.6 J/cm² (12.7 mW/cm²) delivered from a slit lamp using a cut-off filter that transmitted light above 510 nm and another that absorbed all light above 750 nm. They identified an effective therapeutic window for PDT between 40 and 70 minutes after dye injection, which produced damage to the choroidal neovascular membrane (CNV) without damage to retinal vessels. Although there was damage produced to the CNVs, they were not completely destroyed (Fig. 13-5). Using the

same model, Kliman and coworkers [63] used intravenous CASPc, 0.5 mg/kg, followed 24 hours later by 675 nm red light (1–10 mW, 15 seconds to 2 minutes) to produce closure of choroidal neovascularization as judged by fluorescein angiography and histopathology. In our laboratory, we [14] have recently treated experimental choroidal neovascularization in monkeys with intravenous BPD-MA, 1 to 2 mg/kg, using an argon pumped dye laser (692 nm) delivered transcorneally with a slit lamp and fundus contact lens. Angiographically visible CNVs were treated 5 to 120 minutes after dye injection using 75 to 150 J/cm² (150 mW/cm²) with subsequent complete occlusion of both the choriocapillaris and neovascular membrane, documented by fluorescein angiography and confirmed histopathologically.

The primate model of laser-induced choroidal neovascularization has certain limitations that may hinder the direct application of experimental results to choroidal neovascularization associated with human age-related maculopathy. In the primate model, CNVs regress spontaneously so that the incidence of recurrence after PDT cannot be evaluated. In addition, the morphologic changes induced by the production of these membranes coupled with those of PDT renders interpretation of these treatment effects difficult. Photodynamic damage to the primate retinal pigment epithelium and retinal outer segment has been described and is probably related to localization of porphyrin photosensitizers to these structures [13,14,64,65]. Ultrastructural changes after PDT using animal models range from gross disruption of photoreceptors to more subtle findings such as mitochondrial damage [66]. Strategies to decrease collateral retinal and pigment epithelial dam-

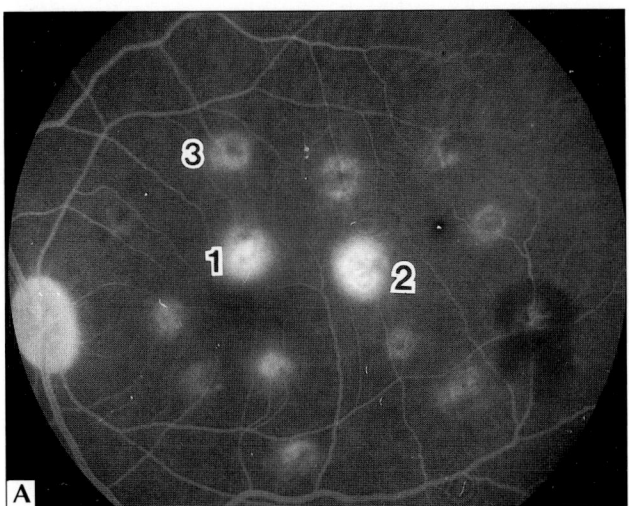
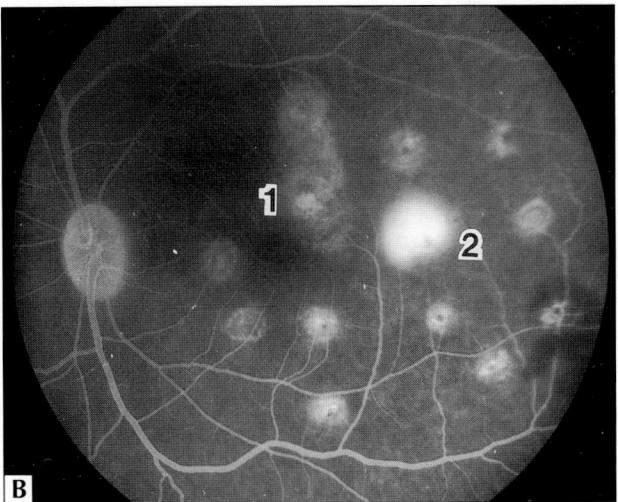

FIGURE 13-5 **A**, Fluorescein angiogram of experimental choroidal neovascular membrane in monkey produced by argon laser photocoagulation. **B**, Two weeks following treatment with rose bengal, 40 mg/kg, and slit-lamp light fitted with filters corresponding to its absorption spectrum, there is only faint staining of the treated lesion. The untreated lesion (1) shows continued leakage and pooling of fluorescein (2). (*From* Miller and Miller [13••]; with permission.)

age after PDT include optimizing the localization and dose of the photosensitizer and the timing of treatment. Further research into these collateral tissue effects is required before PDT for choroidal neovascularization becomes a clinical tool.

CONCLUSIONS

Photodynamic therapy has been used for the treatment of ocular tumors and neovascularization in both clinical and experimental settings. Early clinical trials using these techniques showed mixed or disappointing results. Renewed interest in this form of therapy is related to the development of newer-generation photosensitizers and increasing scientific knowledge regarding basic mechanisms governing successful PDT. These newer photosensitizers show increased efficacy and markedly diminished cutaneous photosensitivity and are currently under investigation. Further refinements in the tissue localization of photosensitizers and treatment protocols for PDT suggest that this therapeutic modality may one day become a standard form of therapy for many ocular disorders, including intraocular tumors and neovascularization.

REFERENCES AND RECOMMENDED READING

Recently published papers of particular interest have been highlighted as:
* Of interest
•• Of outstanding interest

1.•• Liu H, Anderson RR: Photodynamic therapy in dermatology: recent developments. *Dermatol Clin* 1993, 11:1–13.

Excellent overview of the historic development and recent advances in PDT.

2. Daniell MD, Hill JS: A history of photodynamic therapy. *Aust NZ J Surg* 1991, 61:340–348.

3. Diamond I, McDonagh AF, Wilson CB, *et al.*: Photodynamic therapy of malignant tumors. *Lancet* 1972, 2:1175–1177.

4. Dougherty TJ, Grindley GB, Fiel R, *et al.*: Photoradiation therapy II: cure of animal tumors with hematoporphyrin derivative and light. *JNCI* 1975, 55:115–121.

5. Weishaupt KR, Gomer CJ, Dougherty TJ: Identification of singlet oxygen as the cytotoxic agent in photo-inactivation of a murine tumor. *Cancer Res* 1976, 36:2326–2329.

6. Buettner GR, Oberly LW: The apparent production of superoxide and hydroxyl radicals by hematoporphyrin and light as seen by spin-trapping. *FEBS Lett* 1980, 121:161–164.

7. Figge FHJ, Weiland GS, Manganiello LOJ: Cancer detection and therapy. Affinity of neoplastic, embryonic and traumatized tissues for porphyrius and metalloporphyrins. *J Proc Soc Exp Biol Med* 1948, 68:640–641.

8. Gal D, McDonald PC, Porter JC, *et al.*: Cholesterol metabolism in cancer cells in monolayer culture. III. Low density lipoprotein metabolism. *Int J Cancer* 1981, 28:315–319.

9. Jori G, Tomio L, Reddi E, *et al.*: Preferential delivery of liposome-incorporated porphyrin to neoplastic cells in tumour-bearing rats. *Br J Cancer* 1983, 48:307–309.

10. Allison BA, Waterfield E, Richter AM: The effects of plasma lipoproteins on in vitro tumor cell killing and in vivo tumor photosensitization with benzoporphyrin derivative. *Photochem Photobiol* 1991, 54:709–715.

11. Nelson JS, Liaw L-H, Orenstein A, *et al.*: Mechanism of tumor destruction following photodynamic therapy with hematoporphyrin derivative, chlorin, and phthalocyanine. *JNCI* 1988, 80:1599–1605.

12. Castellani A, Pace, GP, Concioli M: Photodynamic effect of hematoporphyrin on blood microcirculation. *J Pathol Bacteriol* 1963, 86:99–102.

13.•• Miller H, Miller B: Photodynamic therapy of subretinal neovascularization in the monkey eye. *Arch Ophthalmol* 1993, 111:855–860.

Recently published study in which experimental choroidal neovascularization was treated with PDT using rose bengal.

14. Walsh AW, Miller JW, Michaud N, *et al.*: Photodynamic therapy of experimental choroidal neovascularization using benzoporphyrin derivative. *Invest Ophthalmol Vis Sci* 1993, 34:1303.

15. Waldow SM, Dougherty TJ: Interaction of hyperthermia and photoradiation therapy. *Rad Res* 1984, 97:380–385.

16. Moulton RS, Walsh AW, Miller JW, *et al.*: Response of retinal and choroidal vessels to photodynamic therapy using benzoporphyrin derivative monoacid. *Invest Ophthalmol Vis Sci* 1993, 34:1169.

17. Bonnet R, Ridge RJ, Scourides PA, *et al.*: On the nature of hematoporphyrin derivative. *J Chem Soc Perkins Trans* 1981, 1:3135–3140.

18. Davidorf J, Davidorf F: Treatment of iris melanoma with photodynamic therapy. *Ophthalmic Surg* 1992, 23:522–527.

19. Nelson JS, Roberts WG, Berns MW: *In vivo* studies on the utilization of mono-l-aspartyl chlorin (NPe6) for photodynamic therapy. *Cancer Res* 1987, 47:4681–4685.

20. Schuitmaker JJ, van Best JA, van Delft JL, *et al.*: Bacteriochlorin a, a new photosensitizer in photodynamic therapy. *Invest Ophthalmol Vis Sci* 1990, 31:1444–1450.

21. Richter AM, Kelly B, Chow J, *et al.*: Preliminary studies on a more effective phototoxic agent than hematoporphyrin. *JNCI* 1987, 79:1327–1332.

22. Liu H, Kollias N, Wimberley J, *et al.*: Photosensitizing potential of benzoporphyrin derivative mono-acid ring A (BPD-MA) in patients undergoing photodynamic therapy. *Photochem Photobiol* 1992, 55(suppl):30.

23. Kreimer-Birnbaum M: Modified porphyrins, chlorins phthalocyanines, and pupurins: second-generation photosensitizers for photodynamic therapy. *Semin Hematol* 1989, 26:157–173.

24. Morgan AR, Skalkos D: Second generation sensitizers: where are we and where should we be going? *SPIE* 1990, 6:87–106.

25. Yoshikawa K, Kurata H, Iwahara S, *et al.*: Photodynamic action of fluorescein dyes in DNA-damage and in vitro inactivation of transforming DNA in bacteria. *Mutation Res* 1978, 56:359–362.

26. Gandin E, Lion Y, Van de Vorst A: Quantum yield of singlet oxygen production by xanthene derivatives. *Photochem Photobiol* 1983, 37:271–278.

27. Wilson CA, Hatchell DL: Photodynamic retinal vascular thrombosis. *Invest Ophthalmol Vis Sci* 1991, 32:2357–2365.

28. Royster AJ, Nanda SK, Hatchell DL, *et al.*: Photochemical initiation of thrombosis. *Arch Ophthalmol* 1988, 106:1608–1614.

29. Nanda SK, Hatchell DL, Tiedeman JS, *et al.*: A new method for vascular occlusion. *Arch Ophthalmol* 1987, 105:1121–1124.

30.•• Miller JW, Stinson WG, Gregory WA: Phthalocyanine photodynamic therapy of experimental iris neovascularization. *Ophthalmology* 1991, 98:1711–1719.
Experimental study demonstrating the feasibility of performing PDT with newer-generation photosensitizers to occlude iris neovascularization.

31. Tse DT, Dutton JJ, Weingeist TA, *et al.*: Hematoporphyrin photoradiation therapy for intraocular and orbital malignant melanoma. *Arch Ophthalmol* 1984, 102:833–838.

32. Sery TW, Shields JA, Augsburger JJ, *et al.*: Photodynamic therapy of human ocular cancer. *Ophthalmic Surg* 1987, 18:413–418.

33. Chambers RB, Arnson DS, Davidorf FH, *et al.*: Treatment of iris melanoma with dihematoporphyrin ether and an ophthalmic laser delivery system. *Contemp Ophthalmic Forum* 1986, 4:79–84.

34. Lewis RA, Tse DT, Phelps CH, *et al.*: Neovascular glaucoma after photoradiation therapy for uveal melanoma. *Arch Ophthalmol* 1984, 102:839–842.

35. Panagopoulos JA, Svitra PP, Puliafito CA, *et al.*: Photodynamic therapy for experimental intraocular melanoma using chloraluminum sulfonated phthalocyanine. *Arch Ophthalmol* 1989, 107:886–890.

36. Liu LHS, Chuo N: Hematoporphyrin phototherapy for experimental intraocular malignant melanoma. *Arch Ophthalmol* 101:901•903.

37. Gomer CJ, Jester JV, Razum NJ, *et al.*: Photodynamic therapy of intraocular tumors examination of hematoporphyrin derivative distribution and long-term damage in rabbit ocular tissue. *Cancer Res* 1985, 45:3718–3725.

38. Sery TW, Dougherty TJ: Photoradiation of rabbit ocular malignant melanoma sensitized with hematoporphyrin derivative. *Curr Eye Res* 1984, 3:519–528.

39. Franken KAP, van Delft JL, Dubelman TMAR, *et al.*: Hematoporphyrin derivative photoradiation treatment of experimental malignant melanoma in the anterior chamber of the rabbit. *Curr Eye Res* 1985, 4:641–654.

40. Gomer CJ, Murphree AL, Doiron DR, *et al.*: Preclinical evaluation of ocular photoradiation therapy. In *Proceedings of the international symposium on porphyrins in tumor phototherapy*. Edited by Andreoni A, Cubeddu R. New York: Plenum Press; 1984.

41. Franken NAP, Vrensen GFJM, van Delft JL, *et al.*: Early morphological changes induced by photodynamic therapy in amelanotic Greene melanoma implanted in the anterior eye chamber of rabbits. *Lasers Med Sci* 1988, 3:27–34.

42. Schmidt U, Birngruber R, Hasan T: Selective occlusion of ocular neovascularizations using photodynamic therapy. *Ophthalmologe* 1992, 89:391–394.

43. Schmidt U, Baumann W, Gragoudas E, *et al.*: Photodynamic therapy of experimental choroidal melanoma using a lipoprotein-delivered benzoporphyrin. *Ophthalmology* 1994, 104:89–99.

44.•• Bruce RA Jr: Photoradiation therapy for choroidal malignant melanoma. In *A clinical manual: photodynamic therapy of malignancies*. Edited by McCaughan JS Jr. Austin: RG Landes Co.; 1993.
Overview of a single investigator's experience treating choroidal melanoma with HPD PDT.

45. Bruce RA Jr: Evaluation of hematoporphyrin photoradiation therapy to treat choroidal melanoma. *Lasers Surg Med* 1984, 4:59–64.

46.• Murphree AL, Cote M, Gomer CJ: The evolution of photodynamic therapy techniques in the treatment of intraocular tumors. *Photochem Photobiol* 1987, 46:919–923.

47.•• Favilla I, Barry WR, Gosbell A, *et al.*: Phototherapy of posterior uveal melanomas. *Br J Ophthalmol* 1991, 75:718–721.
Most recent series of patients with choroidal melanoma treated with HPD PDT.

48. Lingua RW, Parel JW: Photodynamic therapy for ocular tumors. *J Photochem Photobiol B* 1991, 119–122.

49. Gonzalez VH, Hu LK, Gragoudas ES, *et al.*: Photodynamic therapy of pigmented choroidal melanomas. *Invest Ophthalmol Vis Sci* 1993, 34:891.

50. Phillips AMR, Browne BH, Allan D: Haematoporphyrin photosensitisation treatment of experimental choroidal melanoma. *Eye* 1987, 1:680–685.

51.•• Ozler SA, Nelson S, Liggett PE, *et al.*: Photodynamic therapy of experimental subchoroidal melanoma using chloraluminum sulfonated phthalocyanine. *Arch Ophthalmol* 1992, 110:555–561.
Recent study of PDT for experimental melanoma demonstrating increased efficacy using a second-generation photosensitizing agent.

52. Hu LK, Huh K, Gragoudas ES, *et al.*: Establishment of pigmented choroidal melanoma. *Invest Ophthalmol Vis Sci* 1992, 33:1252.

53. Ohnishi Y, Yamana Y, Minei M: Photoradiation therapy using argon laser and a hematoporphyrin derivative for retinoblastoma: a preliminary report. *Jpn J Ophthalmol* 1986, 30:409–419.

54. Murphree AL: Retinoblastoma. In *Retina* vol 1, edited by Ryan SJ, Ogden TE. St Louis: CV Mosby; 1989, 544.

55.• White L, Gomer CJ, Doiron DR, *et al.*: Ineffective photodynamic therapy (PDT) in a poorly vascularized xenograft model. *Br J Cancer* 1988, 57:455–458.

Experimental study that demonstrated the importance of tumor vascularity for successful PDT of experimental retinoblastoma.

56. Winther J, Ehlers N: Histopathological changes in an intraocular-like tumour following photodynamic therapy. *Acta Ophthalmol* 1988, 66:69–78.

57. Winther J, Overgaard J: Photodynamic therapy of experimental intraocular retinoblastomas: dose-response relationships to light energy and photofrin II. *Acta Ophthalmol* 1989, 67:44–50.

58. Winther J: Porphyrin photodynamic therapy in an experimental retinoblastoma model. *Ophthalmic Paed Genet* 1987, 8:49–52.

59. Virdi PS, Hayreh SS: Ocular neovascularization with retinal vascular occlusion. *Arch Ophthalmol* 1982, 100:331–341.

60.• Packer AJ, Tse DT, Gu X-Q, *et al.*: Hematoporphyrin photoradiation therapy for iris neovascularization. *Arch Ophthalmol* 1984, 102:1193–1197.

First report to suggest that experimental iris neovascularization could be inhibited with HPD PDT.

61. Ryan SJ: Subretinal neovascularization. *Arch Ophthalmol* 1982, 100:1804–1809.

62. Thomas EL, Langhofer M: Closure of experimental subretinal neovascular vessels with dihematoporphyrin ether augmented argon green laser photocoagulation. *Photochem Photobiol* 1987, 46:5881–5886.

63. Kliman GH, Stern D, Gregory WA, *et al.*: Angiography and photodynamic therapy of experimental choroidal neovascularization using phthalocyanine dye. *Invest Ophthalmol Vis Sci* 1989, 30:371.

64. Haimovici R, Kramer M, Flotte TJ, *et al.*: Localization of benzoporphyrin derivative in the rabbit eye. *Invest Ophthalmol Vis Sci* 1993, 34:1303.

65. Gomer CJ, Jester JV, Razum NJ, *et al.*: Photodynamic therapy of intraocular tumors examination of hematoporphyrin derivative distribution and long term damage in rabbit ocular tissue. *Cancer Res* 1985, 45:3718–3725.

66. Schmidt-Erfurth U, Jacobs D, Flotte TJ: Photothrombosis of ocular neovascularization using benzoporphyrin derivative. *Invest Ophthalmol Vis Sci* 1993, 34:1303.

SELECT BIBLIOGRAPHY

Ciba Foundation: *Photosensitizing compounds: their chemistry, biology and clinical use.* New York: Wiley & Sons; 1989.

Henderson BW, Dougherty TJ, eds: *Photodynamic therapy.* New York: Marcel Dekker; 1992.

Kessel D: *Photodynamic therapy of neoplastic disease*, vol 1. Boca Raton: CRC Press; 1990.

McCaughan JS Jr: *A Clinical Manual: Photodynamic Therapy of Malignancies.* Austin: RG Landes Co.; 1993.

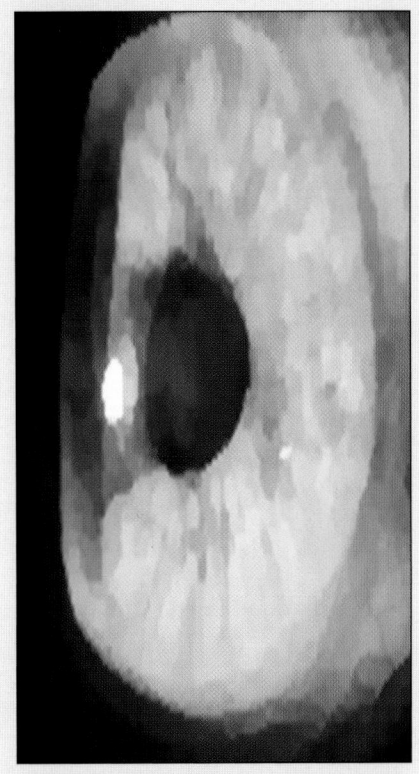

CHAPTER 14

ARGON LASER TRABECULOPLASTY

MARY FRAN SMITH
J. WILLIAM DOYLE

Argon laser trabeculoplasty is a well-tolerated procedure, which has become standard in the treatment of certain cases of progressive primary and secondary open-angle glaucoma. Since its description by Wise and Witter [1] in 1979, treatment technique has changed surprisingly little, although one group presently is investigating significantly lower power application ("trabeculostimulation" vs trabeculoplasty) [2]. Much interest has developed in regard to ALT's place in the glaucoma treatment armamentarium, however, since reports by the Glaucoma Laser Trial Study Group in 1991 and The Normal Tension Glaucoma Study Group in 1992 [3••, 4••]. The use of topical nonsteroidal antiinflammatory drugs as well as apraclonidine after ALT has been gaining popularity as well.

In this review we briefly address the pathophysiologic mechanisms behind successful ALT, and then turn our attention to pertinent clinical points, including patient factors influencing success, variations in technique used, potential complications and drugs aimed at decreasing their incidence, long-term efficacy of ALT, and, of course, the current role of ALT in the care of patients with glaucoma.

PATHOPHYSIOLOGIC CHARACTERISTICS

It is agreed that the major effect of ALT results from increased aqueous outflow through the trabecular meshwork system. Wise and Witter originally postulated that this increased outflow occurred via a mechanical process whereby laser-induced microscars in the trabecular meshwork reversed pathologic laxity and associated collapse of trabecular tissues. Van Buskirk [5] later postulated that ALT eliminates certain relatively unhealthy trabecular endothelial cells. Other, previously dormant, healthy endothelial cells then are stimulated. These cells produce a less outflow-resistant extracellular matrix and are more active from a phagocytic standpoint, thus resulting in a "cleaner" trabecular meshwork more conducive to aqueous outflow. Studies with labelled thymidine support the theory of increased trabecular cell division after ALT [6,7]. Another recent study by Mermoud and coworkers [8] queried as to whether trabecular meshwork–synthesized prostaglandins, stimulated by ALT, might be responsible for some of the effect of lowered IOP.

PATIENT FACTORS INFLUENCING SUCCESS

Generally, ALT results in a short-term (1 year) success rate of approximately 85%. Appropriately chosen eyes average IOP reductions of 6 to 9 mm Hg. Most authorities agree that a 25% to 30% IOP drop is typical in eyes subjected to successful surgery, thus giving greater pressure reductions in eyes with higher preprocedure pressures. However, ALT is not uniformly successful in all patients with open-angle glaucoma. Clearly, some patient groups, *ie*, those patients with quiet eyes and heavily pigmented trabecular meshworks have a better response than do others. In particular, eyes with early pigmentary glaucoma, eyes with pseudoexfoliative glaucoma, and certain eyes with primary open-angle glaucoma (POAG) do well after ALT. In fact, patients in these three groups had the leading success rates after at least 5 years of follow-up (31%, 19%, and 26%, respectively) in a recent report from Germany [9]. Eyes in these patients also are most frequently associated with a lowering of IOP of more than 10 mm Hg after ALT. Points for concern involve several reports on pigmentary glaucoma and one older report regarding pseudoexfoliative glaucoma. Lunde [10] reported worsening of pressure control after ALT in five of 13 eyes with pigmentary glaucoma (although these five eyes generally were in older patients with more advanced glaucoma). Lehto [11] noted a significant diminutive effect on IOP lowering after the first 3 postoperative months (from 53% lower IOP to 14%) in nine eyes with pigmentary glaucoma. Last, a report from Higginbotham and Richardson [12] noted a more rapid, sometimes precipitous failure rate in patients with pseudoexfoliative glaucoma as compared with those with routine POAG.

Another group of patients who may do surprisingly well with ALT are those with eyes with normal- or low-tension glaucoma. Schulzer and the Normal Tension Glaucoma Study Group [4••] anticipated that drug therapy and ALT would generally not achieve adequate pressure lowering in their patients and that filter surgery would soon be required. How-

TABLE 14-1	POSITIVE INDICATIONS FOR ARGON LASER TRABECULOPLASTY
Patient age greater than 40 y	
2–4+ pigmentation of trabecular meshwork	
Phakia	
Absence of ocular inflammation	
Certain diagnoses	
Primary open-angle glaucoma	
Pigmentary (early) glaucoma	
Pseudoexfoliative glaucoma	
Low-tension glaucoma	

ever, of 30 patients with a stable 30% IOP reduction, 57% achieved this lowering with drug treatment or ALT alone (mean follow-up, approximately 1.5 years). In our practice, we now are more prone to try ALT in patients with normal-tension glaucoma (Table 14-1).

Other patient factors influencing ALT success are patient age and, possibly, race. Younger patients (less than 40 years old) frequently do worse with ALT, although some of these patients may have a form of juvenile glaucoma, a diagnosis with a poorer prognosis. As far as race is concerned, Schwartz [13] originally reported a good success rate (97%) in mostly black patients at 18 months follow-up. However, subsequent reports have noted either an insignificant difference in success rates between black and white patients, or even a tendency for treatment in black patients to fail more rapidly than in white patients.

Other negative predictive points for success include certain diagnoses such as uveitis and angle recession. Conditions such as aphakia or pseudophakia and previous failed filter surgery may be associated with

milder (less than 15%), if any, pressure-lowering effects (Table 14-2).

TECHNIQUE

Since Wise and Witter's original description, there has not been a great deal of change in the standard ALT protocol, although research concerning certain treatment variables has been conducted. Most physicians still apply 50-μm spots of 0.1-second duration, with power levels of between 500 mW and 1000 mW (using minimum power to obtain blanching of the trabecular meshwork, with only small bubble formation). Generally, 25 burns per quadrant are applied (Figs. 14-1 and 14-2).

Degree of angle treated

Originally, 360 degrees of the angle was treated with approximately 100 spots in a session. Complications, particularly IOP spikes, led to downward adjustments of the degree of angle treated, ranging from 90 degrees to 180 degrees per session. After Allf and Shields [14] reported that apraclonidine prevented early postoperative IOP elevation after 360-degree ALT, some physicians returned to whole-angle treatment in a single session. There was still debate, however, as to whether 360-degree treatment was any more efficacious than 180-degree treatment. Honrubia and coworkers [15] have recently reported long-term follow-up findings of ALT in eyes with either 180 versus 360 degrees of treatment of the trabecular meshwork. The authors followed 196 eyes, 123 of which received 360-degree ALT treatment and 73 of which received 180-degree treatment. After a mean 5.24 years of follow-up, success

TABLE 14-2	RELATIVE CONTRAINDICATIONS FOR ARGON LASER TRABECULOPLASTY

Patient age less than 35–40 y
Little or no trabecular meshwork pigmentation
Certain diagnoses
  Uveitis
  Angle closure
  Juvenile glaucoma

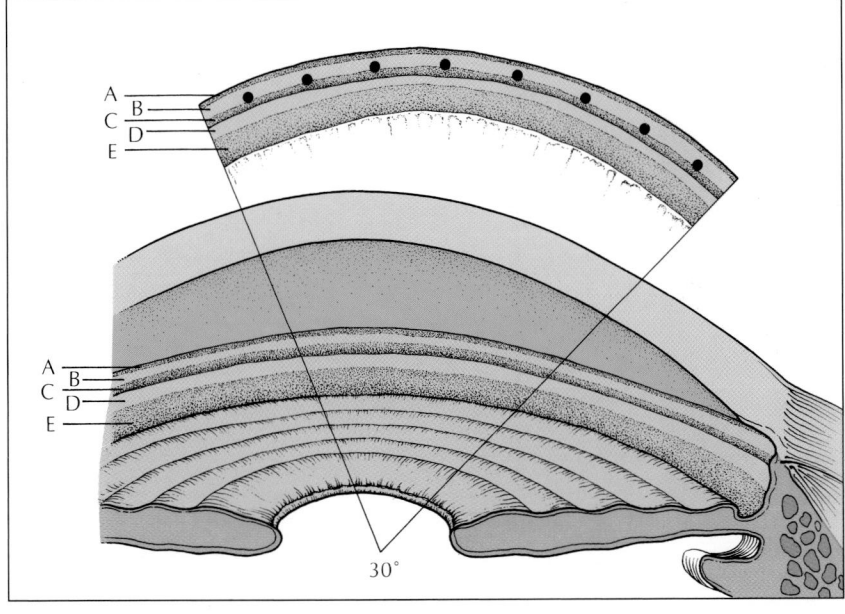

FIGURE 14-1 Gonioscopic view of argon laser trabeculoplasty treatment of the trabecular meshwork. **A**, Schwalbe's line; **B**, Nonpigmented trabecular meshwork; **C**, Pigmented trabecular meshwork; **D**, Scleral spur; **E**, Ciliary body.

was achieved in 58% of the 360-degree–treated eyes versus 38% of the 180-degree–treated eyes (Fig. 14-3). Currently, we treat the entire angle of most eyes in one session and apply apraclonidine after treatment.

Power

As noted, most physicians use power settings in a range between 500 mW and 1000 mW, although there have been successful reports of low-power application (average, 450 mW). Suzuki and coworkers [2] discuss a technique, laser trabeculostimulation, in which they try to avoid cicatrization of trabecular meshwork tissue by using lower-power settings of only 50 mW and exposure times of 1 second. Although they found a drop in IOP after 1 month in 60% of the eyes (n = 40), the long-term overall reduction in IOP with their trabeculostimulation technique was significantly less than with conventional ALT, so we cannot recommend this procedure at this time.

Wavelength

The argon green laser still appears to be the safest and most efficient laser for use in treating ALT. Physician color vision injury may be less likely with argon green than with argon blue-green laser application. The diode laser has received attention as a possible alternative to the argon laser, but there have been no follow-up reports of its use since 1991. The neodymium-yttrium aluminum garnet (Nd:YAG) laser is receiving renewed attention, especially for use in eyes with poorly pigmented angles. Mermoud and coworkers [16•] compared argon laser with Nd:YAG laser treatment in matched eyes of 22 patients. At a 3-month follow-up, there was similar IOP lowering in the two groups (24.5% with Nd:YAG–treated eyes, 32.9% with ALT–treated eyes), although by 6 months there was a tendency for higher IOP in the Nd:YAG–treated group (Fig. 14-4). Interestingly, less inflammation was noted in Nd:YAG–treated eyes.

Repeat treatment

The role of repeat ALT remains at best controversial. Our findings agree with those of Feldman and coworkers [17•]: *ie*, a low success rate (5%) at 4 years, with a significant risk for IOP spike (12%). Therefore, in patients with progressive glaucoma on maximum tolerated drug regimens in whom 360-degree ALT has already been performed, we usually recommend a filter surgery as the next step in management. Of note, Paul and coworkers [18] evaluated diode laser trabeculoplasty in 12 eyes in which ALT had previously failed. The mean duration between the two laser treatments was 46 ± 35 months. A success rate with diode laser treatment of 37% over 4 months was found. Encouragingly, no postoperative pressure spikes occurred. If long-term follow-up proves as favorable, diode laser treatment would be a reasonable option to add to the total treatment protocol.

COMPLICATIONS

As previously noted, IOP spikes are the most serious potential complication after ALT, occurring in approximately 25% of nonpremedicated eyes (Table 14-3). The use of apraclonidine, an α-adrenergic agonist, has dramatically decreased this incidence to less than 3%. Many physicians routinely apply the drug one time before ALT and then immediately after treatment, as described by Robin [19] in 1987. A recent report by Holmwood and coworkers [20•] notes that this dosing

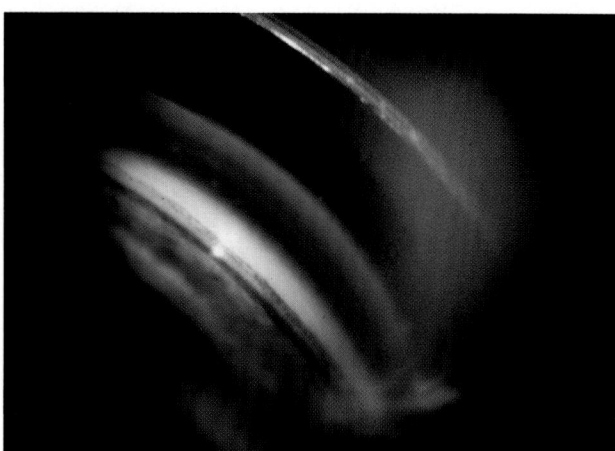

FIGURE 14-2 Application of an argon laser trabeculoplasty spot burn to the anterior pigmented trabecular meshwork.

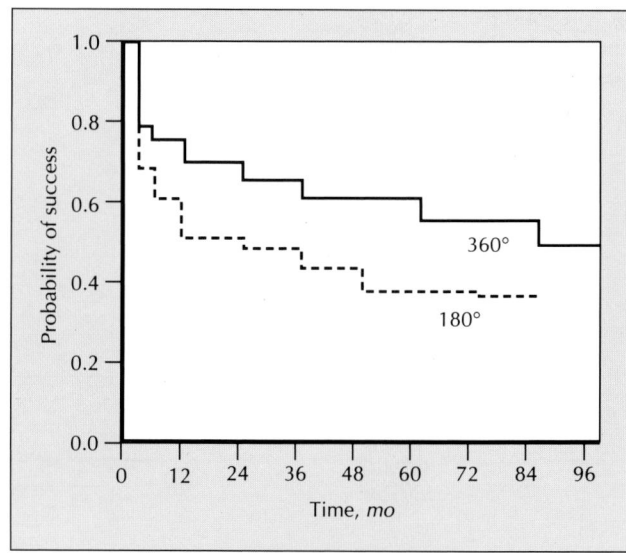

FIGURE 14-3 Survival curves for time to failure after argon laser trabeculoplasty 360 degrees versus 180 degrees of treatment. (*From* Honrubia *et al.* [14]; with permission.)

regimen may not be necessary: they found that, in 60 patients randomly assigned to receive pre- and post-treatment administrations of apraclonidine or to receive post-ALT drug treatment only, there was no significant difference between the two groups in IOP spikes after 360-degree ALT. We have found that because apraclonidine can cause pupillary dilation, which may make ALT slightly more difficult, and rarely, may cause unfortunate systemic side effects such as severe bradycardia, it makes sense based on this study to limit exposure to apraclonidine.

Other less serious complications from ALT include peripheral anterior synechiae (PAS) formation and inflammation. Placing the laser spot on the anterior portion of the pigmented trabecular meshwork has been associated with decreased PAS formation. West [21] noticed a significantly higher incidence of PAS with post-ALT dexamethasone administration compared with fluorometholone or even naphazoline administration (45% vs 22%; n = 109). Thus, it appears reasonable to discontinue routine therapy with dexamethasone after ALT. Perhaps even more interesting is the reported anti-inflammatory effect of diclofenac drops. Herbert and coworkers [22•], in a double-blind placebo-controlled study, used a laser flare-cell meter and found that flare increase after ALT was completely blocked by the topical administration of diclofenac, 0.1%, in 27 eyes. Whether this anti-inflammatory effect can be extrapolated to the formation of PAS remains to be seen. The administration of either fluorometholone or diclofenac for 1 week post-ALT seems appropriate.

LONG-TERM EFFICACY OF ARGON LASER TRABECULOPLASTY

As the results of long-term follow-up studies become increasingly available, it is clear that, in many patients, ALT will only be a temporary solution. Spiegel and coworkers [9] noted a success rate of only 22% in 258 eyes in patients they followed for at least 5 years, defining success as final IOPs of less than 22 mm Hg with stable eye examinations. Filter surgery was required in 13% of eyes. Spaeth and Baez [23•] reported a similar failure rate in 109 eyes in patients they followed for

approximately 5 years; they found a cumulative success rate of only 35%, with subsequent surgery becoming necessary in 32% of eyes within 1 year of performing ALT. Alternatively, as they note, ALT offered 5% of treated patients 10 years of glaucoma control without the need to resort to the expense, risks, and inconvenience of filter surgery. Guzman and coworkers [24] randomly sampled the International Classification of Diseases–9th edition and current procedural terminology codes of 5% of all Medicare beneficiaries to assess how effective ALT was in actually delaying filter surgery. Of those 6954 patients who had undergone ALT in 1986, 1987, and 1988, the cumulative probability of filter surgery at 4 years was only 20%. Certainly, there continues to be a strong role for ALT in future glaucoma management.

CURRENT ROLE OF ARGON LASER TRABECULOPLASTY IN GLAUCOMA MANAGEMENT

Traditionally, at least in the United States where resources are abundant, ALT was believed to be supplemental to maximum medical management. After drug therapy had failed, and before filter surgery, ALT would be performed. The Glaucoma Laser Trial Study reported what on first glance appeared to be favorable data advocating initial ALT over primary medical management. However, concerns with the study have included the relatively short follow-up (2 years) in what is a chronic disease and some incompatibility between the

TABLE 14-3	POTENTIAL COMPLICATIONS AFTER ARGON LASER TRABECULOPLASTY
	IOP elevation (transient)
	Peripheral anterior synechiae
	Iritis or episcleritis
	Hyphema (rare)
	Corneal abrasion (rare)
	IOP—intraocular pressure.

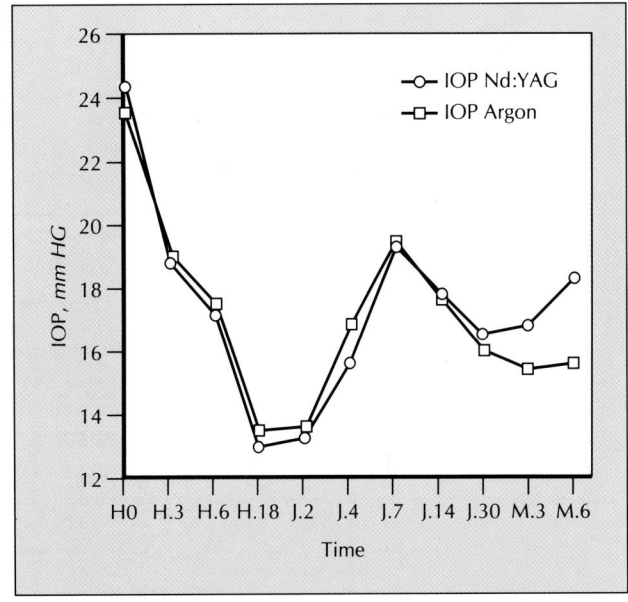

FIGURE 14-4 Intraocular pressure after argon laser trabeculoplasty with either the argon or the neodymium-yttrium aluminum garnet laser over 6 months. H—hour; J—day; M—month. (*From* Mermoud *et al.* [15]; with permission.)

stepped regimens of the two arms of the study. The aforementioned long-term studies raise the question of whether ALT will maintain its advantage over primary medical management after further years of follow-up. Bergea and Svedbergh [25] recently compared primary ALT with pilocarpine administration. This prospective study of 82 eyes with POAG also noted significantly better IOP control in the ALT group (61.5% successful vs 39% in the pilocarpine group), but, again, follow-up was relatively short (2 years). Certainly, long-term studies lasting many years are needed to define better the place of ALT in our treatment protocols. In our practice, patients with POAG, pseudoexfoliative glaucoma, pigmentary glaucoma, low-tension glaucoma, or, occasionally, pseudophakic glaucoma, and with uncontrolled IOPs while receiving some form of topical antiglaucoma therapy, are candidates for 360-degree ALT therapy with post-ALT apraclonidine application and fluoromethalone or diclofenac administration. The performance of ALT before carbonic anhydrase inhibitor administration remains an individual choice. Laser treatment in eyes with high IOP (> 28 mm Hg) and advanced nerve damage is unlikely to provide sufficient control in patients with anticipated long life expectancies, although it may be sufficient in older, unhealthy patients. The only repeat ALTs done in our practice are in patients with inappropriately high IOP who have health factors such that he or she cannot undergo a filter surgery. As future trials unfold, it may become routine to use ALT as an initial procedure in treating newly diagnosed patients with open-angle glaucoma and minimal field loss.

REFERENCES AND RECOMMENDED READING

Recently published papers of particular interest have been highlighted as:
- Of interest
- •• Of outstanding interest

1. Wise JB, Witter SL: Argon laser therapy for open angle glaucoma: a pilot study. *Arch Ophthalmol* 1979, 97:319–322.

2. Suzuki R, Nakayama M, Yoshino H, *et al.*: Laser trabeculostimulation in open-angle glaucoma: a new trial. Part I. *Ophthalmologica* 1992, 205:1–6.

3.•• Beckman H, Meinert CL, Ritch R, *et al.*: The Glaucoma Laser Trial (GLT): results of argon laser trabeculoplasty versus topical medications. *Ophthalmology* 1990, 97:1403–1413.

This study reports the 2-year results of the Glaucoma Laser Trial, in which 271 patients with POAG were prospectively randomized to receive ALT first to one eye, and medical therapy first to the other eye. ALT controlled IOP in 44% of ALT-first eyes, versus 30% of medical therapy-first eyes (timolol only). ALT-first eyes also had a lower mean IOP compared to medical therapy-first eyes.

4.•• Schulzer M, The Normal Tension Glaucoma Study Group: intraocular pressure reduction in normal tension glaucoma patients. *Ophthalmology* 1992, 99:1468–1470.

This report from the Normal Tension Glaucoma Study Group found that 57% (17 of 30) of patients were able to achieve a stable 30% reduction in IOP with topical pilocarpine or ALT (follow-up approaching 1.5 years).

5. Van Buskirk EM: Pathophysiology of laser trabeculoplasty. *Surv Ophthalmol* 1989, 33:264–272.

6. Bylsma SB, Samples JR, Acott TS, *et al.*: Trabecular cell division after argon laser trabeculoplasty. *Arch Ophthalmol* 1988, 106:544–547.

7. Kimpel MW, Johnson DH: Factors influencing in vivo trabecular cell replication as determined by 3H-thymidine labelling: an autoradiographic study in cats. *Curr Eye Res* 1992, 11:297–306.

8. Mermoud A, Pittet N, Herbort CP: Inflammation patterns after laser trabeculoplasty measured with the laser flare meter. *Arch Ophthalmol* 1992, 110:368–370.

9. Spiegel D, Wegscheider E, Lund OE: Argon laser trabeculoplasty: long term follow-up of at least 5 years. *Ger J Ophthalmol* 1992, 1:156–158.

10. Lunde MW: Argon laser trabeculoplasty in pigmentary dispersion syndrome with glaucoma. *Am J Ophthalmol* 1983, 96:721–725.

11. Lehto I: Long term follow-up of argon laser trabeculoplasty in pigmentary glaucoma. *Ophthalmic Surg* 1992, 23:614–617.

12. Higginbotham EJ, Richardson TM: Response of exfoliation glaucoma to laser trabeculoplasty. *Br J Ophthalmol* 1984, 104:52–54.

13. Schwartz AL, Whitten ME, Bleiman B, *et al.*: Argon laser trabeculoplasty in uncontrolled phakic open-angle glaucoma. *Ophthalmology* 1981, 88:202–212.

14. Allf B, Shields MB: Early intraocular pressure response to laser trabeculoplasty 180 degrees without apraclonidine versus 360 degrees with apraclonidine. *Ophthalmic Surg* 1991, 22:539–542.

15. Honrubia FM, Ferrer EJ, Lecinena J, *et al.*: Long term follow-up of the argon laser trabeculoplasty in eyes treated 180 degrees and 360 degrees of the trabeculum. *Int Ophthalmol* 1992, 16:375–379.

16.• Mermoud A, Herbort CP, Schnyder CC, *et al.*: Comparison of argon and Nd-YAG laser trabeculoplasty. *Klin Monatsbl Augenheilkd* 1992, 200:404–406.

This study looks at 22 patients who had ALT (average 1000 mW/shot, 50 shots over 180 degrees) performed in one eye, and Nd:YAG laser trabeculoplasty (average 1 J/shot, 30 shots over

180 degrees) performed in the other eye. There was an average 24.5% reduction in IOP after Nd:YAG laser trabeculoplasty and 32.9% reduction after ALT at 3 months follow-up.

17.• Feldman RM, Katz LJ, Spaeth GL, *et al.*: Long-term efficacy of repeat argon laser trabeculoplasty. *Ophthalmology* 1991, 98:1061–1065.

This study reviewed the effect of repeat 360-degrees ALT in 50 eyes, and found only 35% of eyes to have significant (> 3 mm Hg) IOP reduction with final IOP greater than 22 at 6 months, and only 5% at 4 years. There was also a 12% incidence of IOP elevation after the repeat ALT.

18. Paul AA, Katz LJ, Spaeth GL: Efficacy of diode laser trabeculoplasty in patients previously treated with argon laser trabeculoplasty [Abstract]. *Invest Opthalmol Vis Sci,* 1993, 34(suppl):1069.

19. Robin AL: Argon laser trabeculoplasty medical therapy to prevent the intraocular pressure rise associated with argon laser trabeculoplasty. *Ophthalmic Surg* 1991, 22:31–37.

20.• Holmwood PC, Chase RD, Krupin T, *et al.*: Apraclonidine and argon laser trabeculoplasty. *Am J Ophthalmol* 1992, 114:19–22.

This is a useful study to help dictate apraclonidine prescription with ALT. Thirty eyes received apracionidine, 1%, pre- and post-ALT, and 30 eyes received it only post-ALT. There was no significant difference between the two groups in 1 hour and 2 hour post-ALT IOP.

21. West RH: The effect of topical corticosteroids on laser-induced peripheral anterior synechiae. *Aust NZ J Ophthalmol* 1992, 20:305–309.

22.• Herbort CP, Mermoud A, Schnyder C, *et al.*: Anti-inflammatory effect of diclofenac drops after argon laser trabeculoplasty. *Arch Ophthalmol* 1993, 111:481–483.

This double-blind, placebo-controlled study utilized a laser flare-cell meter to evaluate efficacy of diclofenac, 0.1%, prescription four times a day for 4 days post-ALT. It found complete blockage of flare increase after ALT in the 27 eyes treated with diclofenac.

23.• Spaeth GL, Baez KA: Argon laser trabeculoplasty controls one third of cases of progressive, uncontrolled, open angle glaucoma for 5 years. *Arch Ophthalmol* 1992, 110:491–494.

This report reviewed the effect of ALT over 5 years in 82 eyes with POAG, and noted that after a failure rate in IOP control of 19% in the 1st year, approximately 10% of eyes failed per year, for a final failure rate of 65% after 5 years. Filtration surgery was deferrable in one third of patients for 5 years after ALT.

24. Guzman GI, Javitt JC, Parrish RK, *et al.*: Longevity of argon laser trabeculoplasty: time to trabeculectomy [Abstract]. *Invest Ophthalmol Vis Sci* 1993, 34:897.

25. Bergea B, Svedbergh B: Primary argon laser trabeculoplasty vs. pilocarpine, short-term effects. *Acta Ophthalmol Copenh* 1992, 70:454–460.

SELECT BIBLIOGRAPHY

Coakes R: Laser trabeculoplasty. *Br J Ophthalmol* 1992, 76:624–626.

Migdal C: Rational choice of therapy in established open angle glaucoma. *Eye* 1992, 6:346–347.

Reiss GR, Wilensky JT, Higginbotham EJ: Laser trabeculoplasty. *Surv Ophthalmol* 1991, 35:407–428.

CHAPTER *15*

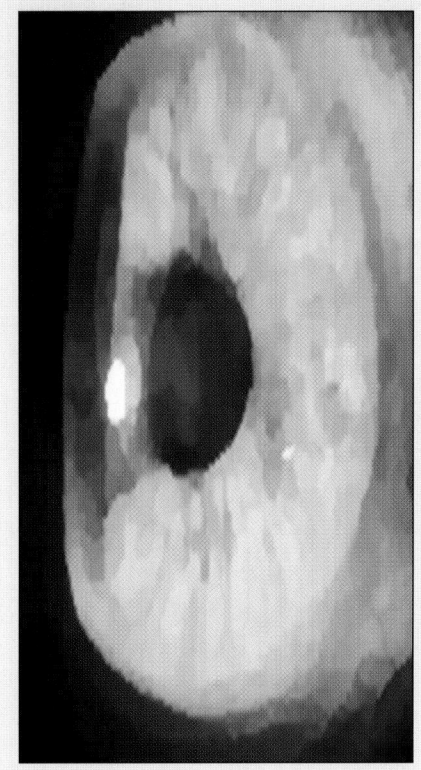

LASER IRIDOTOMY AND PERIPHERAL IRIDOPLASTY

SETH D. POTASH

JEFFREY LIEBMANN

ROBERT RITCH

This review covers recent studies regarding the indications for, and techniques and complications of, laser iridotomy and argon laser peripheral iridoplasty (ALPI). Results from the use of the semiconductor diode laser and the neodymium-yttrium lithium fluoride (Nd:YLF) picosecond laser to perform laser iridotomy are reviewed. ALPI has been proven effective in treating angle-closure glaucoma because of mechanisms other than pupillary block, *ie*, plateau iris syndrome and phacomorphic glaucoma. We review our techniques for performing peripheral laser iridoplasty and document the effectiveness of this procedure *in vivo* with the high-resolution ultrasound biomicroscope. The iris concavity associated with the pigment dispersion syndrome flattens after laser iridotomy, suggesting that a reverse pupillary block mechanism underlies the pathophysiology of this disorder.

LASER IRIDOTOMY

Clinical applications

Laser iridotomy is the procedure of choice for all forms of angle-closure glaucoma in which there is a component of pupillary block. It is also recommended as prophylactic treatment for occludable angles. The efficacy of both the argon and neodymium-yttrium aluminum garnet (Nd:YAG) lasers is well accepted, and attention is now being focused on newer lasers, such as the semiconductor diode laser and the Nd:YLF laser for performing this procedure.

Indications

Angle-closure glaucoma secondary to pupillary block

Laser iridotomy is indicated in the treatment of acute and chronic angle-closure glaucoma, combined-mech-

anism glaucoma, pseudophakic and aphakic pupillary block, nanophthalmos, and as a procedure to follow partial-thickness surgical iridectomy. The Select Bibliography at the end of this chapter provides further materials for an in-depth discussion on these topics.

Prophylactic laser iridotomy

Schwartz and coworkers [1] retrospectively reviewed case records of 114 eyes in 70 patients to assess the long-term outcome of surgical and medical treatment of narrow angles. Comparisons were made between 50 eyes treated with laser iridotomy or surgical iridectomy and 64 eyes treated medically. Eyes subjected to laser iridotomy or surgical iridectomy showed a greater number of improved anterior-chamber configurations (74% vs 28%), had a lower incidence of peripheral anterior synechiae (PAS) (2% vs 10%), and required fewer glaucoma medications. The percentage of eyes with increased intraocular pressure (IOP), abnormal visual field, and decreased visual acuity were similar in the two groups.

Creeping angle closure

Creeping angle closure occurs when PAS develop evenly over 360 degrees and occurs typically in dark brown irides. The angle progressively narrows and the iris appears to develop a more anterior insertion as PAS gradually creep up the ciliary face to the scleral spur and then to the trabecular meshwork. West [2] treated 30 eyes of 16 patients with this condition with either Nd:YAG laser iridotomy or surgical iridectomy. He reported deepening of the anterior chamber in 15 eyes, with a mean increase in depth of 0.05 mm. Deepening of the anterior chamber in these eyes may not represent an improvement of the underlying condition because the change in anterior-chamber depth may be related to a component of pupillary

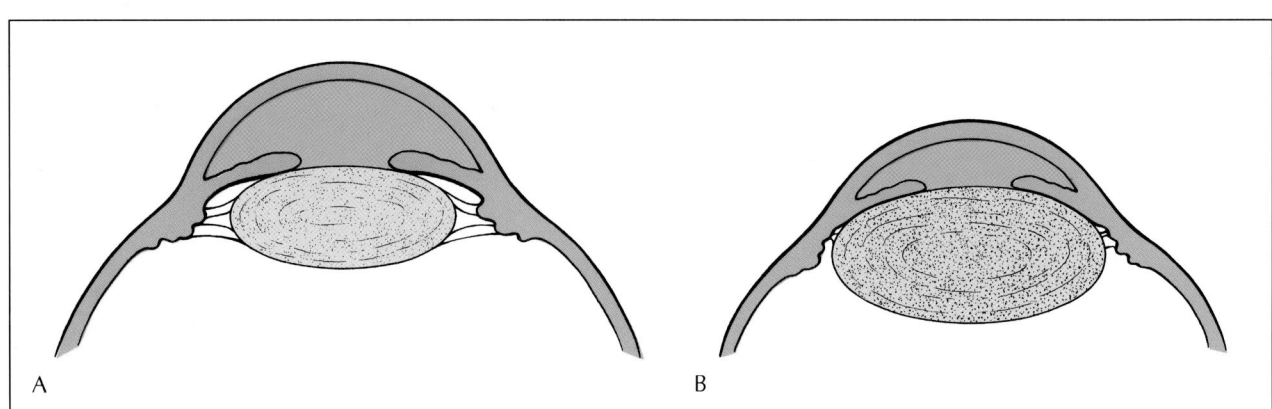

FIGURE 15-1 A, Early phacomorphic glaucoma where pupillary block is primarily responsible for angle closure. Laser iridotomy can be used successfully in this situation because the lens periphery is still away from the iris. **B,** Advanced phaco-morphic glaucoma. Iridotomy is of no benefit in this situation because there is forward displacement of the iris periphery by the intumescent lens. (*From* Tomey and Al-Rajhi [3••]; with permission).

block. A combination of laser iridotomy with laser iridoplasty may be a more effective treatment for creeping angle closure.

Phacomorphic glaucoma

Phacomorphic glaucoma can cause angle closure by a combination of both pupillary block and direct displacement of the peripheral iris by the intumescent lens (Fig. 15-1). Tomey and Al-Rajhi [3••] reviewed the charts of 10 patients who were treated for phacomorphic glaucoma by Nd:YAG laser iridotomy. In some cases, iridotomy in eyes with acute angle-closure glaucoma enabled the eye to become less inflamed before cataract extraction. In others, the fellow eye presented up to years later with a patent iridotomy and a mature cataract, but without acute angle closure. The authors considered that prophylactic iridotomy prevented acute angle closure so that uneventful cataract surgery could be performed. Other benefits of iridotomy in phacomorphic glaucoma include the ability to allow time for corneal edema to resolve, allow safer preoperative mydriasis unless the condition is far advanced, and permit better assessment of IOP control and the extent of PAS so that a decision can be made regarding the possible need for a trabeculectomy at the time of cataract surgery.

The authors point out, however, that if the lens is swollen to the point where the peripheral iris is displaced forward, mechanically closing the angle, laser iridotomy will not prevent the development of glaucoma. In these situations, it has been our experience that ALPI can often open the angle. By using a combination of laser iridotomy to eliminate any element of pupillary block, and iridoplasty, to physically contract the iris stroma at the site of apposition to the trabecular meshwork, we have been able to postpone surgery until the eye is quiet in virtually all patients with acute angle closure caused by phacomorphic

glaucoma and avoid repeat angle closure at the time of dilation before cataract extraction.

Pigment dispersion syndrome and pigmentary glaucoma

Pigment dispersion syndrome results from mechanical rubbing between the concave surface of the iris pigment epithelium and the anterior zonular packets, thereby liberating pigment throughout the anterior segment. Elevated IOP and glaucomatous damage may ensue. For many years, the cause of the iris concavity was not known. Campbell initially proposed that laser iridotomy may reverse the iris concavity by allowing equilibration of the IOP between the anterior and posterior chambers (Fig. 15-2) (Paper presented at The American Glaucoma Society meeting, San Diego, 1991). Karickhoff [4••] reported that the iris concavity present in this disease is consistent with a reverse pupillary block mechanism in which the iris acts as a "flap-valve," draping over the anterior lens capsule and allowing the pressure in the anterior chamber to exceed that of the posterior chamber. He reported on six cases of pigmentary glaucoma treated with laser iridotomy. In all cases, laser iridotomy caused the iris to move forward to assume a planar configuration, thus relieving the iris concavity. Campbell then reported results of a 1.5-year follow-up of 10 eyes with pigment dispersion syndrome treated with laser iridotomy (Paper presented at the Annual Meeting of the Association for Research in Vision and Ophthalmology, Sarasota, FL, 1993). Immediately after treatment he noted resolution of the iris concavity, and, in all cases, the irides have remained flattened and the disease progression has either halted or begun reversal as determined by stabilization of optic nerve and visual field damage and a decrease in pigmentation of the trabecular meshwork.

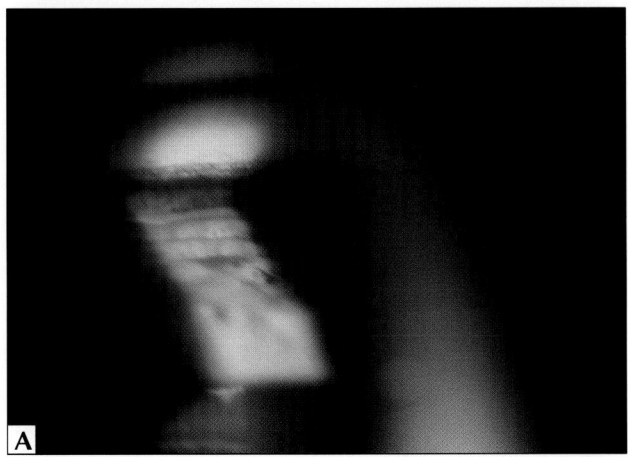 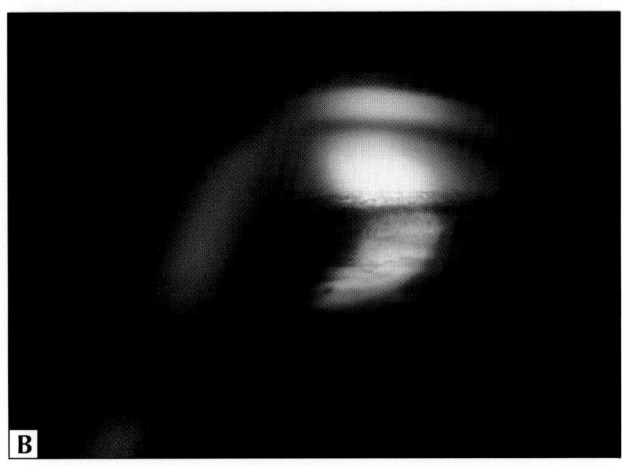

FIGURE 15-2 A, Gonioscopic photograph of an eye with pigment dispersion syndrome before argon laser iridotomy. Note the midperipheral iris concavity. **B,** After laser iridotomy, resolution of an iris concavity is noted.

Fourman [5] has challenged the theory of reverse pupillary block, suggesting that laser iridotomy causes rupture of a membranous zonular matrix, which he postulates causes a relative block in fluid flow across the zonules and results in forward movement of the zonules and contact with the iris pigment epithelium. With the aid of the high-resolution ultrasound biomicroscope, Pavlin imaged *in vivo* a definite iris concavity and its resolution after laser iridotomy, giving further support for a reverse pupillary block mechanism [6••].

Potash and coworkers [7••] examined patients with the pigment dispersion syndrome with the ultrasound biomicroscope. A documented iris concavity was seen in nine of 16 eyes. Reversal of iris concavity was documented in all four eyes treated with laser iridotomy (Fig. 15-3). One eye had a return of the iris concavity after pigment occlusion of the iridotomy. The concavity resolved again after the iridotomy was reopened. Ultrasound biomicroscopic imaging also showed iridociliary process contact, which may prove to be an additional mechanism for pigment release in patients with this disease. This contact is not always relieved by laser iridotomy and may be a reason for persistence of pigment release in some patients despite iridotomy.

Technique

Neodymium-yttrium aluminum garnet laser

The Nd:YAG laser has become the most commonly used laser for performing iridotomy. Ye and coworkers [8] reported a success rate of iris penetration of approximately 97.6% when using the Nd:YAG laser in 80 eyes with primary angle-closure glaucoma. There was a high variability of laser energy (0.9–5.6 mJ) and total number of applications (1–127 applications), which was attributed to differences in iris thickness. The most frequent complication was mild iris bleeding in 39% of treated eyes, which resolved spontaneously. Transient IOP elevations did not correlate with the number of shots or total energy.

In a separate report on the efficacy of the first Nd:YAG laser made in China, a success rate of iris penetration of 100% in 276 eyes treated for primary angle-closure glaucoma was achieved [9].

Sequential argon laser and neodymium-yttrium aluminum garnet laser iridotomy

The large variability of iris thickness and color must always be kept in mind when performing laser iridotomy. Thicker and darker irides are more difficult to penetrate and are associated with higher complication rates. Ho and Fan [10•] performed a prospective clinical study to evaluate the use of the argon and Nd:YAG laser in sequential combination for performing iridotomy on 20 eyes of 13 patients with dark brown irides. Patent iridotomies were achieved in all 20 eyes in one treatment session and only one iridotomy closed during a mean follow-up period of 14 months. The mean total energy delivered per eye by the argon and Nd:YAG lasers was 3.6 J and 9.4 mJ, respectively. The total mean energy used was approximately one third of most studies on pure argon and Nd:YAG iridotomies, suggesting a possible reduction of adverse collateral damage when using the sequential technique [11,12]. The authors noted large, round iridotomies with sharp margins, compared with the slit openings achieved with the Nd:YAG laser alone.

We are able to achieve penetration even through the darkest irides in one session using the argon laser alone. We use a linear incision technique with a spot size of 50 μm, a duration of 0.01 to 0.02 second, and a power of 600 to 1200 mW. The linear incision tech-

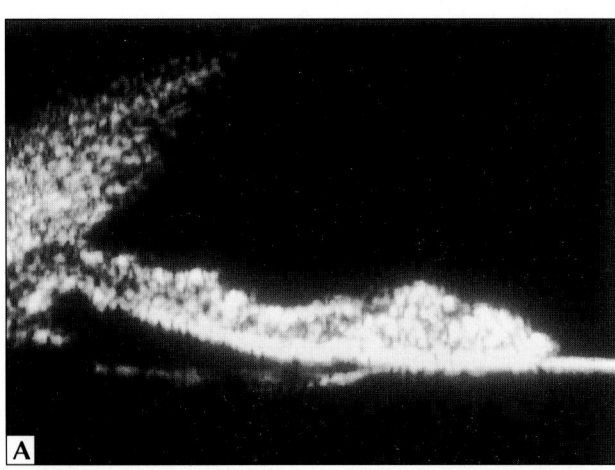
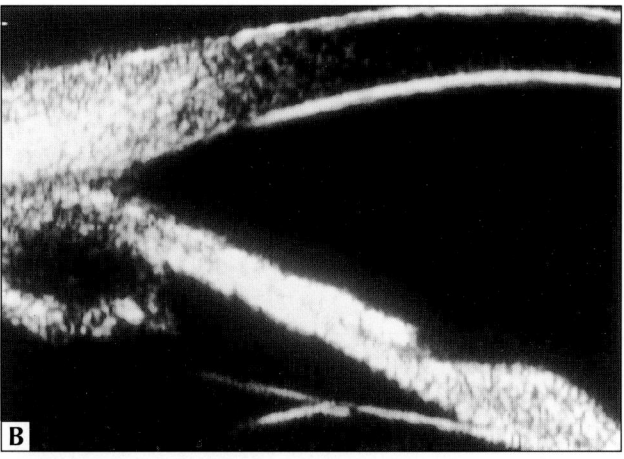

FIGURE 15-3 **A,** High-resolution ultrasound biomicrograph from a patient with the pigment dispersion syndrome. Note the marked iris concavity and presence of iridozonular contact. **B,** Same eye after laser iridotomy. The iris has assumed a planar configuration and iridozonular contact has resolved. The success of laser iridotomy in reversing the iris concavity supports a reverse pupillary block mechanism.

nique allows the dilator muscle to assist in enlarging the opening. Although our technique often requires a higher total energy than that used by Ho and Fan, we have not seen any adverse complications. The short duration of each application results in a decreased incidence of iris charring, which is more common in dark irides. We prefer the argon laser because of efficient energy absorption, lower incidence of iris bleeding, and less pigment dispersion.

Neodymium-yttrium lithium fluoride picosecond laser

The Nd:YLF picosecond laser with a 1053-nm wavelength incises tissue rather than cutting it with photodisruption. Various linear and circular patterns and depth of tissue penetration can be programmed into the computer. Frangie and coworkers [13•] successfully performed Nd:YLF iridotomies in three eyes with a pulse setting of 200 µJ, a delivery of 1000 pulses per second, and a maximum of 5 seconds of laser time (Fig. 15-4). Although the total amount of energy required was greater than that usually used with the neodymium-yttrium aluminum garnet laser, each laser pulse uses a much smaller quantity of energy, providing for a more refined optical breakdown. Because of this feature, the risk for collateral damage with the Nd:YLF picosecond laser may be less than that with the Nd:YAG laser.

Diode laser

With the aid of a semiconductor diode laser, Emoto and coworkers [14•] created iridotomies in 20 rabbit eyes and 40 human eyes. A two-stage method involving stretch burns and penetrating burns was used and complete iris perforation was obtained in all eyes in one session (Fig. 15-5). All human eyes had brown irides. Laser settings for penetrating burns were 75-µm spot size, 0.05-second duration, and 1000-mW power. All iridotomies remained patent at 7 to 9 months of follow-up. Transient complications in the humans included an IOP elevation of more than 10 mm Hg in 20% of eyes, focal corneal endothelial opacification in 5% of eyes, focal lens opacification in 5% of eyes, pupillary distortion in 70% of eyes, and transient lens clouding in 60% of eyes. The compact size, portability, simple construction, and potential low cost of the diode laser make its use an attractive alternative.

Histopathologic findings of neodymium-yttrium aluminum garnet iridotomy

Tetsumoto and coworkers [15] studied iridectomy specimens obtained at the time of cataract extraction from three patients who had undergone previous Nd:YAG laser iridotomies 3 to 5 years earlier for appositional angle closure. The specimens were examined by both light and transmission electron microscopy. In all cases, there was no evidence of fibrinous aggregates, inflammatory response, scarring, or pigment epithelial proliferation. The authors interpreted these findings to indicate a lack of tendency toward late closure of Nd:YAG laser iridotomies in humans.

Complications

Although laser iridotomy is generally a safe procedure to perform, complications do occur. Previously documented complications include peaking of the pupil toward the site of the iridotomy, transient anterior uveitis, formation of posterior synechiae, hemorrhage from iris vessels after Nd:YAG iridotomy, lens opacities, post-laser IOP elevation, closure of the iridotomy, and retinal damage. This past year, some further complications were reported.

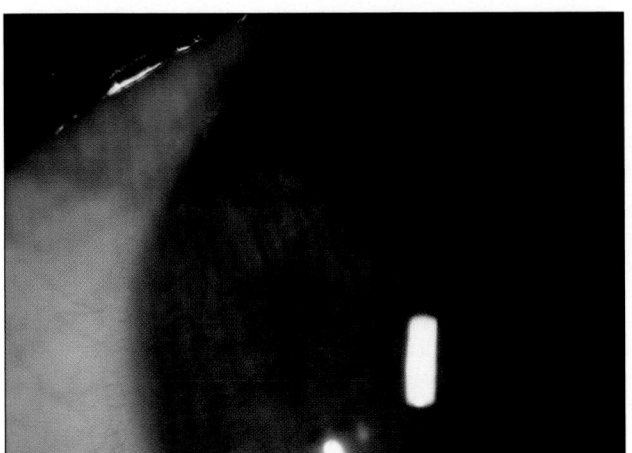

FIGURE 15-4 Clinical photograph of a peripheral iridotomy generated by the neodymium-yttrium lithium fluoride picosecond laser using a 2-mm–long line pattern. (*From* Frangie *et al.* [13•]; with permission).

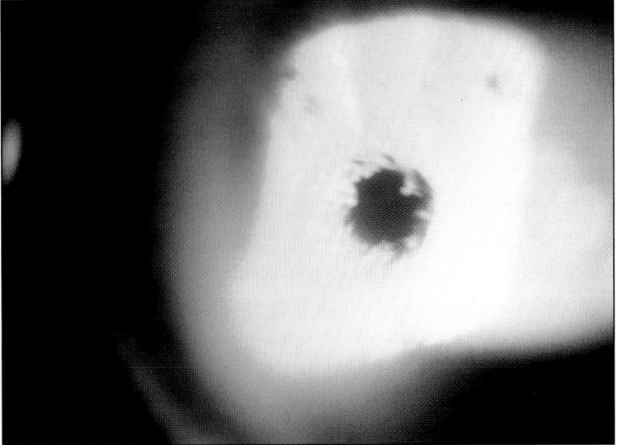

FIGURE 15-5 Diode laser iridotomy in a patient with angle-closure glaucoma. (*From* Emoto *et al.* [14•]; with permission).

Monocular blurring and glare

Causes of transient blurring after laser iridotomy include anterior segment inflammation, pigment dispersion, retinal pigment bleaching, and keratopathy from methylcellulose.

After the procedure, some of our patients have complained of seeing a glaring, horizontal line of light, especially when driving in bright sunlight. Murphy and Trope [16] reported a similar phenomenon in patients after Nd:YAG laser iridotomy when the upper lid only partially covered the iridotomy site. They attributed this phenomenon to possible spherical and chromatic aberration plus the diffractive interaction of the eyelid or lashes with the iridotomy. Weintraub and Berke [17] noted that this phenomenon occurred despite complete coverage of the iridotomy by the upper lid. Their patients' symptoms disappeared when the lid was either raised or lowered sufficiently, and they postulated a base-up prism effect of the tear meniscus formed by the edge of the upper lid, thus causing an upward bending of the light rays and resulting in the perceived extra image being displaced downward. They confirmed their hypothesis by bringing the lid forward away from the globe, dissipating the tear meniscus, with resolution of the symptoms. They suggest placement of the iridotomy in the horizontal meridian to avoid the tear meniscus as a possible solution to the glaring light phenomenon. Another recent report suggested the use of a toric contact lens with an opaque portion to cover the iridotomy as a possible solution for patients with this problem [18].

Corneal endothelial cell damage

Focal damage to the corneal endothelium or Descemet's membrane after laser iridotomy is not infrequently seen, but is usually transient. A small but statistically significant decrease of endothelial cell density has been previously reported in the area of cornea overlying the site of the iridotomy with the use of specular microscopy [19]. Power and Collum [20•] studied the scanning electron microscopic appearance of the corneal endothelium after Nd:YAG laser iridotomy in an enucleated globe from a patient with a uveal melanoma and shallow anterior chamber. A 500-μm-diameter area of denuded endothelial cells was produced when no contact lens was used for the laser procedure. The area of cell loss was reduced by nearly 50% when an Abraham-yttrium aluminum garnet goniolens was used. The authors concluded that the convex-plus lens can help minimize cell loss after Nd:YAG laser iridotomy.

Wilhelmus [21•] reported five patients with shallow anterior chambers and bilateral cornea guttata who developed unilateral progressive corneal edema and visual loss after argon laser iridotomy. Although a direct correlation between total laser energy and the onset of corneal edema was not seen in all patients, the patient who received the most energy for iris penetration (63 J) experienced an immediate decline in vision that never recovered. All five patients eventually underwent penetrating keratoplasty, and histopathologic study revealed generalized endothelial cell loss in all five, as well as thickening of Descemet's membrane and guttata, suggesting that a prior endothelial dystrophy predisposed these patients to corneal decompensation after laser iridotomy. Risk factors cited for intractable corneal edema after laser iridotomy include preexisting guttata, previous angle closure, and high laser energy with multiple applications. Whether the laser energy directly injures the corneal endothelium or the endothelium is secondarily damaged by pigment debris or a thermal increase in the aqueous humor has yet to be determined. Although we have not observed corneal decompensation following laser iridotomy, we have seen one patient with preexisting Fuch's endothelial dystrophy who developed bullous keratopathy after ALPI.

Lens-induced endophthalmitis

Margo and coworkers [22•] reported findings from a patient who developed severe lens-induced endophthalmitis after Nd:YAG laser iridotomy. The patient had been blind for 15 years secondary to chronic angle-closure glaucoma and subsequently developed progressive iris bombé as a result of an advancing cataract, with an elevation of IOP of up to 48 mm Hg. The pressure could not be controlled medically but responded well to laser iridotomy. A fibrinous iritis developed after the laser treatment that worsened despite an hourly administration of topical corticosteroid drops. A hypopyon subsequently developed and the eye became inflamed and painful. After enucleation, histopathologic study revealed several large tears in the anterior lens capsule associated with granulomatous inflammation surrounding exposed lens fibers, dislocation of the lens nucleus inferiorly, and inflammation involving the anterior chamber, uveal tract, peripheral retina, and anterior vitreous.

Aqueous misdirection

Until recently, it was believed that laser iridotomy could eliminate the risk for subsequent aqueous misdirection in eyes with angle-closure glaucoma by avoiding surgical incision of the eye. Cashwell and Martin [23••] reported six cases of aqueous misdirection after laser iridotomy in the absence of incisional surgery. The clinical appearance of a shallow anterior chamber in all six patients and the development of elevated IOP in five patients occurred up to years after iridotomy. The authors ruled out choroidal detachment, nanophthalmos, and plateau iris syndrome as the cause of anterior chamber shallowing in all patients. All six patients had been exposed to miotic agents in the perilaser period; however, in two patients, miotic therapy was discontinued 1 week and 8 months before aqueous misdirection was diagnosed. Four of the patients responded to mydriatic agents with deepening of the anterior chamber and improvement in IOP. Aqueous misdirection recurred in five of the six patients: one following discontinuation of atropine therapy because of an allergy, two following trabeculectomy, one during trabeculectomy, and one after uncomplicated extracapsular cataract extraction with a posterior chamber implant. The authors believed that these patients may have had primary aqueous misdirection that became manifest after miotic therapy or laser surgery.

In response to Cashwell and Martin's findings, Hodes [24] and Fourman [25] pointed out that, given the use of miotic agents in these patients, a causal relationship linking laser iridotomy to the development of aqueous misdirection could not be ascertained. In addition to miotic therapy, other possible contributory factors to the development of a shallow anterior chamber and elevated IOP in these patients included intraocular inflammation, ciliary body spasm, and possible occlusion of the iridotomy by vitreous.

In another case report, a 50-year-old woman developed bilateral aqueous misdirection 4 weeks after successful bilateral laser iridotomies for angle-closure glaucoma [26•]. The condition was worsened by pilocarpine treatment but resolved after the administration of atropine and cyclopentolate, with deepening of the anterior chamber and improvement of IOP. The authors suggested that systemic hydrochlorothiazide therapy may have caused ciliary body swelling in this patient that precipitated ciliolenticular block and aqueous misdirection. This patient was also treated with miotic agents in the perilaser period, which may have also contributed to the development of aqueous misdirection.

Acute post-laser rise of intraocular pressure
The usefulness of topical apraclonidine, 1%, for preventing a post-laser IOP rise after iridotomy has been previously reviewed [27]. Hsieh [28] studied the effect of a combination of timolol maleate, 0.5%, and acetazolamide, 125 mg orally, on IOP elevation after argon laser iridotomy. Treatment was given to 39 patients 1 hour before laser iridotomy. Comparison was made with 29 patients who received no pretreatment. IOP elevation 2 hours after laser iridotomy was significantly less in the timolol-acetazolamide treatment group, with only two of 39 eyes (5%) showing an elevation from the pre-laser baseline IOP. Sixteen of 29 eyes (55%) in the control group had an elevation in IOP.

Effect of pupil dilatation on iridotomy area
Functional failure of both argon and Nd:YAG laser iridotomies may occur. In this situation, the iridotomy is patent, but small and acute angle-closure glaucoma may develop. A large iridotomy should theoretically circumvent this potential problem, and Fleck [29] has previously suggested that the iridotomy should not be less than 200 μm in diameter and 0.31 mm^2 in area. In a follow-up study, this group performed photometric analysis of the effect of pupillary dilation on Nd:YAG laser iridotomy in 21 eyes of 21 patients [30•]. Iridotomy area after dilation correlated with that before dilation but did not significantly correlate with measures of the shape or position of the iridotomies. Two iridotomies became reduced to less than 20% of their initial area, but no data were presented pertaining to a change in IOP or the development of angle closure. Because both of these eyes had a small initial iridotomy area compared with the other eyes, the authors concluded that the only effective method of avoiding an unacceptably small iridotomy after pupil dilatation is to create a sufficiently large iridotomy at the time of initial laser treatment.

PERIPHERAL IRIDOPLASTY

Clinical applications
When laser iridotomy cannot be safely or effectively performed, or does not eliminate appositional angle closure, ALPI can be effective in opening a closed angle [31••]. The technique consists of placing a circumferential ring of contraction burns in the extreme iris periphery to contract the iris stroma between the site of the burn and the angle, thereby widening the angle (Fig. 15-6) [32].

Indications
Angle-closure glaucoma
Argon laser peripheral iridoplasty is usually effective in breaking an attack of angle-closure glaucoma that is unresponsive to drug therapy or in which laser iridotomy is ineffective or cannot be performed because of corneal edema, anterior segment inflammation, or a shallow anterior chamber.

Weiss and coworkers [33••] successfully treated 20 of 32 eyes with ALPI in patients in whom angle-closure glaucoma was not relieved by laser iridotomy. The median duration of angle closure was 12 days in the 20 eyes treated successfully, compared with a median duration of 90 days in the 12 eyes that did not respond well. After a median follow-up period of 18 months, 19 of the 20 successfully treated eyes maintained an IOP of 21 mm Hg or less. In the treated patients, no eye had a diagnosis of plateau iris configuration, and the majority of patients had either pseudophakic pupillary block or primary angle-closure glaucoma. It was not specified whether or not these patients received miotic therapy before ALPI to see how this therapy may have affected the angle; others have noted a permanent lowering of IOP after the temporary use of miotics in cases of persistent angle closure after laser iridotomy [34].

We have found that patients with acute angle-closure glaucoma who respond poorly to drug therapy usually have a component of lens-induced or phacomorphic angle closure, which is made worse by the effect of miotics. In these cases, anterior-chamber shallowing and an increase in axial lens thickness overcome any tendency to open the angle by constricting the pupil. Frequent administration of pilocarpine causes further narrowing of the angle because of an increase in

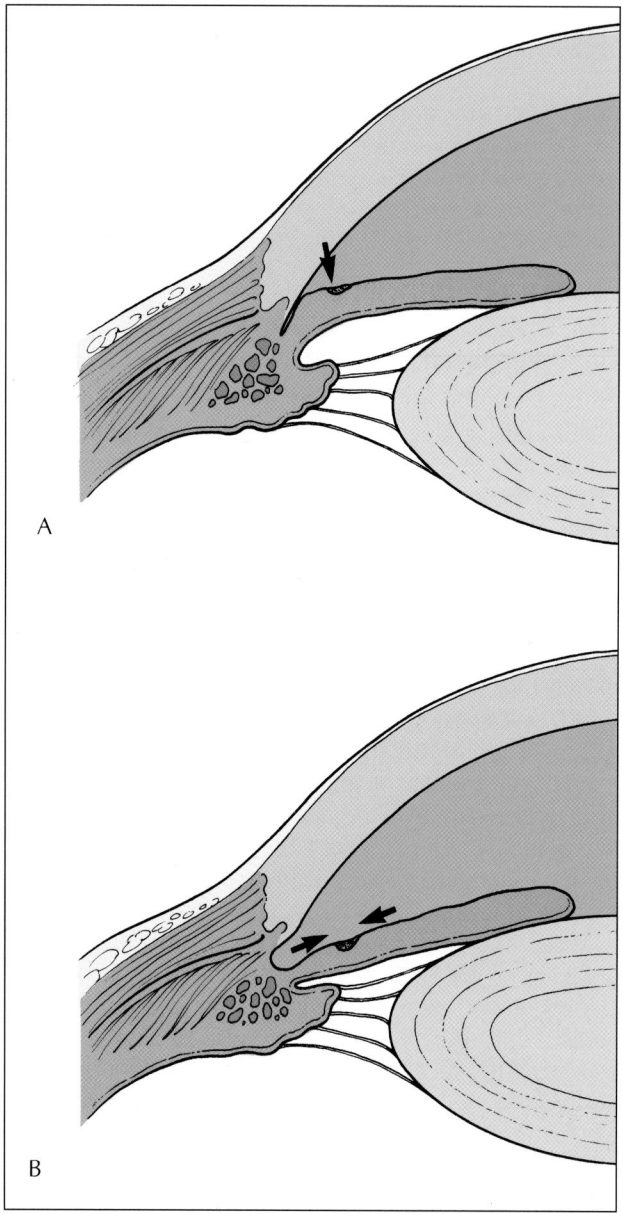

FIGURE 15-6 A, Iridoplasty contraction burns (*arrow*) placed on peripheral iris. **B**, Resulting contraction of peripheral iris stroma, opening the angle and relieving apposition of iris to trabecular meshwork. (*From* Ritch *et al.* [32]; with permission).

relative pupillary block or forward movement of the lens-iris diaphragm. It has been our practice to treat acute angle-closure glaucoma initially with aqueous suppressants and hyperosmotic agents. Once the pressure is lowered, a drop of pilocarpine, 2%, can be administered. If the angle appears more open after the pilocarpine treatment, we will often treat the patient medically until the cornea clears and laser iridotomy can be performed. If the angle closes further or the IOP increases after pilocarpine therapy, we prefer to treat with ALPI at that point to open the angle. Because ALPI does not relieve any associated component of pupillary block, the performance of laser iridotomy is essential once the cornea clears.

Agarwal and coworkers [35] performed ALPI as primary therapy in 40 eyes of 33 patients with angle-closure glaucoma. Ten treated eyes had subacute angle closure and 30 had chronic angle closure. After iridoplasty, IOPs of 22 mm Hg or less were achieved in all eyes with subacute angle closure and in 70% of eyes with chronic angle closure. Their success rate with iridoplasty was directly related to the presence of PAS, optic disc cupping, and preexisting visual field damage.

Wand [36•] treated six eyes of five patients with synechial angle closure of long duration with laser iridoplasty. A goniolens was used to visualize the PAS directly. In each case, 60% to 100% of the synechial closure was anatomically opened and there was a mean decrease in IOP of 5.5 mm Hg. We have not been successful at breaking PAS with this procedure.

Adjunct to laser trabeculoplasty

Argon laser peripheral iridoplasty can be used to widen a narrow angle to allow adequate visibility for spot placement for laser trabeculoplasty. Focal contraction burns may be used when iris irregularities or intraepithelial cysts obstruct the view of the trabecular meshwork [37]. We have also found focal burns useful in cases in which the iris stroma obstructs the internal ostium after trabeculectomy or ab interno sclerostomy. These burns must be applied relatively early in the postoperative course before the formation of permanent synechiae.

Kurdagli and coworkers [38] used a combination of argon laser trabeculoplasty (ALT) alone or combined with ALPI to treat 18 eyes in which trabeculectomy had failed as a result of a blockage of the internal ostium by the iris root 2 weeks to 5 years after surgery. Normalization of IOP was seen in 13 eyes after laser treatment; however, it was not specified how many of the successfully treated eyes received iridoplasty. The authors concluded that ALT alone or in combination with ALPI is an effective treatment that can avoid the risks involved with repeat filtering surgery.

Lens-related angle-closure glaucoma

Angle-closure glaucoma caused by lens intumescence or forward lens movement is often not successfully eliminated after laser iridotomy because pupillary block is not the key mechanism involved. Residual appositional closure after laser iridotomy can often be relieved with peripheral iridoplasty. Following this procedure, the judicious use of cycloplegic agents may help ascertain the mechanism of angle closure.

Plateau iris syndrome

Plateau iris is an anatomic variant of iris structure in which the iris root angulates sharply forward from its insertion point and then again angulates sharply centrally, giving the surface of the iris a normal, flat appearance. Many patients with the plateau iris syndrome are at risk for the development of angle closure despite a patent laser iridotomy. Pupillary dilation may trigger such an attack. Recently, it was demonstrated that large or anteriorly positioned ciliary processes are responsible for the plateau iris syndrome. With the aid of indentation gonioscopy after iridotomy, Ritch [39•] observed a different pattern of iris contour from that found in eyes with primary angle closure on the basis of relative pupillary block and believed this was consistent with anteriorly positioned ciliary processes. The

high-resolution ultrasound biomicroscope confirmed this mechanism and provided images of the iris after ALPI showing that these contraction burns are successful anatomically (Fig. 15-7) [40••].

Nanophthalmos

Patients with nanophthalmos are predisposed to angle-closure glaucoma as a result of anterior-chamber crowding and may demonstrate persistent appositional closure after laser iridotomy that can be relieved by ALPI. No recent studies reporting the efficacy of ALPI in nanophthalmos have been published.

Techniques

Beginning approximately 45 minutes before treatment, pilocarpine, 2%, and apraclonidine, 1%, are applied topically to stretch the iris and prevent a post-laser IOP spike, respectively. Topical anesthesia is administered and an Abraham lens is used. We prefer a spot size of 500 μm, a duration of 0.5 second, and a low power setting of 200 to 400 mW, depending on iris color. These laser parameters allow condensation and compaction of the iris stroma but do not cause tissue vaporization or disruption. The spots are aimed through the periphery of the lens and 20 to 30 spots are placed at 360 degrees, thus leaving two spot-diameters between each

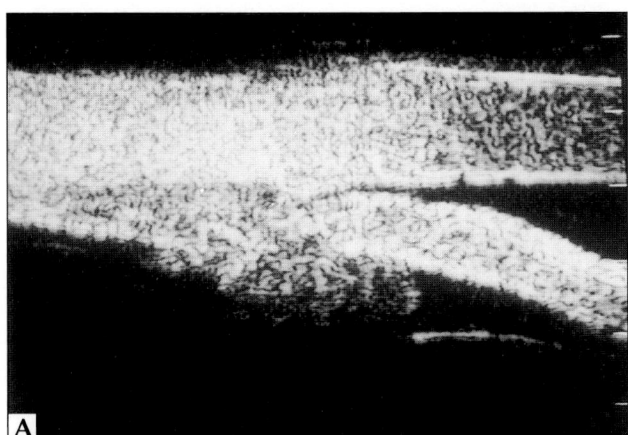

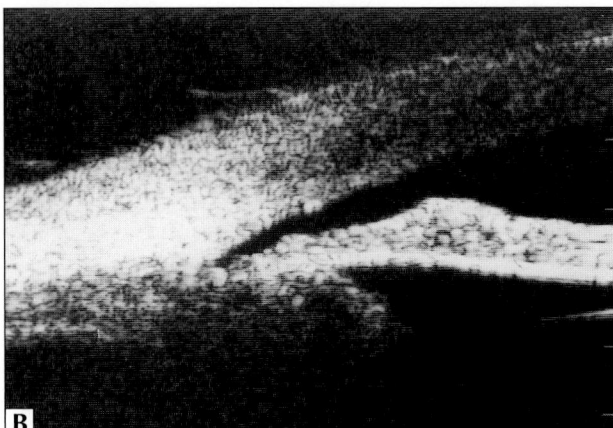

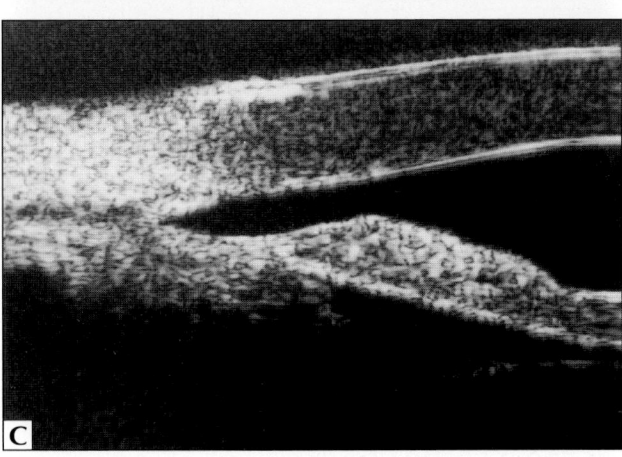

FIGURE 15-7 A, Ultrasound biomicroscopic image of a typical angle cross-section in an eye with the plateau iris syndrome. Ciliary process is positioned forward and appositional closure is present. **B,** After peripheral iridoplasty, the angle is open, but still narrow. **C,** More peripheral burns open the angle further. (*From* Pavlin *et al.* [40••]; with permission).

spot and making certain radial iris vessels are avoided (Fig. 15-8). One should begin with 200 mW of power in dark irides and 300 mW in light irides and adjust the power as necessary to achieve contraction. It is important to treat as far peripherally as possible. It is also useful to allow a thin crescent of the aiming beam to overlap the sclera at the limbus and have the patient look in the direction of the aiming beam to obtain more peripheral spot placement.

We occasionally use a 200-µm spot size of 0.2-second duration and 100 to 250 mW. We find these variables to be more effective for causing contraction in light gray irides and for focal treatment when the iris root is plugging a trabeculectomy ostium or sclerostomy site. During these latter two situations, we prefer to treat the iris by focusing the laser through a goniolens because this procedure provides direct visualization of the problem and enables more accurate spot placement. It is important to realize, however, that when ALPI is performed using a goniolens, a more diffuse burn with less stromal contraction is obtained because the laser strikes the iris surface more tangentially.

Another situation in which a goniolens is useful for iridoplasty is when there is a very sharp plateau configuration to the iris contour. The direct visualization of the area of apposition allows better spot placement. In patients with a very steep plateau, ALPI can be repeated to reach a more peripheral location after the first treatment—burns placed just inside the point of apposition pull the angle open and expose more peripheral iris stroma for a second application (Fig. 15-8).

Immediately after ALPI, a drop of apraclonidine, 1%, and a drop of a topical corticosteroid is applied. Gonioscopy is performed and IOP is checked 1 hour post-laser treatment. Topical steroid therapy is continued for a few days.

Complications

A mild iritis is common but usually transient and responds well to topical steroid treatment. Pupillary distortion rarely occurs and is more evident after focal treatment. Post-laser elevations in IOP may be related to inflammation or extensive synechial closure and usually respond well to drug therapy. Corneal endothelial burns can occur, especially in patients with a very shallow anterior chamber. These burns usually last a few days and are of no major consequence.

CONCLUSIONS

Although laser iridotomy is effective in relieving pupillary block, ALPI can open an appositionally closed angle when pupillary block is not a mechanism or when laser iridotomy cannot be performed. Iridotomy also relieves reverse pupillary block, which may be the mechanism responsible for the development of the pigment dispersion syndrome. The combined use of laser iridotomy and iridoplasty is effective in treating a number of situations, including the plateau iris syndrome and phacomorphic glaucoma. The diode and Nd:YLF picosecond lasers are newer treatment modalities that can successfully achieve a patent iridotomy.

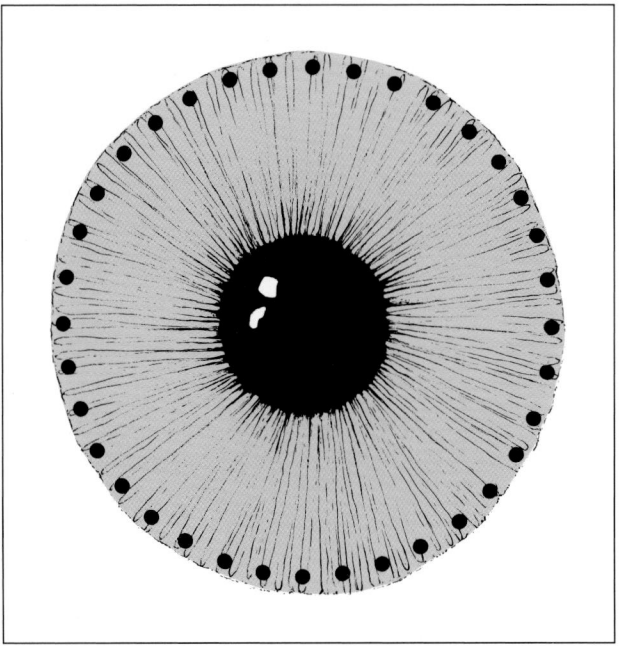

FIGURE 15-8 Technique of peripheral iridoplasty showing placement of contraction burns circumferentially around the iris as far peripheral as possible. (*From* Ritch *et al.* [32]; with permission).

REFERENCES AND RECOMMENDED READING

Recently published papers of particular interest have been highlighted as:

• Of interest

•• Of outstanding interest

1. Schwartz GF, Steinmann WC, Spaeth GL, *et al.*: Surgical and medical management of patients with narrow anterior chamber angles: comparative results. *Ophthalmic Surg* 1992, 23:108–112.

2. West RH: Creeping angle-closure glaucoma: the influence of iridotomy and iridectomy. *Aust NZ Ophthalmol* 1992, 20:23–28.

3.•• Tomey KF, Al-Rajhi AA: Neodymium:YAG laser iridotomy in the initial management of phacomorphic glaucoma. *Ophthalmology* 1992, 99:660–665.

The authors present retrospective data supporting the efficacy of laser iridotomy before cataract extraction in eyes with phacomorphic glaucoma. In all treated eyes, laser iridotomy was effective in either relieving or preventing acute angle-closure glaucoma so that uneventful cataract extraction could be performed.

4.•• Karickhoff JR: Pigmentary dispersion syndrome and pigmentary glaucoma: a new mechanism concept, a new treatment, and a new technique. *Ophthalmic Surg* 1992, 23:269–277.

Reverse pupillary block is proposed as the mechanism responsible for the iris concavity in the pigment dispersion syndrome. After laser iridotomy in six eyes, the iris assumed a permanent planar configuration in all cases. With the use of transillumination defects as a target, iridotomy was achieved using a lower energy pulse.

5. Fourman S: Iridotomy in eyes with pigmentary glaucoma [Letter]. *Ophthalmic Surg* 1992, 23:843–844.

6.•• Karickhoff JR: Iridotomy in eyes with pigmentary glaucoma [Letter]. *Ophthalmic Surg* 1992, 23:844–845.

Karickhoff discusses reverse pupillary block further. The first ultrasound biomicroscope scan documenting the presence of an iris concavity and its resolution after laser iridotomy is provided by Pavlin.

7.•• Potash SD, Tello C, Liebmann J, *et al.*: Ultrasound biomicroscopy in pigment dispersion syndrome. *Ophthalmology* 1993, in press.

Demonstration of the structural relationships among the iris, lens, zonules, and ciliary processes that characterize the pigment dispersion syndrome are presented. The success of miotic therapy and laser iridotomy in relieving the iris concavity associated with this disease is conclusively demonstrated, supporting the hypothesis of reverse pupillary block.

8. Ye T, Ge J, Zhuan W: A preliminary study of short-term efficacy of Nd:YAG laser peripheral iridotomy in patients with primary angle-closure glaucoma. *Yen Ko Hsueh Pao* 1991, 7:115–119.

9. Li J: YAG laser treatment in anterior segment disease of the eye. *Chung Kuo I Hsueh Ko Hsueh Yuan Hsueh Pao* 1992, 14:215–219.

10.• Ho T, Fan R: Sequential argon-YAG laser iridotomies in dark irides. *Br J Ophthalmol* 1992, 76:329–331.

The authors successfully performed laser iridotomy in 20 dark brown irides by using a combination of the argon and Nd:YAG lasers. Penetration was typically achieved with low total energy and minimal complications.

11. Del Priore LV, Robin AC, Pollack IP: Nd:YAG and argon laser iridotomy: long term follow-up in a prospective, randomized clinical trial. *Am J Ophthalmol* 1988, 95:1207–1211.

12. Moster MR, Schwartz LM, Spaeth GL, *et al.*: A controlled study comparing argon and Nd:YAG iridectomy. *Am J Ophthalmol* 1986, 93:20–24.

13.• Frangie JP, Park SB, Aquavella JV: Peripheral iridotomy using Nd:YLF laser. *Ophthalmic Surg* 1992, 23:220–221.

Initial clinical report of the use of the Nd:YLF picosecond laser to perform iridotomy in three patients. Because of the short-duration pulses, the optical breakdown is well refined and tissue incision rather than explosion is achieved. Iris bleeding occurred in one case as a result of direct incision of an iris vessel. No increase in IOP occurred after the laser procedures.

14.• Emoto, Okisaka S, Nakajima A: Diode laser iridotomy in rabbit and human eyes. *Am J Ophthalmol* 1992, 113:321–327.

Successful iridotomies were performed in 20 rabbit eyes and 40 human eyes with the semiconductor diode laser. The portability and cost can potentially make the diode laser an attractive alternative for anterior-segment laser surgery.

15. Tetsumoto K, Kuchle M, Naumann GOH: Late histopathological findings of neodymium:YAG laser iridotomies in humans. *Arch Ophthalmol* 1992, 110:1119–1123.

16. Murphy P, Trope GE: Monocular blurring: a complication of laser iridotomy. *Ophthalmology* 1991, 98:1539–1542.

17. Weintraub J, Berke SJ: Blurring after iridotomy [Letter]. *Ophthalmology* 1992, 99:479–480.

18. Fresco BB, Trope GE: Opaque contact lenses for YAG laser iridotomy occlusion. *Optom Vis Sci* 1992, 69:656–657.

19. Panek WC, Lee DA, Christensen RE: The effects of Nd:YAG laser iridotomy on the corneal endothelium. *Am J Ophthalmol* 1991, 111:505–507.

20.• Power WJ, Collum LM: Electron microscopic appearances of human corneal endothelium following Nd:YAG laser iridotomy. *Ophthalmic Surg* 1992, 23:347–350.

The authors used scanning electron microscopy to study corneal endothelial changes after Nd:YAG laser iridotomies in an eye enucleated for a posterior uveal melanoma. Less endothelial damage was observed when an Abraham lens was used compared with when the laser was focused directly through the cornea.

21.• Wilhelmus KR: Corneal edema following argon laser iridotomy. *Ophthalmic Surg* 1992, 23:533–537.

Five patients with preexisting endothelial dystrophy and shallow anterior chambers developed bullous keratopathy after argon laser iridotomy. High laser energy and multiple applications in patients with corneal guttata may contribute to the development of intractable corneal edema and visual loss.

22.• Margo CE, Lessner A, Goldey SH, Sherwood M: Lens-induced andophthalmitis after Nd:YAG laser iridotomy. *Am J Ophthalmol* 1992, 113:97–98.

A case report of a 50-year-old patient who developed lens-induced endophthalmitis after Nd:YAG laser iridotomy. The patient required enucleation because of intractable pain. Histopathologic examination revealed several large tears in the anterior capsule.

23.•• Cashwell LF, Martin TJ: Malignant glaucoma after laser iridotomy. *Ophthalmology* 1992, 99:651–658.

Six cases of malignant glaucoma are reported to have occurred at varying periods of time after laser iridotomy. A causal relationship could not be demonstrated because all patients had received miotics in the perilaser period. Primary aqueous misdirection manifesting after laser iridotomy could not be ruled out.

24.   Hodes BL: Malignant glaucoma after laser iridotomy [Letter]. *Ophthalmology* 1992, 99:1641–1642.

25.   Fourman S: "Malignant" glaucoma post laser iridotomy [Letter]. *Ophthalmology* 1992, 99:1751.

26.• Aminlari A, Sassani JW: Simultaneous bilateral malignant glaucoma following laser iridotomy. *Graefes Arch Clin Exp Ophthalmol* 1993, 231:12–14.

The authors present a case report of a 50-year-old woman who developed bilateral malignant glaucoma 4 weeks after laser iridotomies for angle-closure glaucoma. Ciliary body swelling caused by the use of hydrochlorothiazide may have attributed to the development of a shallow anterior chamber and the development of ciliolenticular block.

27.   Hurvitz LM, Kaufman PL, Robin AL, *et al.*: New developments in the drug treatment of glaucoma. *Drugs* 1991, 41:514–532.

28.   Hsieh JW: Effects of timolol and acetazolamide on intraocular pressure elevation following argon laser iridotomy. *Taiwan I Hsueh Hui Tsa Chih* 1992, 91:29–33.

29.   Fleck BW: How large must an iridotomy be? *Br J Ophthalmol* 1990, 74:583–588.

30.• Fleck BW, Fairley E, Wright E: A photometric study of the effect of pupil dilatation on Nd:YAG laser iridotomy area. *Br J Ophthalmol* 1992, 76:678–689.

The authors measured the change in iridotomy area after pupil dilatation in 21 eyes previously treated with Nd:YAG laser iridotomy. Two eyes that had initially small iridotomies experienced a significant decrease in iridotomy area after pupil dilatation. The authors suggest that an iridotomy be sufficiently large (200 μm in diameter, 0.31 mm^2 in area) to avoid the potential for functional failure.

31.•• Ritch R: Argon laser peripheral iridoplasty: an overview. *J Glaucoma* 1992, 1:206–213.

An in-depth discussion of the indications for, and techniques and complications of, ALPI. The author presents his own preferences for treatment and several modifications of techniques as well.

32.   Ritch R, Shields MB, Krupin T, eds.: *The Glaucomas*. St. Louis: CV Mosby, 1989:581–603.

33.•• Weiss HS, Shingleton BJ, Goode SM, *et al.*: Argon laser gonioplasty in the treatment of angle-closure glaucoma. *Am J Ophthalmol* 1992, 114:14–118.

The authors performed argon laser iridoplasty in 32 eyes in which angle-closure glaucoma was unrelieved by laser iridotomy. Successful treatment was defined as anatomic opening of 50% or more of the angle. Eyes that responded favorably to the treatment had a significantly shorter duration of angle closure and most eyes maintained adequate IOP control after 18 months of follow-up.

34.• Lowenstein A, Geyer O, Goldstein M, *et al.*: Argon laser gonioplasty in the treatment of angle-closure glaucoma [Letter]. *Am J Ophthalmol* 1993, 115:399–400.

The authors point out that laser iridoplasty may occasionally be superfluous in patients who maintain appositional closure after laser iridotomy because many patients will respond favorably to a short course of miotic therapy, with permanent alteration in the angle.

35.   Agarwal HC, Kumar R, Kalra VK, *et al.*: Argon laser iridoplasty: a primary mode of therapy in primary angle-closure glaucoma. *Ind J Ophthalmol* 1991, 39:87–90.

36.• Wand M: Argon laser gonioplasty for synechial angle closure. *Arch Ophthalmol* 1992, 110:363–367.

Six eyes of five patients with synecial angle closure of varying duration responded well to peripheral iridoplasty, with successful opening of 60% to 100% of the angle in all cases and a mean IOP drop of 5.5 mm Hg.

37.   Metz D, Ackerman J, Kanarek I: Laser trabeculoplasty enhancement by argon laser iridotomy and/or iridoplasty [Letter]. *Ophthalmic Surg* 1984, 15:535.

38.   Kurdagli N, Mamedov NG, Novoderezhkin VV, *et al.*: The laser correction of recurrent elevated intraocular pressure after a surgical operation to control glaucoma complicated by the blocking of the postoperative fistula by the root of the iris. *Vestn Oftalmol* 1992, 108:40–41.

39.• Ritch R: Plateau iris caused by abnormally positioned ciliary processes. *J Glaucoma* 1992, 1:23–26.

Results of indentation gonioscopy of eyes with the plateau iris syndrome after laser iridotomy suggest that abnormally large or anteriorly positioned ciliary processes may be responsible for the anatomic basis of this condition.

40.•• Pavlin CJ, Ritch R, Foster FS: Ultrasound biomicroscopy in the plateau iris syndrome. *Am J Ophthalmol* 1992, 113:390–395.

With the use of high-resolution ultrasound biomicroscopy, the *in vivo* pathophysiologic mechanisms of the plateau iris syndrome are demonstrated for the first time. In eight patients with the clinical diagnosis of the plateau iris syndrome, ciliary processes were situated anteriorly compared with the position in normal subjects and in patients with angle closure caused by pupillary block. These findings suggest that the ciliary processes provide structural support beneath the peripheral iris, thus preventing the iris root from falling away from the trabecular meshwork after iridotomy.

SELECT BIBLIOGRAPHY

Pollack IP: Current concepts in laser iridotomy. *Int Ophthalmol Clin* 1984, 24:153–180.

Ritch R, Liebmann J, Solomon IS: Laser iridectomy and iridoplasty. In *The Glaucomas*. Edited by Ritch R, Shields MB, Krupin T. St. Louis: CV Mosby; 1989:581–903.

Ritch R, Solomon IS: Laser treatment of glaucoma. In *Ophthalmic Lasers*, edn 3. Edited by L'Esperance FA Jr. St. Louis: CV Mosby; 1989:650–748.

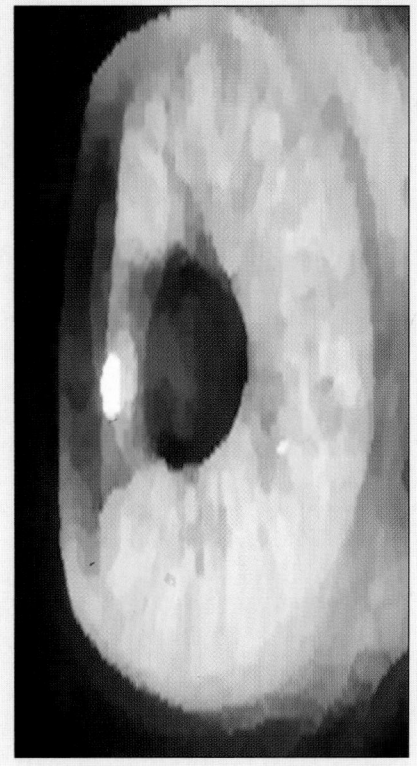

CHAPTER 16

LASER CYCLOPHOTOCOAGULATION

M. BRUCE SHIELDS

When faced with an especially difficult case of glaucoma that has not responded to medical therapy or more conventional surgical intervention, such as laser trabeculoplasty or a filtering operation, many surgeons have turned to a cyclodestructive procedure in the hope of lowering the intraocular pressure (IOP) by reducing aqueous production. This surgical approach, however, is considered by most surgeons to be a "last-resort" effort, because the past techniques of cyclodiathermy and cyclocryotherapy, and even the more recent technique of therapeutic ultrasonography, all cause significant damage to ocular tissues with associated high complication rates. The introduction of the laser has provided an alternative source of cyclodestruction and offers a more precise means by which to damage the ciliary body and create less damage to adjacent structures. Although complication rates remain high with cyclophotocoagulation, they are significantly less than with other forms of cyclodestruction, and continued evaluation of new lasers and new techniques may one day provide a cyclophotocoagulation procedure that is more than a last resort.

ROUTES OF DELIVERY

Unlike other cyclodestructive operations that are limited to the transscleral mode of energy delivery, laser energy can be delivered to the ciliary body by several routines: transpupillary and intraocular, as well as transscleral. Although the first two methods have the theoretical advantage of direct visualization of the ciliary processes being treated, they also have significant limitations. I discuss these two methods briefly first, and follow with the more commonly used transscleral cyclophotocoagulation.

TRANSPUPILLARY CYCLOPHOTOCOAGULATION

The technique of transpupillary cyclophotocoagulation, which was introduced by Lee and Pomerantzeff [1] in 1971, involves the direct application of laser energy to individual ciliary processes with the use of a gonioscopic lens but is limited to those eyes in which a sufficient number of ciliary processes can be visualized gonioscopically. Such visualization is not possible in most glaucomatous eyes, especially those in which long-term miotic therapy prevents wide dilation. However, there are some situations, such as a large iridectomy or retraction of the iris in advanced neovascular glaucoma, that may provide adequate gonioscopic visualization of the ciliary processes (Fig. 16-1) [2]. Typical argon laser settings are 0.1 to 0.2 second, 100 to 200 μm, and an energy level that is sufficient to produce white discoloration as well as a brown concave burn, often with pigment dispersion or gas bubbles (usually, 700 to 1000 mW). Special contact lenses with scleral depressors have been developed to rotate the processes into better view, although the value of this procedure has yet to be established. All visible portions of the ciliary process should be treated, which usually requires three to five applications per process. It is customary to treat all processes for up to 180 degrees at one session, with additional treatment at subsequent sessions if required.

Experience with transpupillary cyclophotocoagulation has been disappointing [3]. The success rate has been low, even in the small percentage of cases in which gonioscopic visualization has allowed treatment of a large number of ciliary processes. These failures may be because of, in part, an inadequate number of ciliary processes that can be visualized and treated or to an insufficient intensity of the laser burns to each process. However, even when all the

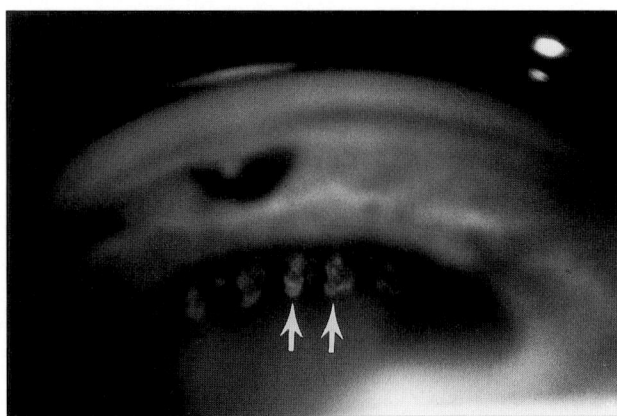

FIGURE 16-1 Gonioscopic view of ciliary processes (*arrows*) during transpupillary cyclophotocoagulation. Exposure of processes in this eye is caused by retraction of iris by fibrovascular membrane of neovascular glaucoma. (*From* Shields [2]; with permission.)

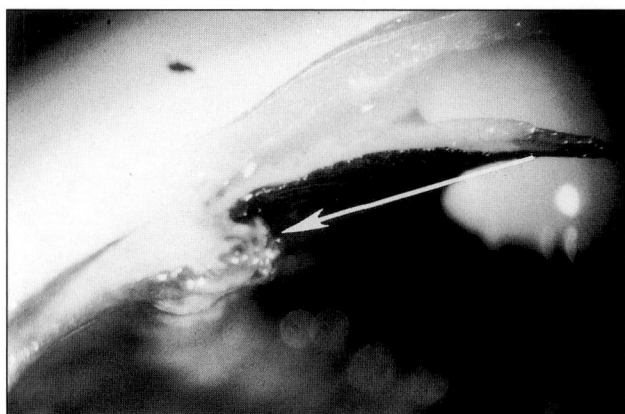

FIGURE 16-2 Section of human autopsy specimen of an eye showing angle of ciliary process visualization during transpupillary cyclophotocoagulation (*arrow*), which provides view of only the anterior tip of the process. (*From* Shields [4]; with permission.)

processes can be visualized for 360 degrees, the treatment is not always successful. Another cause of failure may be the angle at which the processes are viewed gonioscopically, which only allows the anterior tips of the ciliary ridges to be seen and treated, even when scleral indentation is used (Fig. 16-2) [4]. Nevertheless, transpupillary cyclophotocoagulation may be worth trying in some cases, such as refractory neovascular glaucoma, before going to more aggressive therapy.

INTRAOCULAR CYCLOPHOTOCOAGULATION

Another method by which laser energy can be applied directly to individual ciliary processes is with an endophotocoagulator through a pars plana incision. This procedure is most commonly performed in conjunction with vitreous surgery for diabetic retinopathy in eyes with intractable neovascular glaucoma [5•,6]. After performing the vitrectomy (and lensectomy if the eye is not already aphakic) the IOP is lowered and scleral indentation is used to bring the ciliary processes into transpupillary view. The individual processes are then treated under direct visualization with the endophotocoagulator, which is inserted through the same cannula as is used for the vitrectomy instrument (Fig. 16-3). The endophotocoagulator is attached to an argon laser, and the tip of the laser probe is positioned 2 to 3 mm from the processes. Standard laser settings include an exposure time of 0.1 to 0.2 second and a power level that is sufficient to produce a white reaction and shallow tissue disruption (usually, 1000 mW). Three to five laser exposures are then applied to each process in the two quadrants opposite to the entry site. In one large series, 75% of the eyes were found to have an IOP of 21 mm Hg or less with or without medications after one or two treatments in an average follow-up lasting 13 months [5•].

Although the main value of intraocular cyclophotocoagulation is as an adjunct to pars plana vitrectomy, it has also been evaluated as a primary surgical procedure for the treatment of eyes with refractory glaucoma. These operations have used either the transpupillary visualization of the processes during intraocular cyclophotocoagulation, as described previously, or have used an ocular endoscope to which a laser fiberoptic has been attached [6]. These techniques for cyclophotocoagulation have the advantage of allowing precise treatment to individual ciliary processes, which has been confirmed by histologic study in monkey eyes (Fig. 16-4) [7]. However, they have the obvious disadvantage of being invasive procedures with the associated increased risks, which in effect makes their results less promising than those from transscleral cyclophotocoagulation.

A newer ophthalmic laser microendoscope system (Endo Optiks, Little Silver, NJ) has been developed for intraocular cyclophotocoagulation in which fiberoptics for a television monitor, a diode laser delivery system, and an illumination source are all housed in an 18-gauge probe. The probe is introduced through a pars plana incision into an aphakic eye after prior anterior vitrectomy. While visualizing the ciliary processes on the television monitor, the diode laser energy is applied to the processes in the same manner as described previously for argon laser intraocular cyclophotocoagulation. Preliminary experience sug-

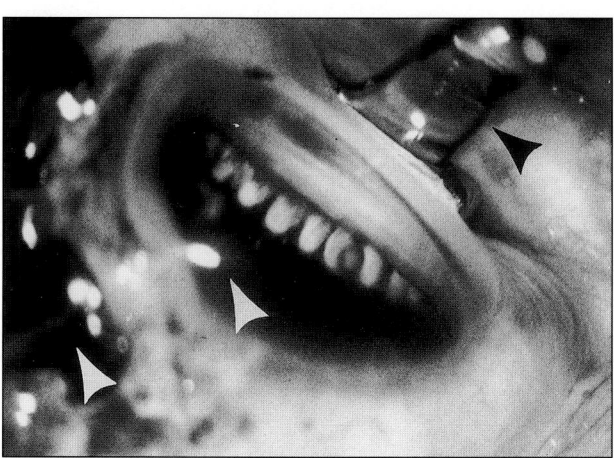

FIGURE 16-3 Intraocular cyclophotocoagulation with transpupillary visualization. Ciliary processes are brought into view with scleral depressor (*black arrow*) and treated with laser endophotocoagulator (*white arrows*) via a pars plana incision. (*From* Shields [4]; with permission.)

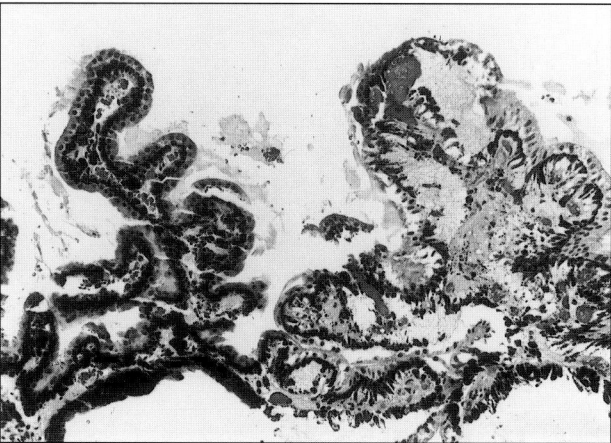

FIGURE 16-4 Light microscopic view of monkey eye, enucleated and fixed immediately after intraocular cyclophotocoagulation with endoscopic visualization. Note extensive disruption of ciliary epithelium and stroma in treated process on the right, compared with relatively normal structure of untreated process to the left. (Hematoxylin & eosin; original magnification, x 125.)

gests that endoscopic-diode cyclophotocoagulation may one day have a role in the management of difficult cases of neovascular glaucoma with aphakia [8•].

TRANSSCLERAL CYCLOPHOTOCOAGULATION

The concept of applying laser energy to the ciliary body by the transscleral route was popularized by the work of Beckman and Waeltermann [9•]. In 1984, they reported a 10-year experience with 241 eyes treated with transscleral ruby-laser cyclophotocoagulation. Although their initial experience was encouraging, it was not until the availability of specially designed neodymium-yttrium aluminum garnet (Nd:YAG) lasers that widespread interest developed in transscleral cyclophotocoagulation.

Instruments

The Nd:YAG lasers that have been evaluated for transscleral cyclophotocoagulation differ according to 1) laser mode (pulsed, thermal mode, or continuous-wave mode), and 2) the delivery system (noncontact, slit-lamp system; or contact-probe, fiberoptic system). The only instrument that is currently available for slit-lamp delivery is the Microruptor II (H-S Meridian Inc., Minneapolis, MN), which operates in the free-running thermal mode of 20-ms pulses. Two additional features that are required to perform transscleral cyclophotocoagulation are 1) an adjustable offset between the focal points of the helium-neon aiming beam and the therapeutic beam, so that the therapeutic beam can be at a predetermined distance inside

the eye while aiming on the conjunctiva, and 2) high energy levels of up to 8 to 9 J.

Several laser units are now available for contact transscleral cyclophotocoagulation, although the one that has been most extensively evaluated is the SLT CL60 (Surgical Laser Technologies, Oaks, PA), which is an Nd:YAG laser that operates in the continuous-wave mode with a range of 0.1 to 10 seconds. A 2.2-mm sapphire-tip, hand-held probe, which is focused at 1.5 to 2 mm in air, is coupled to a fiberoptic delivery system. The unit can provide powers in excess of 10 W (energy in joules = power in watts × duration in seconds).

More recently, the Microruptor III (H-S Meridian) has been introduced, which also provides continuous-wave Nd:YAG laser energy with contact-probe delivery. In addition, semiconductor diode lasers are being evaluated for transscleral cyclophotocoagulation. These lasers operate in a continuous-wave mode and can be delivered by either contact probe with the OcuLight SLX (Iris Medical Instruments, Inc., Mountain View, CA) or slit lamp with the Microlase (Keeler Instruments, Broomall, PA).

Histologic observations

Histologic studies in animal and human eyes have shown that the laser-induced tissue damage is limited primarily to the ciliary epithelium, with minimal damage occurring to other ocular structures. Studies with the noncontact pulsed laser in human autopsy specimens of eyes have revealed a blister-like elevation of the epithelial layers from the adjacent stroma, with marked disruption primarily of the pig-

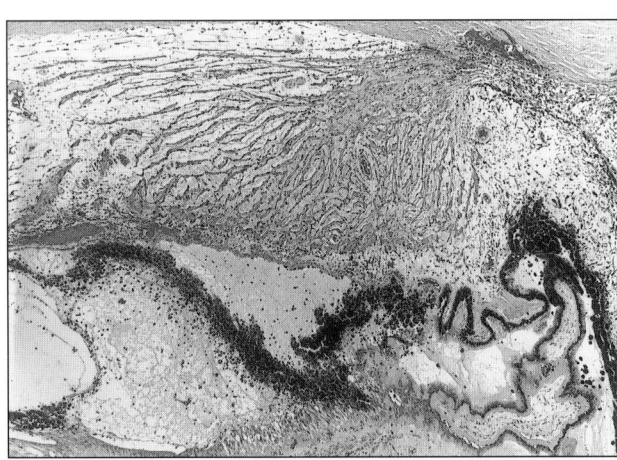

FIGURE 16-5 Light microscopic view of radially sectioned specimen of ciliary body of human eye treated with noncontact, pulsed transscleral neodymium-yttrium aluminum garnet cyclophotocoagulation 2 days before enucleation, showing disruption of ciliary epithelium and separation from underlying stroma with fibrin and a scant number of leukocytes in the blister-like space. (Hematoxylin & eosin; original magnification, x 100.) (*From* Blasini, *et al.* [11]; with permission.)

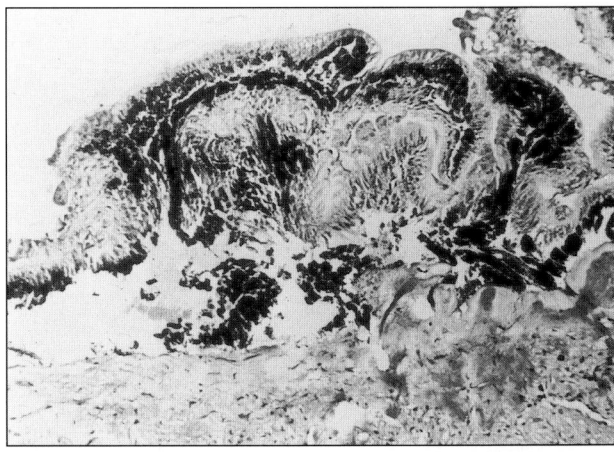

FIGURE 16-6 Light microscopic appearance of cyclophotocoagulation lesion created by continuous-wave neodymium-yttrium aluminum garnet laser at 700 ms and 10 W, with probe 1 mm posterior to limbus and perpendicular to sclera. Note moderate disruption and marked convolution of ciliary epithelial layers with slight separation from underlying stroma and prominent coagulative changes of stromal tissue. (Hematoxylin & eosin; original magnification, x 40.) (*From* Prum, *et al.* [12]; with permission.)

mented epithelium but minimal change in the ciliary muscle and sclera in the path of the laser beam [10]. Similar histologic findings, with the addition of fibrin and scant inflammatory cells between the disrupted epithelial layers and stroma, have been seen in human eyes that were enucleated a few days after the procedure (Fig. 16-5) [11]. In that study, no significant changes were observed in the ciliary body vasculature or adjacent sclera. In contrast to the lesions created by the noncontact pulsed laser, the lesions created by the contact, continuous-wave Nd:YAG laser appeared to have a smaller, more coagulative effect on the epithelium, with less of the blister-like elevation (Fig. 16-6) [12].

The histologic observations in animal and human eyes suggest that the most likely mechanism by which transscleral Nd:YAG cyclophotocoagulation reduces aqueous production is through destruction of the ciliary epithelium. However, because IOP reduction has also been observed when the laser lesions were applied posterior to the pars plicata, alternative mechanisms of pressure reduction have also been considered [13•]. These mechanisms include ciliary vascular disruption, with reduced aqueous production, or chronic inflammation, which could either reduce inflow or increase uveoscleral outflow.

Techniques

Unlike most other laser procedures, the intraoperative pain associated with transscleral cyclophotocoagulation is such that retrobulbar anesthesia is usually required. With the Microruptor II noncontact pulsed technique, the patient is positioned at the slit lamp and the lids are separated manually or with a special contact lens (Fig. 16-7) [14]. The lens also compress-es and blanches the conjunctiva and provides measurements from the limbus. Standard laser settings include a pulse of 20 ms and a maximum offset between the aiming and therapeutic beams, which is 3.6 mm in air. Placement of the laser lesions 1.0 to 1.5 mm behind the limbus is optimum for damaging the pars plicata and is preferred by most surgeons, although some surgeons use a more posterior placement of 2 to 3 mm. Preferred energy levels vary considerably from 2 to 8 J, and the optimum energy level has yet to be established. In a prospective study comparing energy levels of 4 and 8 J, the higher energy level was associated with a trend toward better intraocular control, although this trend did not reach statistical significance and there was no clinical or statistical difference in the final visual outcome [15]. The total number of laser applications also varies among surgeons, with most using 30 to 40 evenly spaced lesions for 360 degrees (Fig. 16-8) [16].

The contact, continuous-wave technique with the SLT CL60 generally uses exposure times of 0.5 to 0.7 second. The laser focus is fixed by the design of the probe tip, which is held perpendicular to the surface of the conjunctiva with the anterior edge of the probe 0.5 to 1.5 mm behind the limbus. As with the noncontact system, preferred power settings vary considerably from 4 to 9 W, with 30 to 40 applications for 360 degrees [17••]. The Microruptor III Nd:YAG laser and the Iris semiconductor diode laser have been evaluated with similar protocols, although durations of exposure of up to 2 seconds have been studied with these units. The duration of laser exposure appears to influence the nature of tissue response even among the continuous-wave units, although the optimal clinical protocol has yet to be established [18].

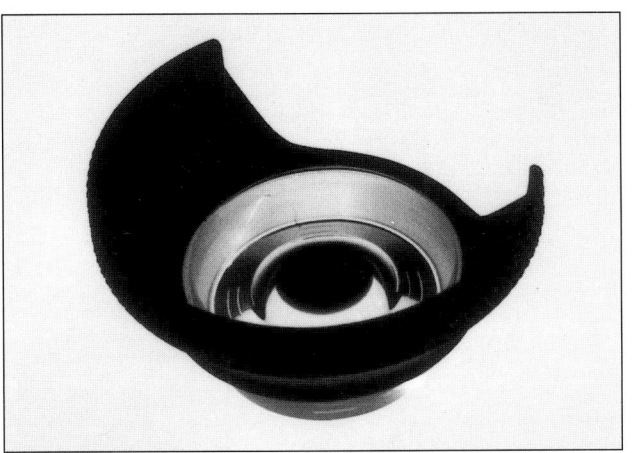

FIGURE 16-7 Contact lens designed for use with noncontact transscleral neodymium-yttrium aluminum garnet cyclophotocoagulation. (*From* Shields, *et al.* [14]; with permission.)

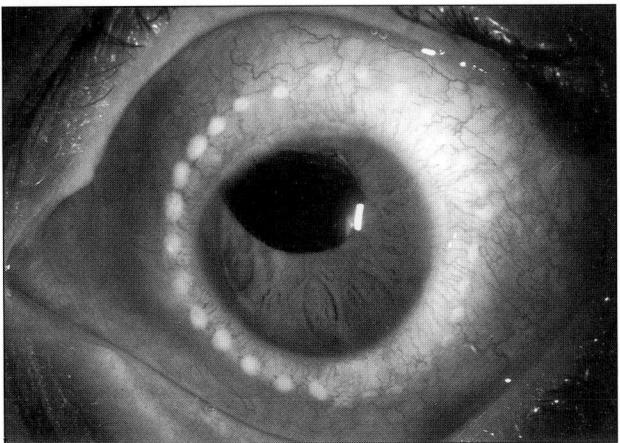

FIGURE 16-8 Slit-lamp appearance of conjunctival burns (*white spots*) immediately following noncontact, pulsed transscleral neodymium-yttrium aluminum garnet cyclophotocoagulation. Note larger diameter of lesions on left side, treated without the contact lens, compared with lesions on right, treated with the lens. (*From* Shields [17]; with permission.)

Postoperative management is directed primarily at inflammation, which is always present and can be severe. One approach is to use a subconjunctival injection of dexamethasone with topical atropine and prednisolone for approximately 10 days [19]. Transient IOP rise is not a common problem, although it is advisable to check the pressure a few hours after the procedure and the following day. Preoperative antiglaucoma drug therapy should be continued postoperatively, with the exception of miotics, and should be gradually discontinued as the decline in pressure allows. Postoperative pain is usually mild and transient, requiring only a mild analgesic.

Clinical experience

Preliminary experience with both the noncontact and contact techniques has shown satisfactory IOP reduction in approximately two thirds or more of the cases after the initial treatment session, with most of the remainder coming under control with one or more repeat treatments [17,19••]. Maximum pressure reduction is typically achieved in 1 month, and it is usually desirable to wait at least this long before re-treating. The contact technique requires less total energy and appears to have slightly better efficacy with lowering IOP and a lower complication rate with regard to reduction in visual acuity. Both techniques have significant advantages over cyclo-cryotherapy, which include less transient IOP rise, less inflammation, and less pain. However, reduced visual acuity remains a significant problem, especially with the noncontact technique, which may be related to the postoperative inflammation and macular edema. Efforts to reduce the visual loss associated with macular edema have included the use of nonsteroidal anti-inflammatory agents such as oral indomethasone or topical ketorolac. However, there have been no controlled studies to evaluate the efficacy of these measures with transscleral cyclophotocoagulation, and the patient must be informed that visual loss is a significant risk with this operation. The surgery should only be recommended when alternative treatments are not believed to offer a better outcome.

PRESENT STATUS AND FUTURE ROLE

At present, there is sufficient evidence to claim that transscleral cyclophotocoagulation is the cyclodestructive procedure of choice. However, whether it will assume a broader role in the treatment of glaucoma than has been the case with cyclodestructive surgery in the past is a question that awaits further evaluation of new lasers and refined techniques.

REFERENCES AND RECOMMENDED READING

Recently published papers of particular interest have been highlighted as:
• Of interest
•• Of outstanding interest

1.   Lee P-F, Pomerantzeff O: Transpupillary cyclophotocoagulation of rabbit eyes: an experimental approach to glaucoma surgery. *Am J Ophthalmol* 1971, 71:911.

2.   Shields MB: *Textbook of Glaucoma*, edn 3. Baltimore: Williams & Wilkins, 1992:622.

3.   Shields S, Stewart WC, Shields MB: Transpupillary argon laser cyclophotocoagulation in the treatment of glaucoma. *Ophthalmic Surg* 1988, 19:171.

4.   Shields MB: Cyclodestructive surgery for glaucoma: past, present and future. *Trans Am Ophthalmol Soc* 1985, 83:285.

5.•• Zarbin MA, Michels RG, de Bustros S, *et al.*: Endolaser treatment of the ciliary body for severe glaucoma. *Ophthalmology* 1988, 95:1639.
This is one of the largest reported series of intraocular cyclophotocoagulation, in which an argon laser endophotocoagulator was used to treat ciliary processes under direct visualization. Seventy-five percent of the eyes had IOP of 21 mm Hg or less after one or two treatments with an average follow-up of 13 months.

6.   Shields MB: Intraocular cyclophotocoagulation. *Trans Ophthalmol Soc UK* 1986, 105:237.

7.   Shields MB, Chandler DB, Hickingbotham D, *et al.*: Intraocular cyclophotocoagulation: histopathologic evaluation in primates. *Arch Ophthalmol* 1985, 103:1731.

8.• Uram M: Ophthalmic laser microendoscope ciliary process ablation in the management of neovascular glaucoma. *Ophthalmology* 1992, 99:1823.
This preliminary study suggests a future role for television-monitored endoscopic cyclophotocoagulation in selected cases of neovascular glaucoma in aphakia or pseudophakia.

9.• Beckman H, Waeltermann J: Transscleral ruby laser cyclocoagulation. *Am J Ophthalmol* 1984, 98:788.
This is the pioneer study in transscloral cyclophotocoagulation. Although the ruby laser never achieved clinical application, the principles established set the stage for application of subsequent lasers.

10.   Hampton C, Shields MB: Transscleral neodymium:YAG cyclophotocoagulation: a histologic study of human autopsy eyes. *Arch Ophthalmol* 1988, 106:1121.

11. Blasini M, Simmons R, Shields MB: Early tissue response to transscleral neodymium:YAG cyclophotocoagulation. *Invest Ophthalmol Vis Sci* 1990, 31:1114.

12. Prum BE, Shields SR, Simmons RB, *et al*.: The influence of exposure duration on transscleral Nd:YAG cyclophoto-coagulation. *Am J Ophthalmol* 1992, 114:560.

13.• Schubert HD: Non-contact and contact pars plana transs-cleral neodymium:YAG laser cyclophotocoagulation in postmortem eyes. *Ophthalmology* 1989, 96:1471.

Based on this and related studies, the author suggests that mech-anisms other than direct ciliary epithelial destruction may be involved in IOP reduction following transscleral cyclophotocoag-ulation.

14. Simmons RB, Blasini M, Shields MB, *et al*.: Comparison of transscleral neodymium:YAG cyclophotocoagulation with and without a contact lens in human autopsy eyes. *Am J Ophthalmol* 1990, 109:174.

15. Shields MB, Wilkerson MH, Echelman DA: A comparison of two energy levels for noncontact transscleral neodymi-um:YAG cyclophotocoagulation. *Arch Ophthalmol* 1993, 111:484.

16. Shields MB: *Textbook of Glaucoma*, edn 3. Baltimore: Williams & Wilkins, 1992:621.

17.•• Schuman JS, Puliafito CA, Allingham RR, *et al*.: Contact transscleral continuous-wave neodymium:YAG laser cyclophotocoagulation. *Ophthalmology* 1990, 97:571.

This is one of the largest reported clinical trials using a continu-ous-wave, contact Nd:YAG laser for transscleral cyclophotocoag-ulation. In 140 eyes, there was a successful reduction in 62% with only 7% losing two or more lines of visual acuity.

18. Echelman DA, Nasisse MP, Shields MB, *et al*.: Influence of exposure time on inflammatory response to Nd:YAG cyclophotocoagulation in rabbits. *Arch Ophthalmol* 1994, in press.

19.•• Hampton C, Shields MB, Miller KN, *et al*.: Evaluation of a protocol for transscleral neodymium:YAG cyclophotoco-agulation in 100 patients. *Ophthalmology* 1990, 94:910.

This is one of the largest reported series of thermal pulsed, non-contact Nd:YAG laser transscleral cyclophotocoagulation. In 100 patients, approximately 67% had a successful pressure reduction with a single treatment and the majority of the remaining patients were brought under control with additional treatments. However, some degree of visual loss was seen in nearly half of the patients.

SELECT BIBLIOGRAPHY

Shields MB: Transscleral Nd:YAG cyclophotocoagulation. In *Color Atlas of Ophthalmic Surgery: Glaucoma*. Edited by Minckler DS and Van Buskirk EM. Philadelphia: JB Lippincott; 1992:210–218.

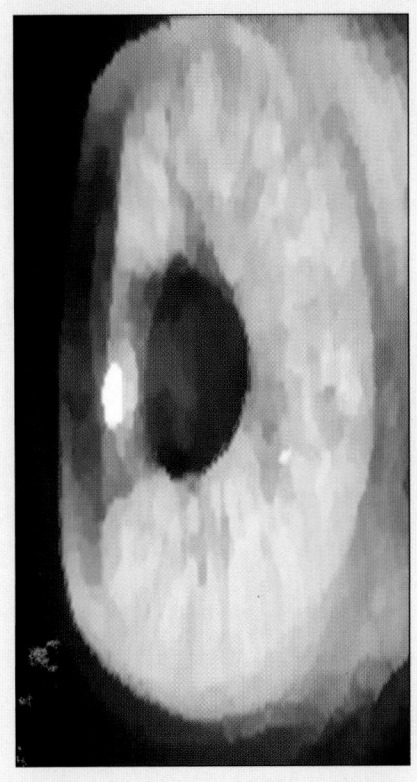

CHAPTER 17

AB INTERNO LASER
SCLEROSTOMY

PAMELA R. HENDERSON
EVE J. HIGGINBOTHAM

Glaucoma filtration surgery done via conventional methods is very successful; however, less invasive techniques, which could minimize intraoperative and postoperative complications, are always being explored. The failure of glaucoma filtration surgery is thought to result from subconjunctival scarring secondary to fibroblast proliferation because platelet-derived factors released during invasive surgery incite an inflammatory response [1,2]. As ophthalmologists have become more proficient in the use of lasers in the treatment of various ocular conditions, attention has been turned to the use of laser energy for the creation of a filtering fistula between the anterior chamber and the subconjunctival space. This technique would minimize or eliminate conjunctival manipulation, thereby reducing the stimulus for fibroblast proliferation. In addition, laser modalities are attractive options because they provide hemostasis and cause minimal trauma to adjacent tissues.

There are several approaches to the creation of ab interno sclerostomies. Success has been reported with the use of an automated-trephine, ab interno laser sclerostomy involving fiberoptics and gonioscopic noninvasive ab interno laser sclerostomy techniques [3]. This chapter focuses on ab interno laser sclerostomy.

GONIOSCOPIC DELIVERY

Gonioscopic delivery of laser energy in the creation of a sclerostomy offers significant advantages compared with conventional surgery, as well as invasive methods of performing ab interno laser sclerostomy. This technique requires minimal conjunctival manipulation, so no dissection is necessary. It does not require anterior chamber instrumentation, and it provides good access to all four quadrants. Drawbacks include the fact that success is dependent on media clarity. Accurate focusing of the laser is therefore not always optimal in this technique, which makes it difficult to superimpose multiple laser applications, a key factor in achieving patency (Fig. 17-1).

March and coworkers [4•] were able to create laser sclerostomies by using a modified neodymium-yttrium aluminum garnet (Nd:YAG) goniolens in six human cadaver eyes. The minimal total energy required for perforation was 3.3 J and a total of 26.6 J was required to create an "optimal" fistula. Gherezghiher and coworkers [5] were able to create patent fistulae when using an Nd:YAG laser in primates via gonioscopic delivery. Two monkeys treated required high energies for fistula formation (23 and 24 J) and two required lower energies (12 and 14 J). Sclerostomies remained patent for 180 days as determined by tonographic and histologic examination. Endothelial cell damage was noted at the site of laser treatment.

In an early summary of results from an uncontrolled series of 70 patients with sclerostomies formed by a variety of permutations of Q-switched Nd:YAG laser, dye enhancement, and pulsed krypton laser, March [6] was able to demonstrate that 50 of the 70 patients maintained some permanent filtration and lowering of intraocular pressure (IOP). The other 20 patients had prompt sealing of the fistulae. The complication rate was reportedly very low.

DYE ENHANCEMENT

Latina and coworkers [7••] were able to create sclerostomies *in vitro* in the eyes of 54 Dutch-belted rabbits and *in vitro* in human eyes obtained postmortem. Iontophoresis of methylene blue into the sclera at the limbus was performed to enhance laser light absorption. Pulse durations of 1.5 and 2.0 µs required 20 pulses or fewer to perforate human sclera with pulse energies of 75 to 100 mJ. Full-thickness fistulae were successfully

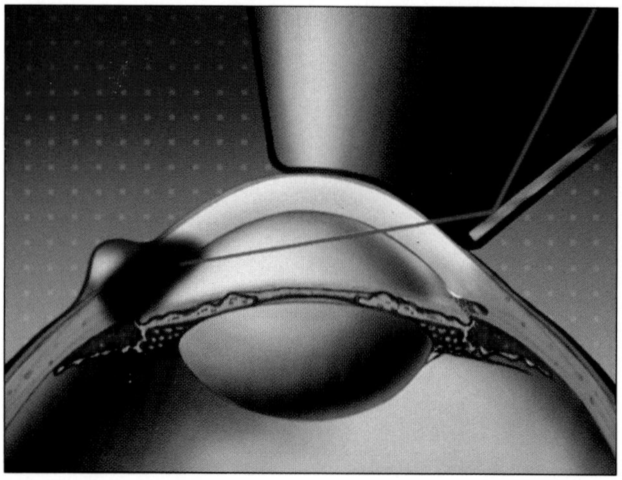

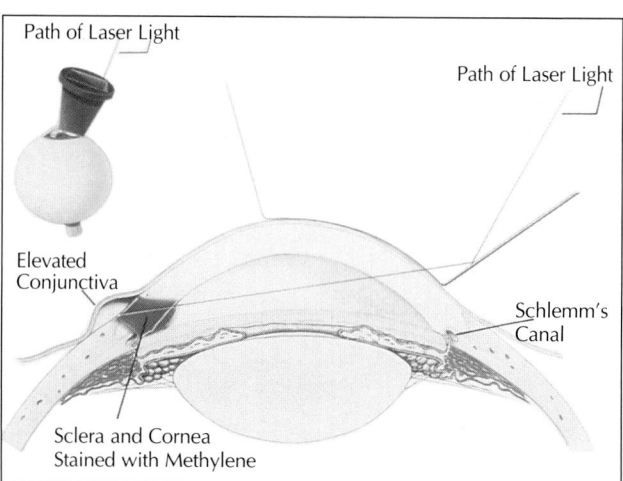

FIGURE 17-1 Gonioscopic ab interno laser sclerostomy. (Courtesy of Surgical Laser Technologies, Malvern, PA.)

FIGURE 17-2 Gonioscopic ab interno laser sclerostomy with methylene-blue dye enhancement. (Courtesy of Surgical Laser Technologies, Malvern, PA.)

created in 80% of rabbit eyes at pulse durations of 1.5 and 2.0 μs (Fig. 17-2).

Latina and coworkers [8••] also reported completion of successful sclerostomies in 21 of 35 eyes (55%), with an associated acute mean reduction in IOP of 23 mm Hg. The technique used was methylene blue dye–enhanced gonioscopic ab interno laser sclerostomy. A partial fistula was created in 24% of eyes and no fistula was formed in 21% of eyes. At 1 year, 50% of eyes with an optimal sclerostomy had an IOP of less than 22 mm Hg.

Twelve patients with refractory glaucoma were treated by Melamed and coworkers [9] with internal sclerostomy involving laser ablation of dyed sclera. The technique involved iontophoretic impregnation of sclera at the limbal region with methylene blue, 1%, and delivery of a pulsed-dye laser beam to the stained area through a goniolens. Successful complete sclerostomy was achieved in 58% of eyes, but there was reduction of IOP in all cases.

Saraff and Lee [10] have been working on iontophoretic delivery of Reactive Black 5 (RB5) stain into sclera. RB5 is stable over time and does not bleach upon exposure to laser light, as is the case with methylene blue. Bleaching prevents further absorption of laser energy, resulting in incomplete fistula formation; the use of RB5 could eliminate this complication.

INTRACAMERAL TECHNIQUES

The other approach to ab interno laser sclerostomy is via intracameral techniques with a fiberoptic delivery system coupled to a laser source. The contact endoscope is passed through a corneal incision across the anterior chamber to the proposed sclerostomy site. Gaasterland and coworkers [11] used a 200-μm-diameter fiberoptic probe to create sclerostomies in bovine eyes with an argon laser set at 333- to 363-nm wavelengths.

Jaffe and coworkers [12] also were able to create ab interno laser sclerostomies with a high-powered argon endolaser that delivered via a 300-μm fiberoptic system in rabbits. Fistulae of approximately 400 μm in diameter were successfully created in all eyes. The mean energy requirement was 1.7 J. IOP decreased by an average of 12±5 mm Hg on postoperative day 1.

Shahinian and coworkers [13••] used a 300-μm quartz fiberoptic probe attached to a potassium titanyl phosphate crystal Nd:YAG laser with output to an argon laser and were able to create an ab interno sclerostomy through a limbal stab incision in a human eye *in vivo*. Three pulses of 8 W for 0.1 second were used. The sclerostomy failed in 1 year. Infrared lasers such as the continuous-wave Nd:YAG laser coupled to a fiberoptic probe attached to a synthetic sapphire-tipped laser scalpel have also been widely used. Higginbotham and coworkers [14••] demonstrated the effectiveness of this approach versus thermal sclerostomy in the rabbit model. Fifteen rabbits underwent internal Nd:YAG sclerostomy while 12 rabbits underwent conventional external thermal sclerostomy. The fellow eye in each animal served as a control. By the 13th day, all of the standard thermal sclerostomies had failed, but 80% of the laser sclerostomies were still functioning at 21 days. Complications, however, were more common in the laser-treated group (Table 17-1).

Liu and Higginbotham [15] performed ab interno laser sclerostomy with an Nd:YAG laser carrying a

TABLE 17-1	DURATION OF FUNCTIONAL BLEBS AND IOP REDUCTION* IN LASER VERSUS SURGERY GROUP			
	Duration, *d*			
Group	**≤ 7**	**8–14**	**≥ 14**	***p†***
	Number of eyes with functional blebs			
Surgery, *n*=12(%)	9(75)	3(25)	0	0.0340
Laser, *n*=15(%)	4‡(27)	8§(53)	3(20)	
	Number of eyes with IOP reduction			
Surgery, *n*=11(%)	6¶(55)	5(45)	0	0.0013
Laser, *n*=15(%)	2‡(13)	2(13)	11§(73)	

*The decrease in IOP greater than 2 mm Hg compared with the contralateral untreated eye after digital massage.
†Chi-square test.
‡This number includes one rabbit that died before meeting the criteria for failure.
§This number includes four rabbits that died before meeting the criteria for failure.
¶One rabbit never demonstrated a pressure reduction and therefore was excluded.
IOP—intraocular pressure.

synthetic sapphire-tipped probe in four aphakic human eyes. They found an average decrease in IOP of 14 mm Hg. Two patients without blebs achieved successful control through taking glaucoma medications. One patient was excluded from study due to hypotony. Long-term follow-up of these patients is discussed later (Fig. 17-3).

Javitt and coworkers [16] also demonstrated the ability to produce ab interno sclerostomies in rabbits via intracameral techniques. They used between 1.6 and 2.4 J of total energy to create full-thickness fistulae. All blebs failed within 3 to 7 days. Histologic examination revealed that the fistulae were plugged with fibrin.

Five patients with glaucoma, uveitis, and severe scarring of the superior conjunctiva were treated by Wilson and Javitt [17] via Nd:YAG laser ab interno sclerostomy with a sapphire-tipped probe. Between 2.4 and 4.8 J were required to complete the procedure. At 25 months, 60% of patients had an average IOP of 15 mm Hg.

In terms of cutting accuracy and atraumatic perforation, the excimer laser at 193 nm is unmatched. Unfortunately, light at 193 nm is not transmitted by the cornea or aqueous material and cannot be passed through an endoscope. Therefore, investigation of laser sclerostomy techniques involving the excimer laser has centered on delivery at 308 nm, which can be passed through an endoscope. The peak absorption wavelength of sclera is 193 nm; hence, excimer energy delivered at 308 nm is less well absorbed, resulting in degradation of cutting performance.

Berlin and coworkers [18] were able to use ab interno endoscopic delivery of excimer laser energy at 308 nm in rabbits to create sclerostomies. Fistula patency was maintained for up to 4 months. Less than 100 pulses at a fluence of 3.5 J/mm^2 were required.

Yttrium aluminum garnet lasers doped with other elements have been successfully used in the creation of sclerostomies via the intracameral ab interno approach. Hill and coworkers [19] used a rabbit model to compare erbium-yttrium aluminum garnet (Er:YAG) with Nd:YAG laser sclerostomies and found that the filtering bleb and IOP reduction lasted longer in the Er:YAG group. Collateral thermal damage was also less with the Er:YAG sclerostomies (Fig. 17-4 and Table 17-2).

Our technique of ab interno laser sclerostomy is an invasive procedure in which we use an air-cooled continuous-wave Nd:YAG laser (Surgical Laser Technologies, Malvern, PA) connected to a quartz optical fiber and laser scalpel. After preoperative preparation and retrobulbar anesthetic administration, the patient is prepped and draped in the usual sterile fashion. The operating room microscope is brought into position. With the aid of a 30-gauge disposable needle, the conjunctiva is ballooned up at the site of the proposed sclerostomy with either viscoelastic substance or balanced salt solution. A beveled corneal incision is made just inside the limbus in the inferotemporal quadrant. The anterior chamber is deepened with a viscoelastic substance. The synthetic sapphire-tipped laser scalpel with a tip diameter of 200 to 400 µm is introduced through the clear corneal incision, keeping it parallel to the iris. The tip is advanced across the chamber and positioned at the level of the anterior trabecular meshwork. With the help of the Zeiss four-mirror goniolens, the procedure can be monitored wherever corneal clarity permits. The focusing beam is evident at the tip of the laser scalpel and once it is in proper place, the laser is armed and discharged by pressing the foot pedal. The operating room and microscope lights are dimmed to aid in visualization of the laser scalpel. The endpoint is visualization of the

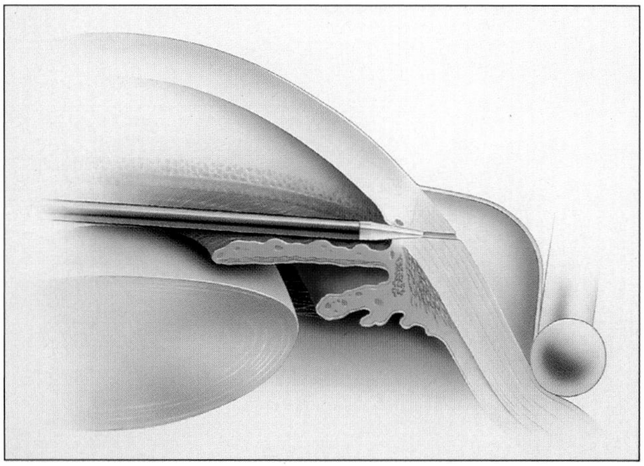

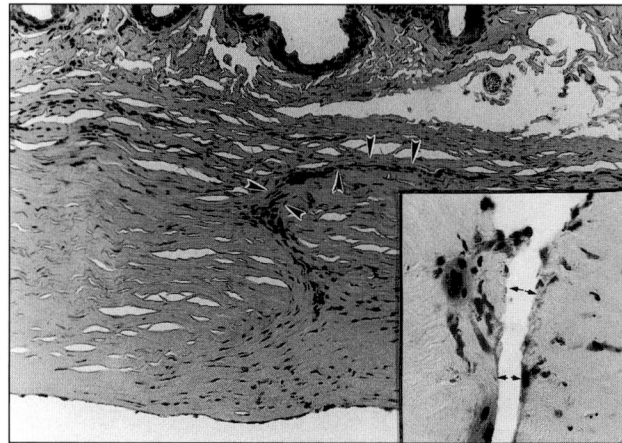

FIGURE 17-3 Invasive ab interno laser sclerostomy with sapphire-tipped laser scalpel. (Courtesy of Surgical Laser Technologies, Malvern, PA.)

FIGURE 17-4 Microphotograph showing site of closed internal sclerostomies 49 days after treatment.

tip in the subconjunctival space, and during withdrawal, the foot pedal is depressed again so that the tissue surrounding the tip undergoes further shrinkage, thus facilitating withdrawal of the laser. The average duration of time for creating a sclerostomy is 1 to 2 seconds and 9 to 10 J of energy is usually required to create a patent fistula. To prevent iris incarceration and to perform an iridoplasty, adjacent iris is usually treated with several laser applications. Bleb formation confirms free flow of fluid from the anterior chamber to the subconjunctival space.

The sapphire-tip probe is removed from the eye and the corneal incision is closed with one or two interrupted 10-0 nylon sutures. Subconjunctival 5-fluorouracil may also be injected in the quadrant 180 degrees from the fistula site. Five mg of dexamethasone phosphate may also be injected subconjunctivally. One drop of atropine sulfate, 1%, is also given. The eye is patched and shielded after application of a steroid antibiotic ointment (Figure 17-5).

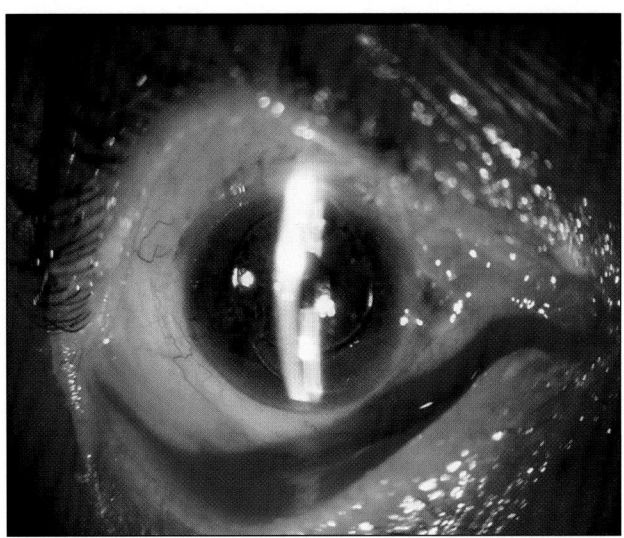

FIGURE 17-5 Immediate postoperative photograph of patient after undergoing ab interno Nd:YAG laser cycloablation.

TABLE 17-2   TECHNIQUE GUIDELINES FOR CONTACT LASER AB INTERNO SCLEROSTOMY

1. The patient is prepared and draped as for standard intraocular surgery.
2. Local or general anesthesia with a retrobulbar or peribulbar block is administered.
3. A 1.5-mm slit incision is made into the posterior edge of the cornea 180 degrees away from the site of the planned sclerostomy.
4. The anterior chamber is filled with a viscoelastic agent delivered through the slit incision.
5. The conjunctiva is ballooned up over the area of the stroma site through a balanced salt solution delivered through a 30-gauge needle.
6. The stainless steel sleeve and distal tip of the contact laser sclerostomy probe is introduced through the slit opening and passed across the anterior chamber to the angle 180 degrees away from the opening.
7. The tip of the sclerostomy probe is placed in contact with the angle anterior to the scleral spur and posterior to the insertion of the conjunctiva externally.
8. A muscle hook is used to pull the ballooned-up conjunctiva over the area of the stroma and to indent the sclera to make the sclerostomy perpendicular to the sclera. This procedure assures as short a sclerostomy tunnel as possible.
9. The power setting and time of duration of the power release depend on the size of the opening desired, patient considerations, tissue condition, and reaction of the tissue to the laser energy. When using the contact laser sclerostomy probe with a 200-μm tip diameter, it is recommended that the user begin each case with a power setting of 10 W and pulse duration of 0.2 s. If the desired tissue effect is not achieved at these settings, the user may elect to increase the power level by 1 or 2 W, but the power setting should not exceed 15 W. If the desired tissue effect is not observed at these settings, another contact laser sclerostomy probe should be used.
10. Typically, the sclerostomy should be achieved in two to three firings of the laser. After each firing, the sclera should be inspected externally for penetration. If thickness of the conjunctiva prevents visualization, use of the muscle hook to feel the probe may be helpful. Insertion of a cannula through the opening can be helpful in the final inspection. Further enlargement of the opening can be made at the discretion of the physician. The probe can be applied to the iris to perform an iridoplasty. Two to three applications should be adequate.
11. The contact laser sclerostomy probe is removed.
12. The corneal incision should be closed with one 10-0 nylon suture. If the surgeon feels that there is a high leakage rate and wishes to use a compression shell, this may be done.
13. The anterior chamber should be repressurized with viscoelastic delivered through the corneal incision.
14. 5-fluorouracil usually should be given at the time of surgery 180 degrees away from the sclerostomy site.
15. Injections of subconjunctival steroids and antibiotics can be given at the discretion of the surgeon.

Postoperatively, prednisolone acetate, 1%, is given every hour while the patient is awake. Atropine sulfate, 1%, drops are given twice a day. Subconjunctival 5-fluorouracil injections may be given daily for 5 to 7 days, then every other day for an additional 7 days. 5-fluorouracil injections should be discontinued if corneal epithelial defects manifest as a result of the injections. Digital pressure may be used if IOP rises above approximately 12 mm Hg or when bleb shrinkage is noted. Therapy with atropine drops is discontinued after 4 weeks and topical steroid therapy should be tapered over the next several weeks.

We performed Nd:YAG laser internal sclerostomy via the intracameral technique with 5-fluorouracil injection by the method just described in a pilot study. Nine patients with uncontrolled, advanced glaucoma participated in the study. All were aphakic or pseudophakic with poor vision. Each had previous failed filters with severe scarring.

Success was defined as an IOP of less than 21 mm Hg or a 20% reduction in IOP if the baseline pressure was less than 21 mm Hg. Good IOP control was achieved in four of the nine patients with gonioscopically visible internal sclerostomy openings and functioning blebs as evidenced by digital pressure. The mean preoperative IOP was 29 mm Hg (SD = 7.70). The mean postoperative IOP was 19 mm Hg at 3 months (SD = 2.59), 17 mm Hg at 6 months (SD = 3.03), 17 mm Hg at 12 months (SD = 2.67), and 18 mm Hg (SD = 3.10) at 18 months. The mean percentage change in IOP for all cases compared with baseline values was -40.17% (SD = 18.95%). The mean fall in IOP was 12 mm Hg (SD = 5.49). The follow-up period for all cases ranged from 14 weeks to 181 weeks, with a mean of 94.78 weeks (SD = 60.08 weeks). The difference in IOP compared with postoperative levels was statistically significant at 3, 6, 12, and 18 months.

No significant intraoperative complications were noted except mild-to-moderate hyphema in two cases, which cleared within the first postoperative week. A small sterile hypopyon developed in one patient (who had a previous history of uveitis and cyclocryotherapy) on postoperative day 2; the hypopyon subsequently cleared. Two patients developed choroidal detachments in postoperative week 2. However, neither of the patients required drainage. All of the patients received varying dosages of 5-fluorouracil injections and one patient developed a corneal epithelial defect due to the 5-fluorouracil injections that subsequently healed after patching of the eye and termination of the injections. The same patient developed a wound leak on postoperative week 37, which was successfully treated with cyanoacrylate glue, a symblepharon ring, and a glaucoma shield.

As stated earlier, four of the nine cases were considered successes (44.4%) and five were considered failures (55.6%). Three of the four patients with suc-cessful surgery required the addition of timolol, pilocarpine, or phospholine iodide for good IOP control. Out of the five patients with unsuccessful surgery, three opted for further surgical treatment with Nd:YAG laser cycloablation. Two of the three had subsequent good IOP control following the cycloablative procedure and one had to undergo repeat cycloablation during the following year. One patient declined further surgical intervention. One patient had pigmentation of the sclerostomy opening for which a repeat sclerostomy was unsuccessfully performed. All of the patients who had unsuccessful surgery had severe subconjunctival scarring with flat nonfunctioning blebs.

In our series, two types of probes with tip diameters of 200 µm and 400 µm were used. Interestingly, two of the three patients in whom 400-µm probes were used had successful outcomes, indicating that larger-sized probes have some bearing on the long-term success of maintaining a patent fistula. Retrospectively, it was also noted that patients who had successful surgery had been advised to perform digital pressure in the early postoperative period. This maneuver likely had a beneficial effect on fistula patency.

All of these patients were at high risk and all had had previous surgery, which contributed to the low success rate. Findings from our series of patients with complicated and advanced glaucoma are similar to those reported by Wilson and Javitt [17], who reported a successful outcome in three of five cases. In addition, the procedure is technically simpler and faster to perform than is conventional glaucoma filtration surgery in eyes with severe conjunctival scarring and previously failed filter surgery. In such eyes, seton surgery is also a viable option. However, considering the fact that pressure control can be achieved without the placement of hardware, in selected cases laser sclerostomy may be the preferred method of treatment.

Laser sclerostomy is a full-thickness procedure and has the attendant complications typically seen with conventional filtration surgery such as hypotony, serous, and hemorrhagic choroidal detachments. In addition, one may encounter the added complication of thermal tissue damage, however, this technique still provides many advantages over conventional filtering surgery. The procedure is much quicker than conventional glaucoma surgery. Filtration can be achieved without conjunctival dissection and its associated scarring. Multiple filtration fistulae can be created at one operative session and most sites around the lumbus are accessible. From the first day, the bleb is water tight, hence flat chambers occur less frequently. It is also easy to do iridoplasty following the completion of the sclerostomy, thereby minimizing the chance for failure because of iris incarceration.

The preliminary results of our pilot study are encouraging as are reports from other investigators discussed previously in the chapter. Clearly, however, our experience is limited and further refinement of the technique is required as well as studies on larger series of patients with longer follow-up periods before this procedure can be routinely recommended.

In the future, we can expect other laser modalities such as the diode laser as well as the adjunctive use of antimetabolites, such as mitomycin C to enhance survivability. Karp and coworkers [20] used the diode laser to compare the success of ab externo, ab interno, and conventional posterior sclerectomy techniques. Twenty-five New Zealand rabbits underwent filtration surgery in one eye and the fellow eye remained unoperated. Ab externo diode laser sclerostomy was performed in 10 rabbits; 10 other rabbits underwent ab interno laser sclerostomy and five rabbits underwent posterior sclerostomy procedures. The mean time to failure (defined as IOP difference measuring less than 4 mm Hg) for the ab externo, ab interno, and conventional techniques were compared. The respective times to failure were 17.4 (±11.5) days, 13.1 (±6.7) days, and 6.0 (±3.1) days respectively. The ab externo laser group was statistically more successful than the conventional group ($P = 0.02$), however the ab interno group was not statistically significant ($P = 0.15$). This finding may result from more frequent complications in the ab interno group, which included conjunctival and corneal burns.

In a subsequent experiment, mitomycin C was applied transconjunctivally on rabbits before performing ab externo diode laser sclerostomy [21]. This technique used a sponge that had been previously soaked in a 0.5 mg/cm^3 solution of mitomycin C. The sponge was then placed on top of the conjunctiva for 7 minutes. The ab externo surgery was then performed. Succulent blebs were seen in this group of rabbits beyond 7 days that were not seen in a group of rabbits that did not receive mitomycin C. Theoretically, mitomycin C can be used in a transconjunctival manner for ab interno surgery. The advantage of this modality is that the mitomycin C can be readily irrigated away, is unlikely to enter the eye, and is easily controlled by the surgeon. Future use of this antimetabolite or others may enhance the success of ab interno laser sclerostomy.

REFERENCES AND RECOMMENDED READING

Recently published papers of particular interest have been highlighted as:
- Of interest
- •• Of outstanding interest

1. Maumenee AE: External filtering operation for glaucoma; the mechanisms of function and failure. *Trans Am Acad Ophthalmol Soc* 1960, 58:319.

2. Addicus EM, Quigley HA, Green WR, *et al.*: Histologic characteristics of filtering blebs in glaucomatous eyes. *Arch Ophthalmol* 1983, 101:795.

3. Brown RH, Lynch MG, Denlam DB, *et al.*: Internal sclerostomy with an automated trephine for advanced glaucoma. *Ophthalmology* 1980, 95:728.

4.• March WF, Gherezghiher T, Koss MC, *et al.*: Experimental YAG laser sclerostomy. *Arch Ophthalmol* 1985, 103:1543.
In this study, a Q-switched Nd:YAG laser was used to create a corneoscleral perforation in human cadaver eyes. Minimal total energy required for perforation was 3.312 mJ, but "optimal" perforation required 26.676 mJ.

5. Gherezghiher T, March WF, Koss MC, *et al.*: Neodymium:YAG laser sclerostomy in primates. *Arch Ophthalmol* 1985, 103:1543.

6. March WF: Long-term follow-up of patients undergoing laser sclerostomy. *Ophthalmic Laser Therapy* 1987, 2:161.

7.•• Latina MA, Dobrogowski M, March WF, *et al.*: Laser sclerostomy by pulsed dye laser and goniolens. *Arch Ophthalmol* 1990, 108:1745.
Methylene blue dye, 1%, with an absorption peak of 668 nm was used to enhance the optical absorption of sclera via iontophoresis in 54 Dutch-belted rabbit eyes. Using a µs pulse-dye laser full-thickness fistulae were successfully created in 80% of treated eyes.

8.•• Latina MA, Melamed S, March WF, *et al.*: Gonioscopic ab interno laser sclerostomy. A pilot study in glaucoma patient. *Ophthalmology* 1992, 99:1736.
Gonioscopic delivery of pulsed laser energy to methylene blue enhanced sclera achieved complete sclerostomies in 55% of eyes with an acute mean reduction in IOP of 23 mm Hg.

9. Melamed S, Solomon A, Neumann D, *et al.*: Internal sclerostomy using laser ablation of dyed sclera in glaucoma patients. A pilot study. *Br J Ophthalmol* 1993, 77:139.

10. Saraff D, Lee DA: Iontophoresis of reactive black 5 for pulsed dye laser sclerostomy. *J Ocul Pharmacol* 1993, 9:25.

11. Gaasterland DE, Hennings DR, Boutacoff TA, *et al.*: Ab interno and ab externo filtering operations by laser contact surgery. *Ophthalmic Surg* 1987, 18:254.

12. Jaffe GJ, Mieler WF, Radius RF, *et al.*: Ab interno sclerostomy with a high-powered argon endolaser. *Am J Ophthalmol* 1988, 106:391.

13.•• Shahinian L, Eabert PR, Williams S: Histologic study of healing after ab interno laser sclerostomy. *Am J Ophthalmol* 1992, 114:216.
Histologic characteristics of a healing ab interno laser sclerostomy created in a human eye by a KTP 532 green laser coupled to a

300-µm quartz fiberoptic probe were studied. A 300-µm zone of acellular thermal damage was observed. A thick episcleral scar capped the sclerostomy.

14.•• Higginbotham EJ, Kao G, Peymen G: Internal sclerostomy with the Nd:YAG contact laser versus thermal sclerostomy in rabbits. *Ophthalmology* 1988, 95:385.

Fifteen rabbits underwent internal laser sclerostomy in one eye. The cumulative probability of success was greater in the laser-treated group than the standard surgical group.

15. Liu SF, Higginbotham EJ. Contact Nd:YAG laser internal sclerostomy in aphakic eyes. Initial experience. *Ophthalmology* 1989, (suppl):125.

16. Javitt JC, O'Connor SC, Wilson RP, *et al.*: Laser sclerostomy ab interno using a continuous wave Nd:YAG laser. *Ophthalmic Surg* 1989, 20:552.

17. Wilson RP, Javitt JC: Ab interno laser sclerostomy in aphakic patients with glaucoma and chronic inflammation. *Am J Ophthalmol* 1990, 110:178.

18. Berlin MS, Rajacich G, Duffy M, *et al.*: Excimer laser photoablation in glaucoma filtering surgery. *Am J Ophthalmol* 1987, 103:713.

19. Hill RA, Ozler SA, Baerveldt G, *et al.*: Ab interno Er:YAG laser sclerostomies in a rabbit model. *Ophthalmic Surg* 1992, 23:192.

20. Karp CL, Higginbotham EJ, Edward DP, *et al.*: Diode laser surgery: ab interno and ab externo versus conventional surgery in rabbits. *Ophthalmology* 1993, 100:1567.

21. Karp CL, Higginbotham EJ, Griffin EO, *et al.*: Adjunctive use of mitomycin-C in ab externo diode laser sclerostomy surgery in rabbits. *Invest Ophthalmol Vis Sci* 1992, 33(suppl):1267.

SELECT BIBLIOGRAPHY

Latina MA, Charles J-B: Laser filtration surgery. In *Principles and Practice of Ophthalmology*. Edited by Albert DM, Jakobiec FA. Philadelphia: WB Saunders; 1994:1609–1618.

Ledderer CM Jr, Thomas JV: Laser surgery for glaucoma. In *Glaucoma Surgery*. Edited by Thomas JV, Belcher CD III, Simmons RJ. St. Louis: Mosby Year Book; 1992:157–194.

Oh YG, Rosenquist RC. Laser treatment in glaucoma. In *Management of Difficult Glaucoma*. Edited by Higginbotham EJ, Lee DA. London: Blackwell Scientific Publications; 1993:299–315.

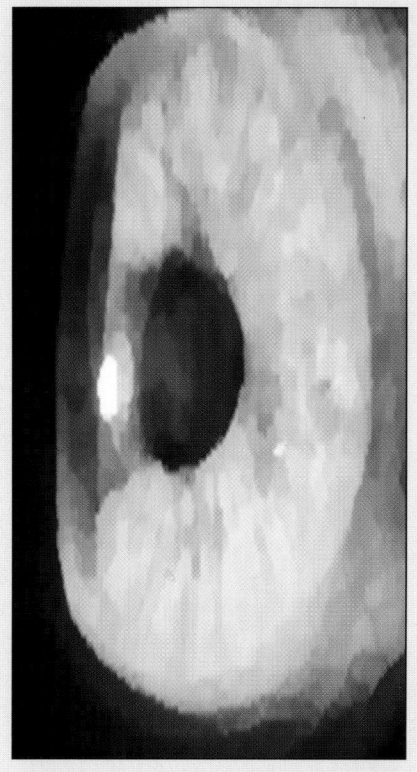

CHAPTER 18

AB EXTERNO LASER SCLEROSTOMY

HOWARD S. BARNEBEY

Over the past decade, various approaches have been proposed to use light energy via a laser to create a sclerostomy. Argon, neodymium-yttrium aluminum garnet (Nd:YAG), diode, and, more recently, holmium-yttrium aluminum garnet (Ho:YAG) lasers have been used to fashion fistulas. Although open to controversy, the Ho:YAG laser has achieved the greatest acceptance to date. Before detailing the current experience with this new laser technology, a review of literature affords a balanced perspective to understand why laser sclerostomy has such universal appeal.

COMPARISON WITH TRABECULECTOMY

The traditional standard of surgical glaucoma care is the trabeculectomy modified by Cairns [1]. The trabeculectomy technique championed a guarded opening that reduced the frequency of complications that were experienced with unguarded procedures (thermal sclerostomy, Scheie procedure, posterior lip sclerectomy, or trephine procedures). Postoperative problems such as flat chambers, choroidal effusions, and choroidal hemorrhage occurred less frequently. This advantage was offset by the observation that postoperative control of intraocular pressure (IOP) was not good [2–4].

As surgeons became more experienced with trabeculectomy procedures, it became apparent that many of the surgical failures were related to scarring external to the scleral flap at the level of tendons and conjunctival tissues [5]. This discovery of external fibrosis provoked a significant interest in reducing the postoperative healing response, which culminated with the introduction of wound-healing modulation [6]. Heparin,

colchicine, corticosteroids, and, more recently, 5-fluorouracil and mitomycin C have been used intraoperatively and postoperatively to reduce the acute and delayed postoperative inflammatory response. The use of these medications, in particular 5-fluorouracil and mitomycin C, have reintroduced many of the complications that the trabeculectomy procedure was designed to avoid; however, the success rate has improved significantly.

APPEAL OF AB EXTERNO LASER SCLEROSTOMY

The appeal of using lasers to create a small full-thickness opening is the opportunity to minimize the manipulation of conjunctival tissues and thus, the stimulus for wound healing. The creation of a 200 to 300 µm opening may be small enough to obviate the complications of other full-thickness procedures where the opening is much larger.

Current technologic advances allow the trained surgeon to create a full-thickness opening using either an internal or external approach. However, the scope of this article will be limited to the Ho:YAG laser using an external approach.

PHYSICAL PROPERTIES OF HOLMIUM-YTTRIUM ALUMINUM GARNET LASER

The Ho:YAG laser probe delivers energy in the infrared region with a 2100 nm wavelength via a 23-gauge probe (Fig. 18-1). This particular wavelength has the advantage of cutting tissue with a high water content, such as sclera, by using a thermal response that mini-

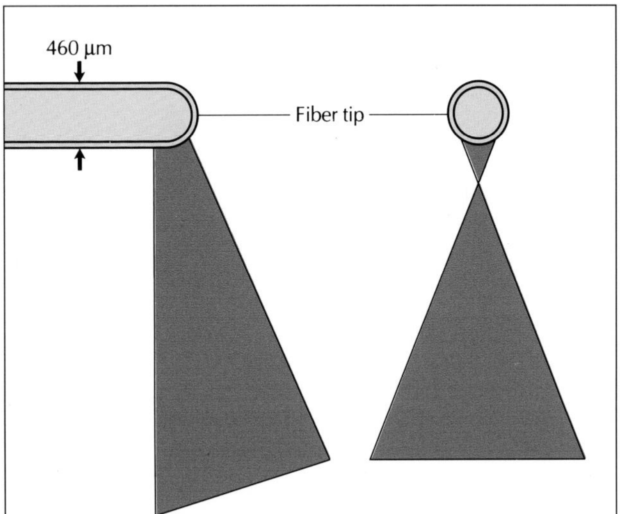

460 µm

Fiber tip

FIGURE 18-1 Schematic of holmium-yttrium aluminum garnet laser probe. This probe delivers energy nearly perpendicular to the probe axis.

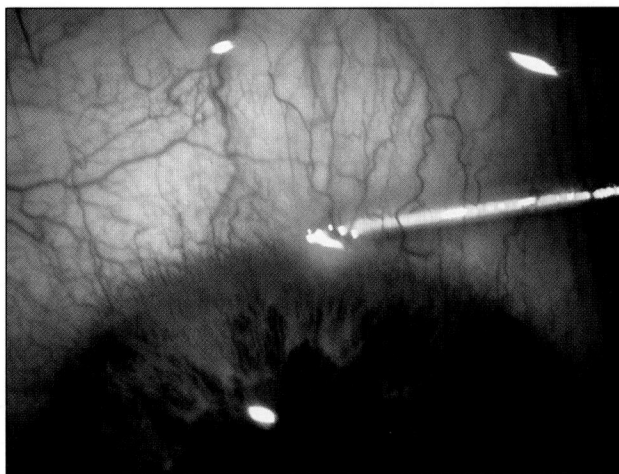

FIGURE 18-2 Holmium-yttrium aluminum garnet laser probe in proper position at the limbus.

mizes bleeding. The probe is introduced subconjuncti-vally through a needle-tract opening or a small incision and directed tangentially to the limbus (Fig. 18-2). A full-thickness opening is created with 20 to 40 applications with power ranging between 100 to 120 mJ with the 5 Hz solid state laser (Fig. 18-3).

ADVANTAGES OF LASER SCLEROSTOMY

Laser sclerostomy offers significant advantages over other glaucoma surgical procedures. The small size of the probe allows the surgeon to create an opening from the subconjunctival space to the anterior chamber with a minimal amount of tissue disturbance and bleeding. Eyes postoperatively treated with the Ho:YAG laser have less anterior segment inflammation than eyes undergoing trabeculectomy or posterior lip sclerecto-my. With less manipulation of conjunctival tissue, there is less inflammation induced from the procedure, and therefore, theoretically less risk of surgical failure from subconjunctival scarring (Fig. 18-4).

The design of the probe allows the surgeon to create openings in areas of the surgical limbus that are difficult to assess. This ability is especially helpful for patients who have conjunctival scarring from prior surgeries or trauma. In these patients, it is possible to create a sclerostomy where only a limited area of conjunctiva can be mobilized (Fig. 18-5).

One clear-cut advantage of laser sclerostomy is the reduced postoperative inflammation observed in eyes treated with the Ho:YAG laser. These eyes have less anterior chamber cells and flare as well as less conjunctival vascular injection in the immediate postoperative period compared with eyes treated surgically with a trabeculectomy. Following surgery, most patients experience a transient period of visual blurring. Visual

recovery is quicker than following trabeculectomy procedures. This procedure can be performed in less time than trabeculectomy and can be done in the office setting as well as in ambulatory surgical centers, which reduces intraoperative time and provides significant cost savings.

DISADVANTAGES OF LASER SCLEROSTOMY

Despite the advantages of laser sclerostomy, there are understandingly disadvantages as well. The procedure as currently performed creates a full-thickness opening into the anterior chamber. Therefore, the complications occurring from a full-thickness opening are present. These complications include hypotony, flat chamber, and choroidal effusions. The occurrence of these problems is less frequent than observed following other surgical procedures. It has been suggested that a smaller sclerostomy opening created with the laser compared with sclerostomies formed with a trephine, punch, or cautery minimizes the likelihood of these complications.

It has been surprising that the most consistent aspect of the procedure, in my experience, is formation of the sclerostomy opening. The creation of a full-thickness opening has not been a significant impediment, but rather, the problem has been maintaining the patency

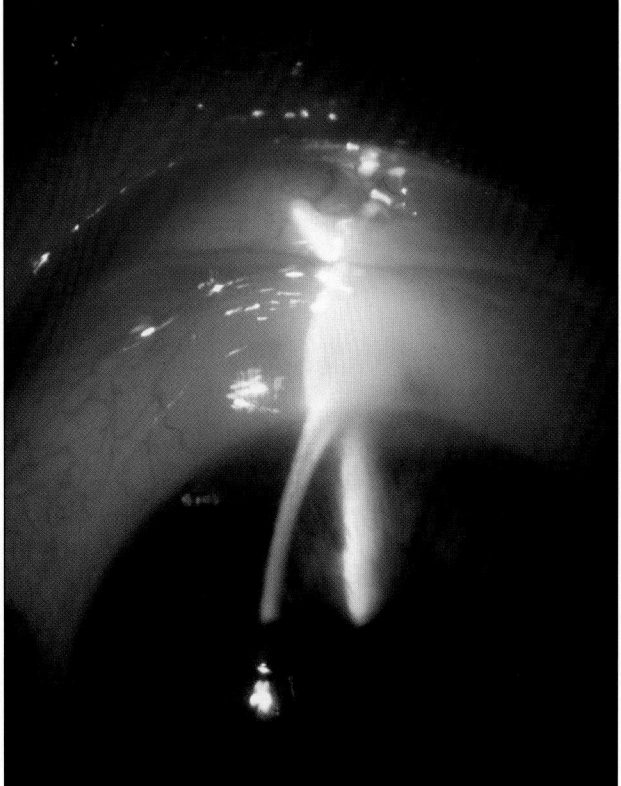

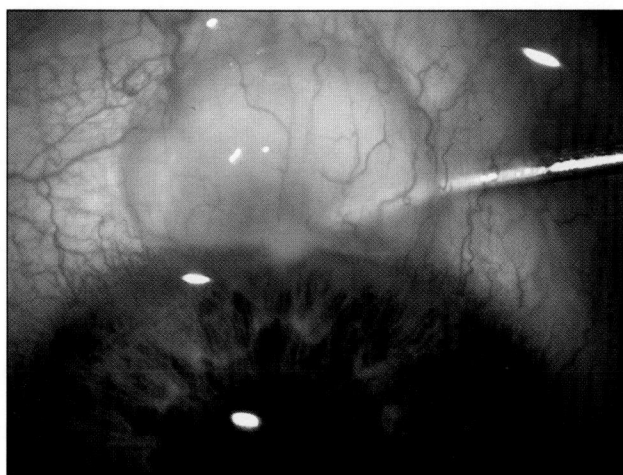

FIGURE 18-3 Conjunctival filtering bleb developed immediately following removal of laser probe, which confirms patency of sclerostomy.

FIGURE 18-4 Diffuse conjunctival filtering bleb in a pseudophakic eye. The sclerostomy site is located at the 12 o'clock position, slightly right of the slit lamp beam at the limbus.

of the fistula in selected patients. The published experiences have demonstrated a failure rate of 40% over a 2-year period of follow-up. The laser procedure had a comparable success rate with trabeculectomy in patients who had increased risk for surgical failure, such as prior surgery, young age, or aphakia [7••]. The explanation for failure appears to be similar for both laser and trabeculectomy procedures, namely, external scarring at the episcleral level [8•]. Thus, the hope that less tissue manipulation following laser treatment would translate into a more successful outcome has not been the initial experience of some ophthalmologists.

MAINTAINING A PATENT SCLEROSTOMY

Another factor to be considered is management of internal sclerostomy incarceration. Because the laser makes a small opening, aqueous fluid dynamics require that the iris remain as far away from the internal opening as possible. Because of the close approximation of the iris to the opening, fluid flow through the relatively small opening is capable of drawing the iris into the sclerostomy opening (Fig. 18-6). When the iris is drawn into the opening, IOP rises dramatically, and unless the opening is reestablished, the sclerostomy opening will occlude externally as well. To prevent this problem from occurring, several approaches have been tried, including pretreating the iris with laser photoretraction or iridotomy, intraoperative iridotomy or photoretraction, a second adjacent sclerostomy, or external compression with oversized bandage contact lens (Fig. 18-7). No one approach is foolproof, and eyes undergoing treatment need to be watched carefully during the first

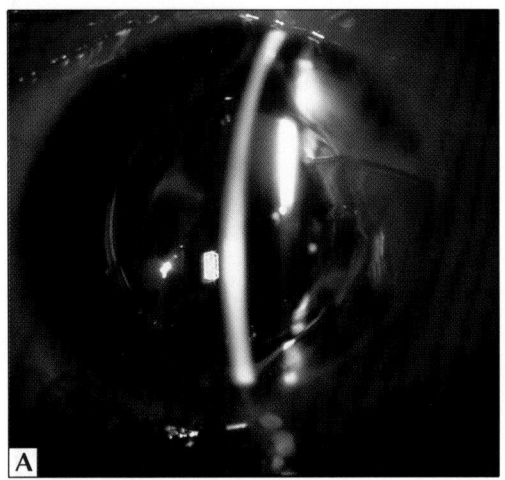
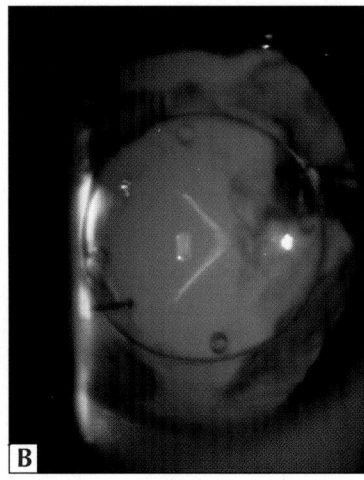
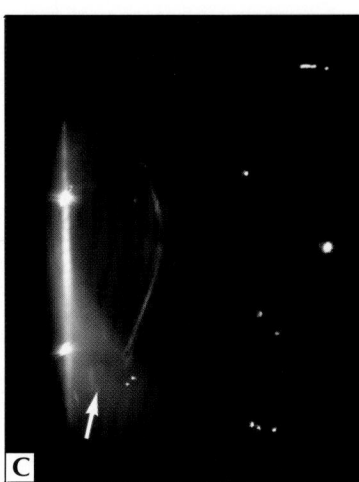

FIGURE 18-5 A, Slit-lamp appearance of eye following trauma and subsequent intraocular lens implantation.
B, Extensive conjunctival scarring left only 1-clock hour of available conjunctiva for a filtering bleb to develop.

C, Appearance of focal bleb temporally inferior 1 year following laser sclerostomy (*arrow*). Vision improved to 20/20 with an intraocular pressure of 9 mm Hg.

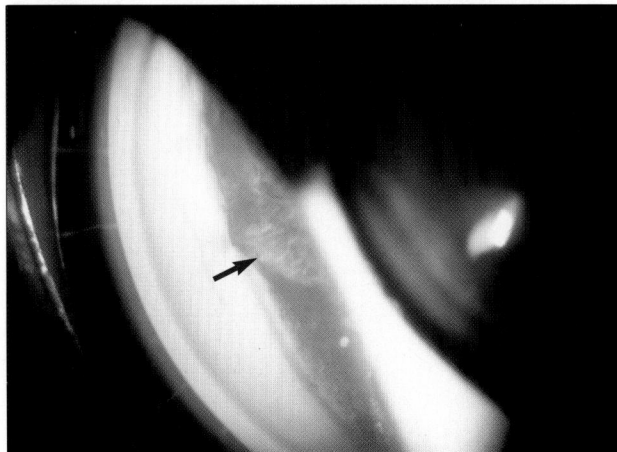

FIGURE 18-6 Gonioscopic view of sclerostomy with peripheral iris incarcerated into opening (*arrow*).

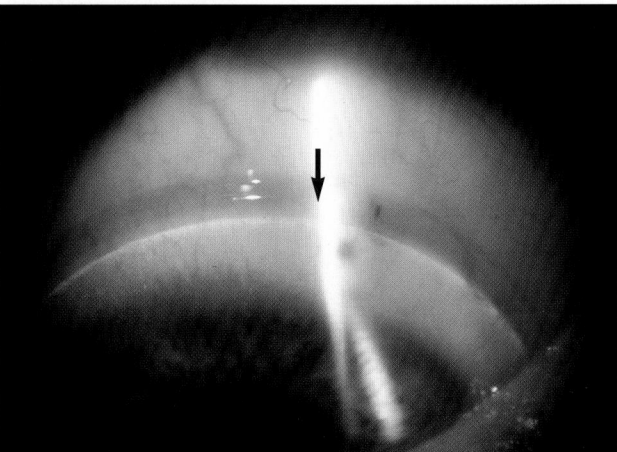

FIGURE 18-7 Oversized bandage soft contact lens positioned to bridge over the sclerostomy fistula, gently compressing conjunctival and tendon's tissues, thus minimizing hyperfiltration and hypotony. *Arrow* shows position of sclerostomy.

few weeks following treatment because iris incarceration can occur without warning. In my experience I have found it is unusual for this problem to occur beyond the first postoperative month, although it has been reported.

The sclerostomy opening may become occluded with other tissues. Although rare, a flap of Descemet's membrane, created at the time of the original procedure, can drift back to cover the internal opening with a transparent membrane (Fig. 18-8). If recognized as a potential factor leading to elevation of IOP, the problem can be solved by perforating the flap with the Nd:YAG laser. Finally, the Ho:YAG laser is capable of thermally inducing corneal striae and irregular astigmatism (Fig. 18-9). These striae can be quite striking, especially if the IOP is low. The effect is transient and diminishes as hypotony resolves. The Ho:YAG sclerostomy procedure has been carefully scrutinized since its introduction several years ago. In the process, much

has been learned about the limitations of the technique (*eg*, the iris needs to be treated to prevent postoperative sclerostomy incarceration). The result has been refinement of a procedure with success rates comparable to standard trabeculectomy.

Antimetabolites

I have discovered that the preoperative use of antimetabolites has profoundly improved the success rate of the procedure. Before creation of the sclerostomy, 5-fluorouracil has been used subconjunctivally in the selected sclerostomy site. Other surgeons have cautiously used mitomycin C in a similar manner preoperatively.

Future Development

Laser sclerostomy is an evolving procedure. This evolution is similar to what we have witnessed with conventional trabeculectomy surgery. There is little question among glaucoma specialists that the trabeculectomy of today is completely different than the similar procedure 5 years ago. Pharmacologic wound modulation (5-fluorouracil, mitomycin C), releasable sutures, and laser suturolysis are examples of the changes that are now part of the standard trabeculectomy procedure.

The intense postoperative monitoring differs little between the laser sclerostomy and trabeculectomy procedures. Initially, it was hoped that laser sclerostomy would require less postoperative vigilance because less manipulation was performed intraoperatively. Initial beliefs have not been proven; however, as new aspects of laser sclerostomy are refined, the postoperative requirements are becoming more predictable.

The experience with the Ho:YAG laser is rapidly maturing. As a by-product of this rapid learning curve, new questions are evolving (*eg*, laser-tissue

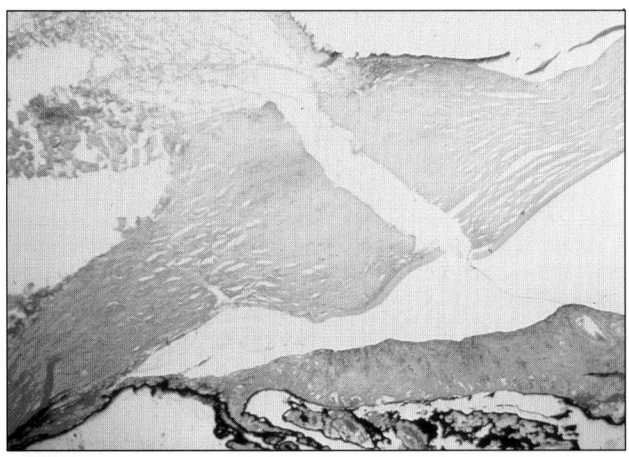

Figure 18-8 Histopathologic appearance of sclerostomy in a rabbit eye 3 days after procedure. In addition to scleral edema, there are areas of coagulative necrosis adjacent to the fistula. A small incomplete flap of Descemet's membrane is present at the internal opening.

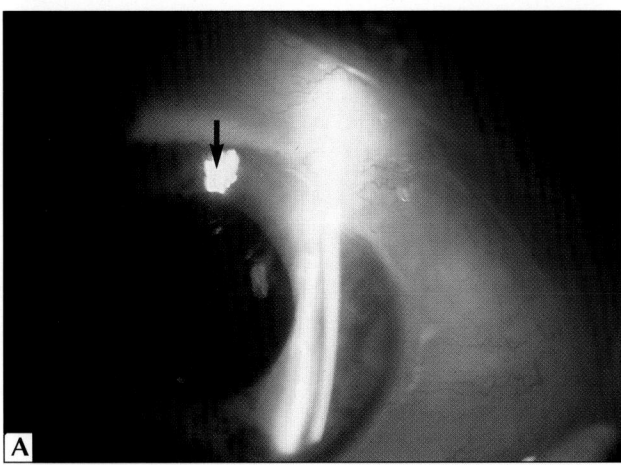
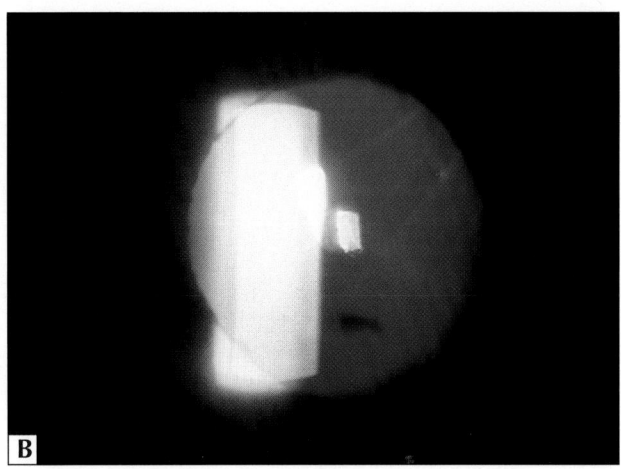

Figure 18-9 Corneal striae induced by sclerostomy. **A,** Direct illumination. **B,** Retro illumination.

interaction). The ideal tissue response has yet to be determined. Some surgeons believe that a laser capable of creating an opening with a thermal response will provide the best outcome, whereas others present cogent arguments for laser systems capable of establishing sclerostomy openings with little or no thermal effect. It is clear that whatever laser selected, the ultimate effect on success rate may be a function more of preventing external and internal failure, and less a factor of tissue response generated by the laser (assuming that the opening is of adequate proportions).

Conclusions

The Ho:YAG laser can successfully create a full-thickness sclerostomy via an ab externo approach. The success of the procedure is equally dependent on modulating wound healing as well as preventing internal occlusion of the sclerostomy opening.

References and Recommended Reading

Recently published papers of particular interest have been highlighted as:
- Of interest
- • Of outstanding interest

1. Cairns JE: Trabeculectomy: preliminary report of a new method. *Am J Ophthalmol* 1968, 66:673.

2. Lamping Ka, Bellows AR, Hutchinson BT, Afran SI: Long term evaluation of initial filtering surgery. *Ophthalmology* 1986, 93:91.

3. Spaeth GL: A prospective, controlled study to compare the Scheie procedure with Watson's trabeculectomy. *Ophthalmic Surg* 1980, 11:688.

4. Blondeau P. Phelps CD: Trabeculectomy cvs. thermoslerostomy: a randomized prospective clinical trial. *Arch Ophthalmol* 1981, 99:810.

5. Marmenee AE: External filtering operations for glaucoma: the mechanism of function and failure. *Trans Am Ophthalmol Soc* 1960, 58:319.

6. Gressel MG, Parrish RK II, Folberg R: 5-FU and glaucoma filtering surgery. I. An animal model. *Ophthalmology* 1984, 91:378.

7.•• Schuman JS, *et al.*: Holmium laser sclerostomy. *Ophthalmology* 1993, 100:1060–1065.
Success rate for Ho:YAG laser sclerostomy is identical to results for 5-fluorouracil trabeculectomy (73%). As expected, the laser sclerostomy complication profile is similar to other full-thickness glaucoma procedures. These authors noted a higher rate of choroidal hemorrhage (7/49) with 4/7 occuring in aphakic eyes. This rate is higher than other surgeons experienced in Ho:YAG laser sclerostomy have noted.

8.• Feldman RM, *et al.*: Histopathologic characteristics of failed holmium sclerostomy. *Am J Ophthalmol* 1993, 116:767.
Case report of patient who underwent a trabeculectomy 3 months after a laser sclerostomy. The site where the sclerostomy was created was patent internally, but occluded intrasclerally, thus inferring that healing occluded from the episcleral surface.

Select Bibliography

March W, ed: Practical laser surgery. *Ophthalmological Clinics of North America* Philadelphia: WB Saunders; 1989.

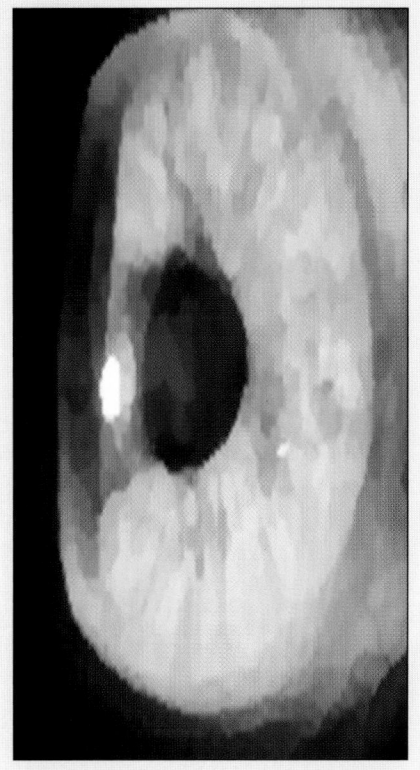

Chapter 19

Excimer Laser Filtering Surgery

Carlo Enrico Traverso
Massimo Corazza
Ugo Murialdo

This chapter briefly reviews the main technical and biophysical issues relevant to excimer laser surgery for the treatment of glaucoma. Results of recent research in animals and humans are summarized, and possible developments of these techniques are discussed.

Excimer laser radiation is able to remove submicroscopic layers of target tissue, with little or no damage to adjacent structures. Seiler and coworkers [1] and Berlin and coworkers [2] were the first to use the excimer laser for the treatment of glaucoma. Since their pioneering work, and despite the widespread availability of such laser systems around the world, a limited amount of clinical research on glaucoma has been published.

Ultraviolet radiation at 193 nm cannot be transmitted efficiently through fiberoptics and water. The target tissue must therefore be reached directly by the beam through air as it exits from the delivery system. Ultraviolet radiation at 308 nm can be transmitted by fiberoptic laser and allows delivery of the beam both ab interno, through the use of intracameral instrumentation, or ab externo, with or without dissection of the conjunctiva.

Collagen has spectral absorption that increases rapidly at wavelengths lower than 240 nm [3]. Peptide and carbon-to-carbon bonds have an energy of 3.0 eV and 3.5 eV, respectively; the 193-nm photon, with its energy of 6.4 eV, has sufficient energy to break those bonds. For glycosaminoglycans, absorption peaks at around 190 nm, and is not significant at 248 nm [4]. In the cornea, after exposure to a 193-nm radiation beam at 10 Hz, with up to 1 J/cm^2 fluence, a narrow zone of damage forms immediately adjacent to the tissue removed by photoablation. This area was measured between 0.06 and 0.3 µm in width and is called pseudomembrane (Fig. 19-1) [5,6].

Thermal damage can occur with excimer laser irradiation and is dependent on the target material as well as on wavelength, fluence, and repetition rate. A 193-nm radiation beam with a fluence of 200 mJ/cm^2 and a maximum repetition rate of 76 Hz will not cause a temperature rise of more than 11°C [7]. Energy levels commonly used for photoablative filtration surgery can therefore be kept within a thermally safe range. In nonpenetrating corneal ablations reaching as deep as 40 µm from Descemet's membrane, endothelial cell damage has been observed and attributed to acoustic waves [6]. In other studies, at the bottom of a photoablative filtration crater obtained at the limbus, such damage has not been visible in the trabecular meshwork of eyes from a human eye bank (Fig. 19-1) [1,8]. In another study of a rabbit model, 5 months after 193-nm excimer laser trabeculectomy, no mechanical or thermal damage was observed with scanning electron microscopy [9].

The 308-nm xenon chloride excimer laser can be transmitted via fiberoptic delivery systems. In human cadaver lenses, cataractous nuclei and cortical material could be ablated in one model, and a sharp decrease in fluence was observed as soon as the distance between probe tip and target reached 1 mm [10]. Laboratory work has shown that absorption of the excimer laser radiations of 193-nm argon fluoride and 308-nm xenon chloride in balanced salt solution, sodium hyaluronate, and human cadaver eyes are considerably different [11]. In balanced salt solution, the 308-nm light was reduced by a factor of 10 after traveling 12 cm, whereas the 193-nm radiation was reduced by the same amount after traveling only 0.016 cm. Similar results were observed for sodium hyaluronate. When the excimer laser was applied to the cornea in cadaver aphakic eyes, incomplete corneal absorption causing diffusion to the posterior pole was noted with wavelengths of 308 nm, and complete corneal absorption was noted with those of 193 nm. With 308 nm, the intensity of the light was reduced by a factor of 10 after traveling the first 5.5 mm; fluorescence at the posterior pole has been observed, however, indicating that the 308-nm wavelength was also transformed into other (longer) wavelengths that traveled through the eye with minimal absorption. This experiment proves that the use of the 308-nm wavelength may expose surrounding eye structures to unintended radiation, with possible undesirable side effects.

INTRACAMERAL INSTRUMENTATION

Ab interno approach with full-thickness sclerostomy

A 308-nm excimer laser with a 400-µm-diameter fiberoptic was used to perform sclerostomies in human cadaver eyes and in rabbits [12]. In human eye bank eyes, scleral perforation at the angle occurred after the delivery of 1.4 to 1.75 J, ie, 80 to 100 pulses at a 20-Hz repetition rate, with 35 mJ/mm^2 fluence. In rabbits, after deepening the anterior chamber with viscoelastics, the fiberoptic was passed across the anterior chamber and the tip was applied to the angle opposite to the entrance site. The probe was slowly advanced as the sclera was perforated. When the instrument was withdrawn, the conjunctiva became elevated by the viscoelastic flowing from the anterior chamber. In this study, filtering blebs continued to function for up to 3 months postoperatively; sclerostomies remained patent throughout the study. The ab interno ablation of trabecular meshwork, with the purpose of creating an open pathway between Schlemm's canal and the anterior chamber, was successfully achieved in enucleated eyes [13]. When using a quartz fiber, both 308- and 248-nm radiation beams were directed to the trabecular meshwork; histologically confirmed pores were obtained with energy levels of 0.3 to 1.5 mJ.

Although ab interno techniques require intraocular maneuvers, their use might be advantageous, especially because the surgical manipulation of conjunctiva is avoided. Ideally, radiation damage should be limited to the target area, with no thermal effects on iris, lens, or conjunctiva. One drawback, common to all photoablation procedures, is the lack of hemostasis with the possibility of intraoperative or postoperative hemorrhage. Also, excimer lasers with wavelengths longer than 193 nm have increasing thermal effects and depth of penetration; their potential for genetic material damage, absent when using the 193-nm radiation beam, has also been demonstrated [14,15].

Ab externo approach with partial-thickness sclerostomy and photoablative sinusotomy

The idea of removing layers of limbal tissue overlying Schlemm's canal, leaving the trabecular meshwork in place, was first adopted for use in sinusotomies and nonpenetrating trabeculectomies [16–18]. Both techniques aimed at a causal treatment of elevated intraocular pressure (IOP) in open-angle glaucoma by removing the sites of aqueous outflow resistance in the sclera, the juxtacanalicular tissue, and the outer wall of Schlemm's canal. Also, both techniques avoided penetration of the anterior chamber and sudden globe decompression during surgery. Although success rates were similar to those with trabeculectomy, flat anteri-

or chamber and choroidal detachment were reported as absent or rare [16–18]. The difficulty in manually dissecting limbal and juxtacanalicular tissue was probably the factor that limited the widespread adoption of this surgical approach.

The availability of excimer lasers to perform a no-touch removal of thin layers of eye tissue renewed the interest for this type of cause-oriented glaucoma surgery. The early work involving partial-thickness filtration surgery with the 193-nm excimer laser showed, on perfused human eyes, a threefold increase in outflow capacity obtained with the photoablative removal of limbal tissue extended down to but not through the trabecular meshwork; considering the small size of the crater (0.8 x 2 mm), the localized increase in outflow obtained experimentally was about 60 times greater [1]. Histologic and electron microscopic samples from 193-nm excimer laser photoablative sinusotomies have shown well-defined craters, with their bottoms reaching the Schlemm's canal area without perforation of the meshwork and no distortion of adjacent structures; the typical "pseudomembrane" of electron-dense deposits was seen covering the walls of the crater (Fig. 19-1) [19••]. The first clinical trials of this procedure gave encouraging results. The surgical technique, displayed in Figure 19-2, is as follows. After topical proparacaine anesthesia is administered, a peribulbar or subconjunctival injection of plain xylocaine 2% is given, and the eye is prepped and draped. After positioning a lid speculum, a bridle silk suture is passed under the superior rectus muscle or intracorneally. A conjunctival flap, limbus or fornix based, is then dissected; the episclera is cleaned bluntly, and bleeders are

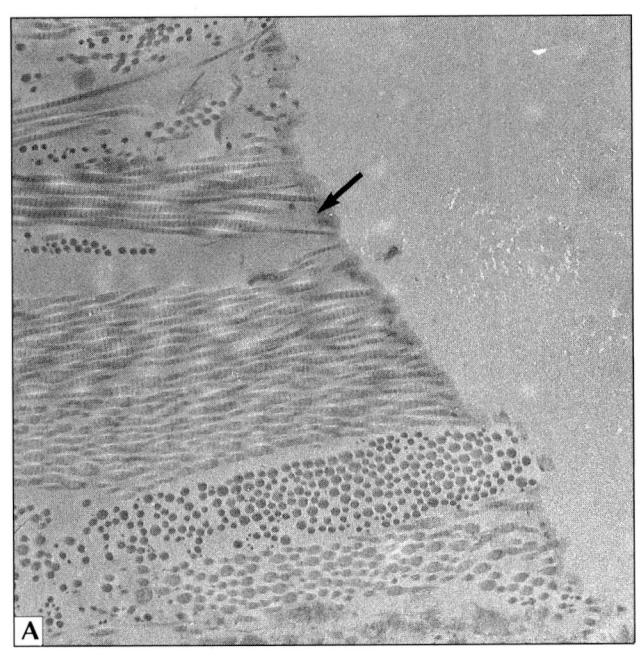

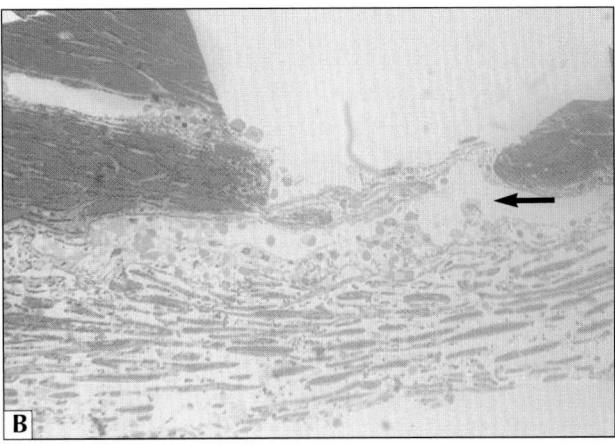

FIGURE 19-1 Photoablative sinusotomy. **A**, On freshly enucleated human eyes, the walls of the crater, examined with transmission electron microscopy, show a smooth surface lined with the typical electron-dense "pseudomembrane" (*arrow*). **B**, At the bottom of the crater, light microscopy shows the removal of limbal tissue down to Schlemm's canal (*arrow*); inner trabecular meshwork is undistorted.

cauterized. The laser beam needs to be shaped in the appropriate rectangular fashion; this can be done either with a built-in diaphragm or by using a custom-made metal mask with a rectangular central opening. The mask is eventually applied so as to leave its window on the limbal area to be treated. A 193-nm argon flouride excimer laser with 180 mJ/cm^2 fluence at 10 Hz is used. Photoablation is started while the field is kept dry with surgical sponges. When aqueous material appears percolating through the juxtacanalicular tissue at the bottom of the crater at such a rate as to hinder effective drying with sponges, the photoablation procedure is

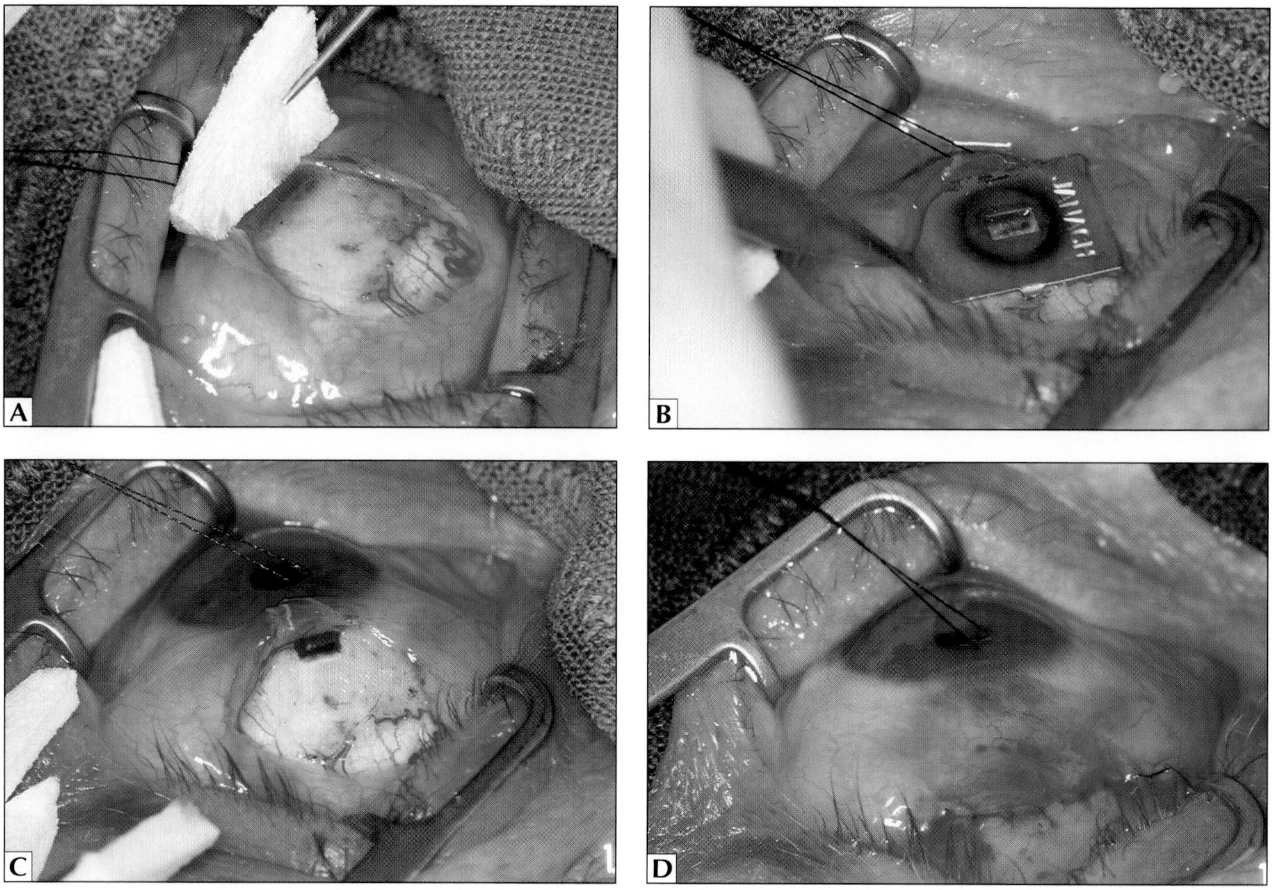

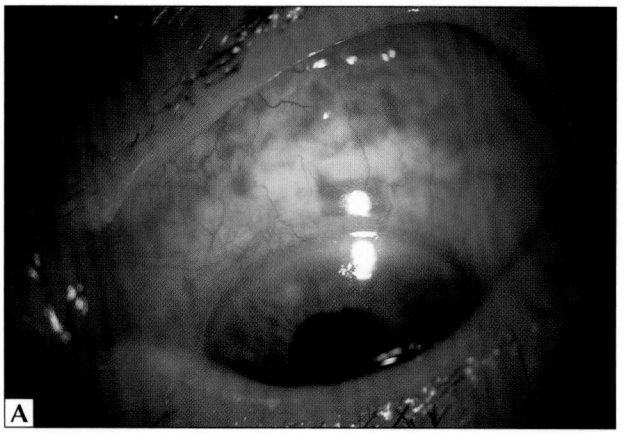

FIGURE 19-2 Photoablative sinusotomy. **A**, After placement of a corneal traction suture, a limbus-based conjunctival flap is fashioned. **B**, Photoablation is performed through a metal mask with a central 1.2 × 2.5 mm opening and is continued until aqueous percolates through the bottom. **C**, At the end, photoablation is partial thickness. **D**, The conjunctiva is closed water-tight, as in trabeculectomy. Note the normal depth of the anterior chamber throughout the procedure.

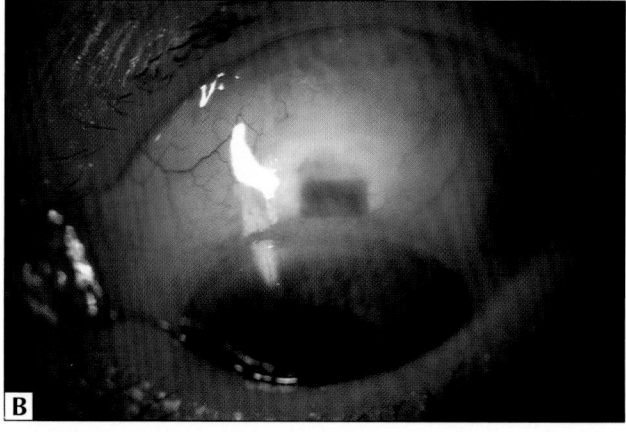

FIGURE 19-3 Photoablative sinusotomy. **A**, The day after surgery the intraocular pressure (IOP) was 2 mm Hg, the anterior chamber was deep with no reaction, and the conjunctiva was diffusely elevated. **B**, Eighteen months later the same eye has an IOP of 12 mm Hg with the patient taking no medication; the conjunctival filtration bleb is thin and diffuse.

discontinued. At the end, the conjunctiva must be closed water-tight.

In phakic primary open-angle glaucoma (POAG), short-term studies have reported success rates, defined as IOPs of 18 mm Hg or less with the patient receiving no medications, varying from 93% to 84%, with final pressures reported in the low teens [20–22,23•]. Despite average IOPs of well below 10 mm Hg during postoperative week 1, a maximum 6% incidence of

FIGURE 19-4 Photoablative sinusotomy, gonioscopic view. The rectangular area corresponding to the photoablative crater (*arrow*) has a ground-glass appearance. Note the integrity of the meshwork.

flat-chamber or choroidal detachment has been reported (Fig. 19-3). No anterior chamber penetration was observed gonioscopically in any case, and in all eyes that had successful results, an obvious conjunctival filtration bleb developed (Figs. 19-4 and 19-5). Inadvertent intraoperative photoablation or rupture of the conjunctival flap was also reported. To date, the most frequent complication is the adhesion of the iris to the trabecular meshwork in the area photoablated ab externo; this complication occurred initially in up to 30% of the cases during the first postoperative week (Fig. 19-6) [23•]. When iridotrabecular adhesion developed, the IOP suddenly rose and the conjunctival bleb disappeared; at gonioscopy, the iris had the typical pulled-up appearance (Fig. 19-6). In our experience, argon fluoride iridoplasty and neodymium-yttrium aluminum garnet (Nd:YAG) iridotomy were successful in detaching the iris from the meshwork; the conjunctival bleb immediately reformed and IOP returned to the low teens in all such patients.

Ab externo approach with full-thickness sclerostomy

A modified open-mask system incorporating an enface air jet to dry the target area during ablation and a conjunctival plication mechanism, allowing ab externo delivery of the 193-nm excimer laser beam to the lim-

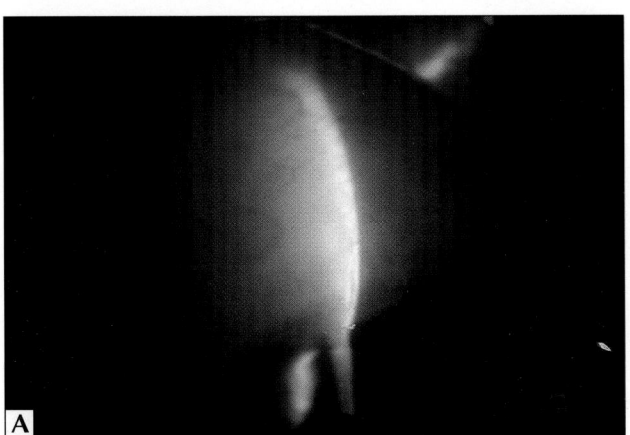

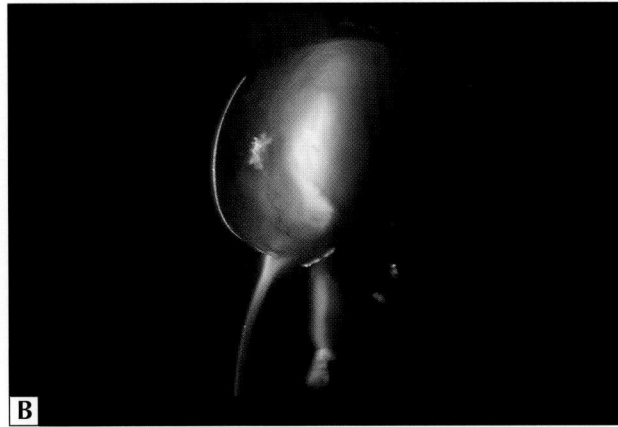

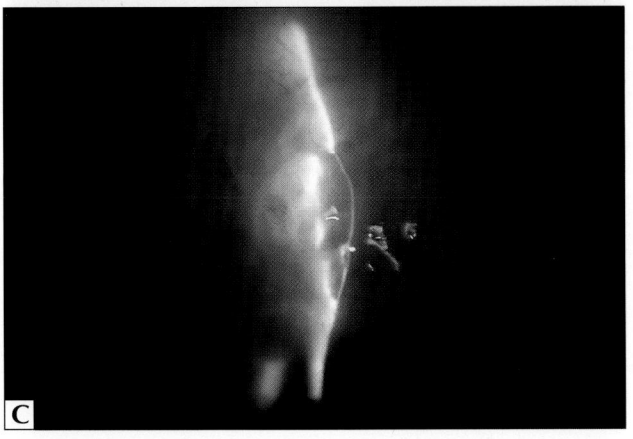

FIGURE 19-5 Photoablative sinusotomy: conjunctival filtration bleb remodeling. In successful cases the conjunctival filtration bleb can become **A,** succulent and diffuse; **B,** thin and elevated; or **C,** micropolycystic.

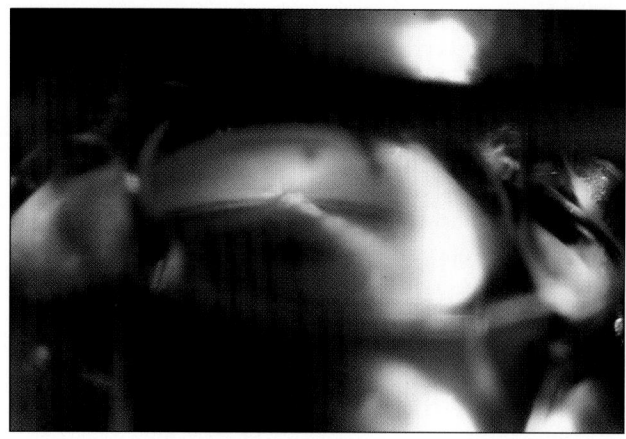

FIGURE 19-6 Photoablative sinusotomy, gonioscopic view. Early postoperative adhesion of the peripheral iris to the treated area.

bus without prior conjunctival dissection, was used to perform small-bore sclerostomies in experimental animals (Fig. 19-7) [24,25]. A subsequent therapeutic trial was conducted in pseudophakic patients with advanced open-angle glaucoma [26]. Six full-thickness sclerostomies (200-µm and 400-µm diameter) and three sclerostomies guarded by a smaller internal ostium were created in nine patients by 193-nm excimer laser ablation (fluence per pulse, 400 J/cm^2; pulse rate, 16 Hz; air jet pressure equal to IOP + 25 mm Hg). After a 6-month follow-up, IOP was controlled (≤ 16 mm Hg) in eight of the nine patients (six of nine without medication). Early postoperative complications included hyphema (from trace to 2.5 mm) in six of the nine patients, temporary fibrinous occlusion in four, and suprachoroidal hemorrhage in one. Con-

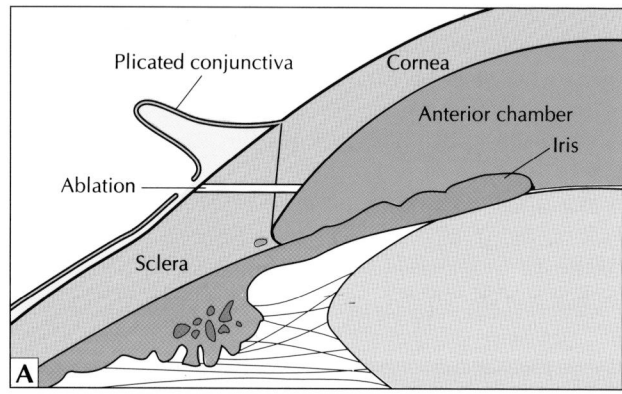

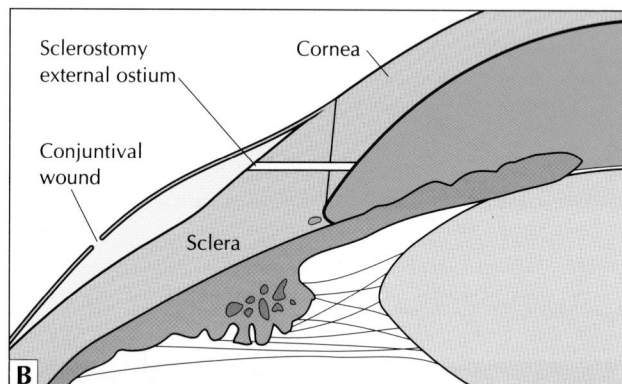

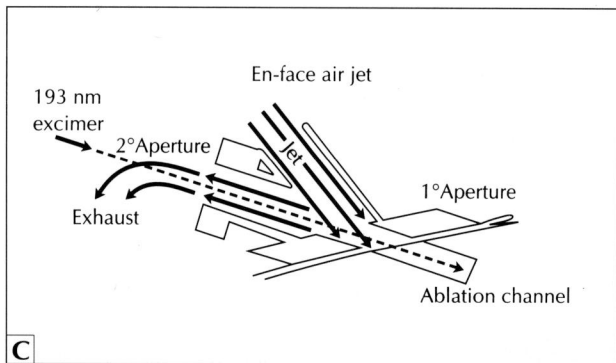

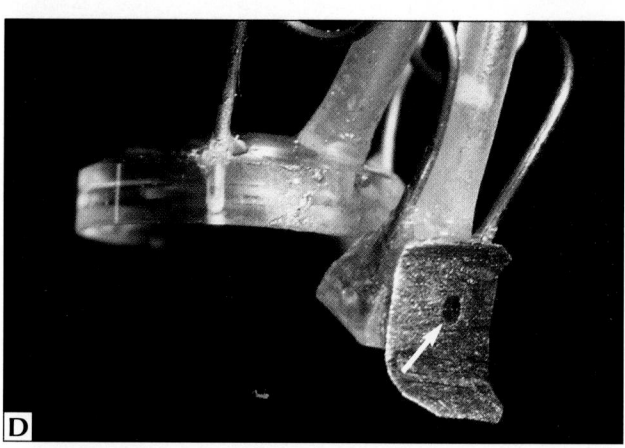

FIGURE 19-7 Ab externo full-thickness sclerostomy with conjunctival plication. **A,** The principle of conjunctival plication and through-and-through photoablation allows the photoablation at the limbus without dissection of the conjunctiva. **B,** The conjunctival hole is self-sealing. **C,** Because a 193-nm argon flouride excimer laser is used, an en-face air jet kept at 25 mm Hg above intraocular pressure is necessary to keep the target dry, remove photoablation byproducts, and promote hemostasis. **D,** The mask has a corneal vacuum fixation ring and suction tube connected to the main body where the outer aperture (*arrow*) is seen beneath the air jet tube. **E,** Another view shows the inner aperture (*arrow*) in the main body. To photoablate, the outer and inner aperture must be aligned over the target. (*Adapted from* Allan *et al.* [26]; with permission.)

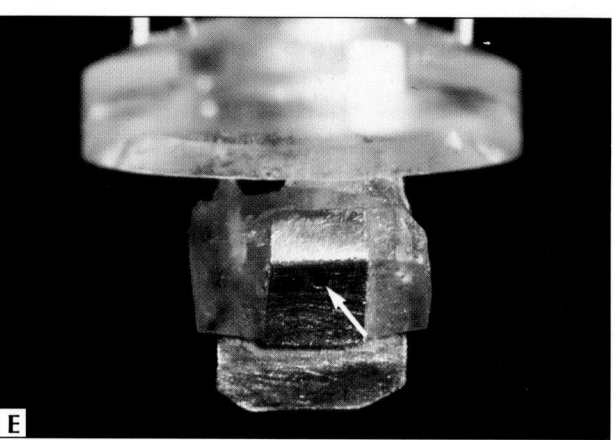

junctival laser wounds were self-sealing. This method introduces the concept of conjunctival plication rather than dissection, which has obvious theoretical advantages. Because small-bore laser sclerostomy procedures are functionally equivalent to full-thickness procedures, they can produce early postoperative hypotony, with an increased risk for suprachoroidal hemorrhage. For this reason, in three cases ablation was ceased at the moment of perforation in an attempt to leave a thin layer of tissue at the bottom of the 400-µm sclerostomy, where only a smaller-diameter internal ostium was obtained. This internal guarding, however, was not sufficient to prevent massive aqueous outflow. Any opening larger than 20 to 50 µm gives very little resistance to the aqueous flow, which is nil for all practical purposes. An interesting possible development will be the ab externo photoablative drilling of non-penetrating sclerostomies, to be eventually opened with ab interno Q-switched Nd:YAG laser applications via a gonioprism, thus allowing for a gradual and adjustable increase in outflow (Fig. 19-8).

In a clinical trial, the ab externo approach with minimal conjunctival dissection was used to perform sclerostomy in seven patients affected by secondary glaucoma [27]. A fiberoptic applicator of 0.32-mm diameter, introduced subconjunctivally and pushed toward the limbus, was used to transmit a 308-nm xenon chloride excimer laser radiation beam with 4 mJ per pulse at 80 Hz. Patients in this sample were awaiting enucleation for severe intractable pain caused by elevated IOP. In all cases the IOP decreased immediately and remained lower than before surgery with the patients receiving no medications, as reported at follow-ups ranging from 3 to 36 weeks.

CONCLUSIONS

In all types of full-thickness filtering procedures, it is important to prevent sudden decompression of the globe, anterior chamber flattening, and hypotony. Viscoelastics can be used to substitute for the aqueous material, thereby filling and deepening the anterior chamber; they facilitate intracameral manipulations, decrease unwanted contacts between instruments and eye structures, and favor hemostasis. From the purely hydrodynamic point of view, viscoelastics increase the time interval before the anterior chamber pressure reaches atmospheric pressure (Fig. 19-9). An injection in the sub-Tenon's space of viscoelastics before surgery dissects and elevates a bleb; a tense, full bleb may be the ideal environment in which to make the through-and-through sclerostomy, both ab interno and ab externo. Should the intrableb pressure be the same as the intracameral pressure, then the problems related to hypotony will eventually be eliminated (Fig. 19-9). The need for a paracentesis would be a drawback in cases of ab externo techniques, which are usually performed without anterior chamber penetration.

The ab interno approach is technically feasible with both the fiberoptic-guided 308-nm xenon chloride excimer laser or needle-guided 193-nm argon fluoride laser [28]. The latter, with an outer probe diameter of 1.1 nm and the need to be aimed at the target, might prove too cumbersome for intracameral use. For transmission of the xenon chloride 308-nm radiation beam, the tip of the fiberoptic must be kept in contact with the target because the energy level declines rapidly in water. Because the glycosaminoglycans are nearly transparent to 308 nm, most viscoelastics will also be unaffected [4]. It remains to be seen whether 308-nm

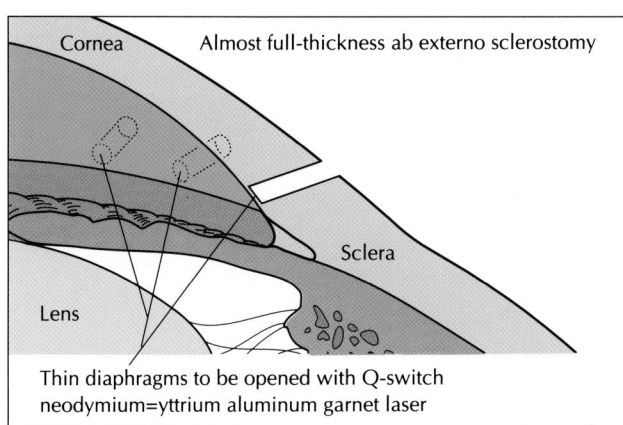

FIGURE 19-8 Staging of guarded photoablative filtration. First, partial-thickness sclerostomies are obtained. The thin diaphragms can then be opened sequentially with a Q-switched neodymium-yttrium aluminum garnet laser via a gonioprism.

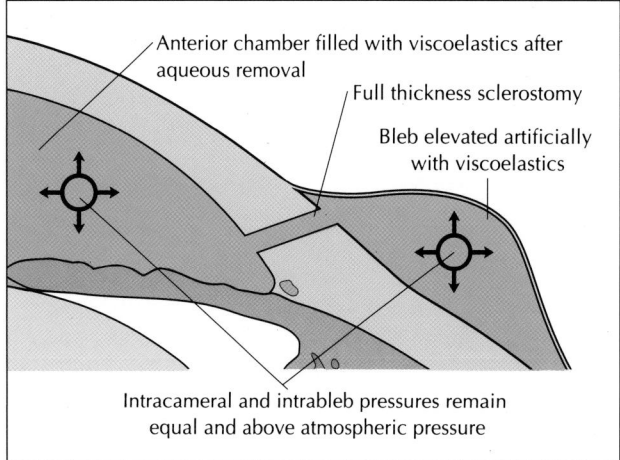

FIGURE 19-9 Possible uses of viscoelastics. Aqueous material is aspirated and substituted with viscoelastics, which are also used to elevate a tense conjunctival bleb. Even with full-thickness procedures, intracameral and intrableb pressures might remain equal and above atmospheric pressure, preventing or delaying hypotony.

xenon chloride lasers are safe enough to be used for ophthalmic surgery.

It is not clear whether ab interno ablation of trabecular tissue will only be effective in lowering IOP in POAG [13]. For primary developmental glaucomas with trabecular dysgenesis, this surgery should work similarly to a goniotomy or trabeculotomy.

Photoablative sinusotomy with the 193-nm excimer laser allows the controlled and progressive removal of 0.2-µm layers of tissue with no collateral damage to adjacent structures. The procedure is extremely precise and self-limiting. Collagen and glycosaminoglycans are efficient chromophores for the 193-nm radiation beam and the penetration depth of the photons is minimal. Because water does not transmit this wavelength, photoablative sinusotomy has a built-in safety feature: as soon as the aqueous material starts percolating from the bottom, further ablation is hindered, thus decreasing the possibility of having unwanted full-thickness penetration.

Photoablative sinusotomy or partial external trabeculectomy is the procedure that has been most extensively studied so far [1,19–22,23•]. Laboratory and clinical data clearly show the feasibility of excimer-laser photoablative sinusotomy for the treatment of uncontrolled POAG. The development in all successful cases of a conjunctival bleb supports the hypothesis of bulk filtration of aqueous material occurring at the site of surgery. When compared with our experience with trabeculectomy, short-term results have shown fewer postoperative complications—in particular, less flat chambers were seen despite the very low IOP recorded during the first postoperative days. At present we are treating failed cases at first with up to six subconjunctival injections of 5-fluorouracil, 5 mg; when the antimetabolite is not effective we resort to ab interno Nd:YAG laser treatment via a gonioprism, converting the procedure to a full-thickness operation (Fig. 19-10). Even though results are promising so far, problems are far from being totally solved or prevented. Cataract formation, long-term IOP control, and visual-field changes need to be addressed. Also, most patients operated on so far by us were excellent candidates for any kind of filtration surgery. The use of tissue plasminogen activator to avoid fibrinous occlusion of the filtration area as well as the titrated use of antimetabolites, already mentioned, also deserve to be explored in detail.

One interesting concept is the possibility of staging the filtering procedure. Several partial-thickness small-diameter sclerostomies or one sinusotomy with a larger bed could be made with precise and atraumatic photoablation techniques. Once the inflammation has settled down, the thin diaphragms remaining at the bottom of the craters could be perforated ab interno with an Nd:YAG laser, thereby creating small inner openings. An adjustable increase of outflow might be then obtained (Figs. 19-9 and 19-10). Antimetabolites could also be used to enhance bleb formation and further adjust the hydrodynamic result.

ACKNOWLEDGMENT

Vanna Re for bibliography assistance and Roberta Parodi for preparing the manuscript.

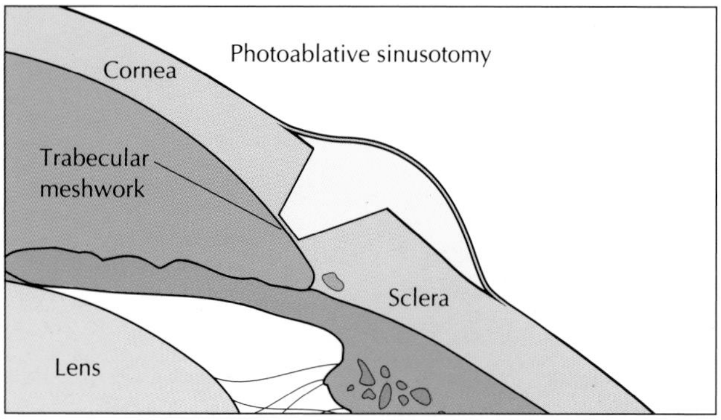

Photoablative sinusotomy
Cornea
Trabecular meshwork
Sclera
Lens

FIGURE 19-10 Photoablative sinusotomy. This procedure, also termed *partial external trabeculectomy*, or PET, is based on the ab externo removal of limbal tissue overlying Schlemm's canal. Photoablation is carried down to but not through the trabecular meshwork. If needed, a Q-switched neodymium-yttrium aluminum garnet laser can be used to increase the outflow further.

REFERENCES AND RECOMMENDED READING

Recently published papers of particular interest have been highlighted as:
• Of interest
•• Of outstanding interest

1.   Seiler T, Kriegerowski M, Bende T, et al.: Partielle externe trabeculektomie. *Klin Monatsbl Augenheilk* 1989, 195:216–220.

2.   Berlin MS, Rajacich G, Duffy M, *et al.*: Excimer laser photoablation in glaucoma filtering surgery. *Am J Ophthalmol* 1987, 103:713–714.

3. Loofbourov JR, Gould BS, Sizer IR: Studies of the ultraviolet absorption spectra of collagen. *Arch Biochem* 1949, 22:406–411.

4. Stone AL: Optical rotary dispersion of mucopolysaccharides: III. Ultraviolet circular dichroism and conformational specificity in amide groups. *Biopolymers* 1971, 10:739–751.

5. Puliafito CA, Steinert RT, Deutsch TF, *et al.*: Excimer laser ablation of the cornea and lens. *Ophthalmology* 1985, 92:741–748.

6. Marshall J, Trokel S, Rothery S, *et al.*: An ultrastructural study of corneal incisions induced by an excimer laser at 193 nm. *Ophthalmology* 1985, 92:749–758.

7. Bende T, Seiler T, Wollensak J: Side effects in corneal surgery: thermal corneal gradients. *Graefe's Arch Clin Exp Ophthalmol* 1988, 226:246–280.

8. Bertagno R, Murialdo U, Giordano G, *et al.*: Ultrastructural findings of photoablative filtration surgery in human eyes. *Exp Eye Research* 1992, 55:S44.

9. Aron-Rosa D, Maden A, Ganem S, *et al.*: Preliminary study of argon fluoride (193 nm) excimer laser trabeculectomy. Scanning electron microscopy at five months. *J Cataract Refract Surg* 1990, 16:617–620.

10. Maglen E, Martinez M, Grindfest W, *et al.*: Excimer laser ablation of the human lens at 308 nm with a fiberoptic delivery system. *J Cataract Refract Surg* 1989, 15:409–414.

11. Keates RH, Bloom RT, Schneider TR, *et al.*: Absorption of 308 nm excimer laser radiation by balanced salt solution, sodium hyaluronate, and human cadaver eyes. *Arch Ophthalmol* 1990, 108:1611–1613.

12. Müller-Stonzelburg N, von Haebler M, Buchwald HJ, *et al.*: Ab interno sclerostomy with the excimer laser via a quartz fiber in albino rabbits. *Fortschr Ophthalmol* 1991, 88:762–769.

13. Vogel M, Schever G, New W, *et al.*: Ablation of trabecular meshwork. *Klin Monatsbl Augenheilk* 1990, 197:250–253.

14. Green HA, Boll J, Parrish JA, *et al.*: Cytotoxicity and mitogenicity of low intensity 248 and 193 nm excimer laser radiation in mammalian cells. *Cancer Res* 1987, 47:410–416.

15. Trentecoste J, Thompson K, Parrish RK III, *et al.*: Mutagenic potential of a 193 nm excimer laser on fibroblasts in tissue culture. *Ophthalmology* 1987, 94:125–129.

16. Krasnov MM: Updated technique of sinusotomy (externalization of Schlemm's canal without scleral resection). *Glacoma* 1987, 9:166–168.

17. Zimmermann TJ, Mandelkorn RM, Kooner KS, *et al.*: Effectiveness of nonpenetration trabeculectomy in aphakic patients with glaucoma. *Ophthalmic Surg* 1984, 15:44–50.

18. Zimmermann TJ, Mandelkorn RM, Kooner KS, *et al.*: Trabeculectomy vs nonpenetrating trabeculectomy: a retrospective study of two procedures in phakic patients with glaucoma. *Ophthalmic Surg* 1984, 15:734–737.

19.•• Seiler T, Kriegerowski M, Patmore A, *et al.*: Partial external trabeculectomy with the excimer laser: an experimental investigation of a new treatment for glaucoma. *Lasers Light Ophthalmol* 1990, 3:97–109.

A landmark paper outlining the principle of partial external trabeculectomy. Light and transmission electron microscopy of human specimens are also shown.

20. Kuwayama Y, Takagi T, Tanaka M, *et al.*: 193 nm excimer laser partial external trabeculectomy [Abstract]. *Invest Ophthalmol Vis Sci* 1992, 33:1017.

21. Traverso CE, Murialdo U, Venzano D, *et al.*: Excimer laser photoablative filtration surgery for primary open-angle glaucoma. *Invest Ophthalmol Vis Sci* 1992, 33:1017.

22. Traverso CE, Murialdo U, Gandolfo E, *et al.*: Ab externo photoablative filtration surgery with the excimer laser for the treatment of primary open-angle glaucoma [Abstract]. *Ophthalmology* 1992, 100:134.

23.• Traverso CE, Murialdo U, DiLorenzo G, *et al.*: Photoablative filtration surgery with the excimer laser for primary open-angle glaucoma: a pilot study. *Int Ophthalmol* 1992, 16:363–365.

Results on 19 eyes are reported in this prospective clinical trial on POAG patients. With a median follow-up of 9 months (range 4–15) an IOP of 18 mm Hg or less on no medication was obtained in 84% of the patients.

24. Allan BD, van Saarlos PP, Cooper RL, *et al.*: Excimer laser microsclerostomy: an in vitro study of dimensional reproducibility [Abstract]. *Invest Ophthalmol Vis Sci* 1992, 33:1017.

25. Allan BD, Van Saarlos PP, Russo AV, *et al.*: Excimer laser sclerostomy: the in vivo development of a modified open mask delivery system. *Eye* 1993, 7:47–52.

26. Allan BD, Van Saarlos PP, Cooper RL, *et al.*: 193 nm excimer laser sclerostomy in pseudophakic patients with advanced open-angle glaucoma. *Br J Ophthalmol* 1994, in press.

27. Kampmeier J, Schutte E, Schroider D, *et al.*: Excimer laser sclerostomy for secondary glaucoma. *Ophthalmologe* 1993, 90:35–39.

28. Lewis A, Palanker D, Hemo I, *et al.*: Microsurgery of the retina with a needle-guided 193 nm excimer laser. *Invest Ophthalmol Vis Sci* 1992, 33:2377–2381.

SELECT BIBLIOGRAPHY

Allan BDS, van Saarlos PP, Cooper RL *et al.*: Laser microsclerostomy for primary open-angle glaucoma: a review of laser mechanisms and delivery systems. *Eye* 1992, 6:257–266.

Krauss JM, Puliafito CA, Steinert RF: Laser interactions with the cornea. *Surv Ophthalmol* 1986, 31:37–53.

Olson RA: The altar of high technology and the excimer laser. *Arch Ophthalmol* 1991, 109:489–490.

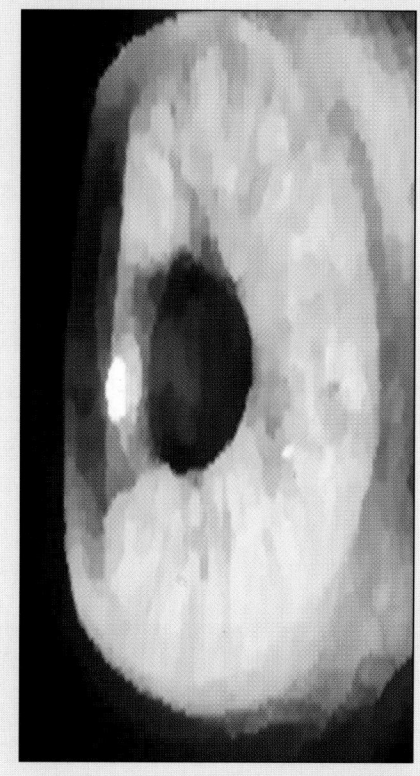

CHAPTER 20

REVISION OF FAILING
FILTERING BLEB

YOUNGHYUN G. OH

The success of glaucoma filtering surgery requires an intact conjunctiva and a patent fistula with constant flow of aqueous humor to maintain elevated conjunctival bleb postoperatively. The cause of filtering bleb failure can be classified as intraocular, scleral, or extraocular [1]. Late postoperative failure of filtering surgeries is most often the result of subconjunctival fibrosis over the fistula. However, failure can occur at the level of sclerostomy by proliferating membranes or intraocular tissues such as vitreous, capsular lens material, or the iris.

Numerous methods of reopening occluded fistula have been described [2,3]. Swan [2] advocated an internal approach with a goniotomy knife or needle to reestablish filtration. Since then, both argon and neodymium-yttrium aluminum garnet (Nd:YAG) lasers have been used either transconjunctivally or by gonioscopic internal approach with varying rates of success [3–11]. During the early postoperative phase, a patent fistula can be maintained by increasing filtration by laser suture lysis, with a minimal chance of a flat chamber. Various techniques of laser

application for failing blebs and the importance of careful patient selection are discussed with suggested guidelines.

ARGON LASER SUTURE LYSIS

Failing filtering bleb in the early postoperative period after trabeculectomy can be managed with either digital massage or laser suture lysis by increasing flow through the fistula. Laser suture lysis is not reserved only for eyes with signs of bleb failure, but is preplanned and used routinely to maximize filtration. This procedure allows a surgeon to titrate the aqueous filtration after trabeculectomy, reducing the incidence of early postoperative hypotony and flat chamber.

Indication

When there is inadequate filtration with elevated intraocular pressure (IOP) from tight closure of the scleral flap, dark nylon or proline sutures are selectively and serially lysed through an intact conjunctiva using the argon laser. It is safer to delay suture lysis until postoperative days 2 or 3 to minimize hypotony and flat anterior chambers. On the other hand, the immediate pressure-lowering effect is greatest for laser suture lysis during the first 2 postoperative weeks, and rarely after the 4th week unless antimetabolites are used in conjunction with glaucoma filtering surgery [11]. Suture lysis should be performed early in eyes with increased risk of early subconjunctival fibrosis, especially after reoperations, combined procedures, or with significant postoperative inflammation.

Technique

Whenever possible, it is better to preplan laser suture lysis at the time of trabeculectomy. If, in the surgeon's judgment, any of the individual sutures seemed to restrict fluid flow more than another, the "key" suture should be noted in the chart to aid in the selection of sutures for later lysis to achieve or avoid its maximum

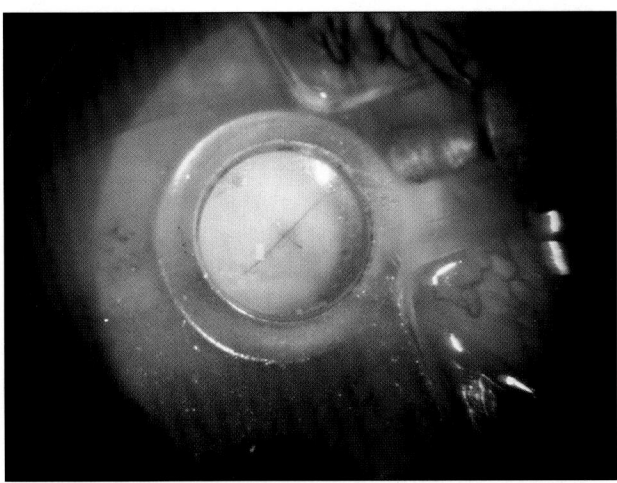

FIGURE 20-1 The Hoskins lens is applied to the conjunctiva overlying the scleral flap suture. (Photograph by Chris Oeinck)

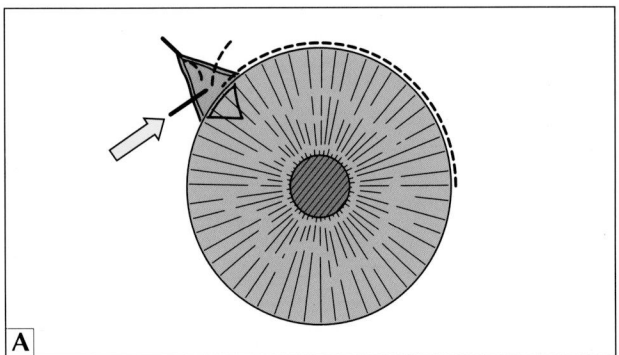

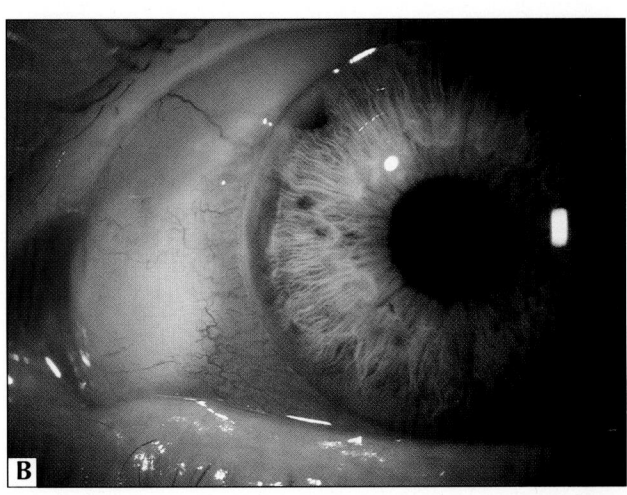

FIGURE 20-2 A, Laser suture lysis. Selecting a suture that is either too temporal or nasal may result in development of dellens. **B,** Laser lysis of a nasal suture resulted in excessive nasal filtering bleb with significant ocular irritations.

IOP lowering effect. Sometimes lysis of the "key" suture, which contributes more to aqueous flow resistance, may result in postlaser hypotony and flat anterior chamber.

The patient is seated at the argon laser and topical proparacaine drops are instilled. The Hoskins lens (Ocular Instruments, Inc., Bellevue, WA) or a rounded corner of a Zeiss four-mirror lens (Ocular Instruments, Inc.) is applied to the conjunctiva overlying the scleral flap sutures (Fig. 20-1). Gentle pressure against the sclera with the lens blanches the conjunctival vessels, allowing a clear view of the underlying sutures. Topical phenylephrine also improves visibility by constricting overlying vessels. After the tight suture is selected for cutting and the aiming beam is sharply focused on it, avoid focusing the laser too superficially on the conjunctiva. I prefer to cut the suture that is closer to the 12 o'clock position, especially when the fistula is located in the nasal or temporal quadrant (Fig. 20-2). When the aqueous flow is directed nasally or temporally, excessive filtering blebs in these locations may create a dellen with significant ocular irritations. Argon laser settings of 0.1 second, 50 μm, and 300 to 500 mW are used, gradually increasing the power to 1000 mW if needed. The suture is lysed with one or two applications (Table 20-1).

If the overlying conjunctival blood vessels are dilated or subconjunctival hemorrhage or conjunctival pigment is present, lower power settings should be used to minimize thermal injury to the conjunctiva. When there is conjunctival hemorrhage obscuring the suture, I have been using the krypton laser for suture lysis to minimize conjunctival burn because the red wavelength of the krypton laser usually does not affect conjunctival vessels unless very high powers are used.

The IOP is remeasured 15 to 30 minutes after each laser suture lysis session. When the IOP is not changed significantly after the procedure, focal pressure on the scleral edge of the incision using a digital massage potentiates the effect of suture lysis by separating the flap from the underlying sclera, thus encouraging outflow. Cutting more than one suture would increase the risk of hypotony and flat chamber.

The use of antimetabolites usually prolongs the effective period of laser suture lysis up to several months. Pappa and coworkers [12] reported that with adjunctive mitomycin C therapy, laser suture lysis was effective even 5 months after trabeculectomy. Postoperative 5-fluorouracil injections are not as effective as mitomycin C in potentiating the effect of the laser suture lysis, especially after the 4th postoperative week. As a general rule, I wait at least 1 week before laser suture lysis if 5-fluorouracil has been used, and 2 weeks for mitomycin C. However, if there are signs of early subconjunctival fibrosis with elevated IOP, laser suture lysis should be performed earlier, even if antimetabolites have been used.

Complications

The most common complication after laser suture lysis is hypotony with a shallow anterior chamber. Savage and coworkers [11] reported that the seven cases of postlaser flat anterior chamber in their series of 43 eyes occurred after lysis of two or more sutures in a single session or during the first 2 postoperative days. The delay in the healing process caused by antimetabolites would also increase the incidence of hypotony after laser suture lysis. A significant reduction of IOP can result in choroidal hemorrhages in susceptible eyes.

The risk factors for conjunctival perforation include high power setting of the laser, conjunctival hemorrhage, and very thin, ischemic bleb. Most cases of conjunctival perforation occurs when the power of the argon laser is set at a level greater than 500 mW, or with longer duration especially in the presence of significant conjunctival injection or hemorrhage. Eyes with conjunctival hemorrhage can be treated with a krypton laser to minimize the risk of wound leak. The leak tends to become persistent in ischemic, thin filtering bleb where mitomycin C has been used. Suture lysis with the Nd:YAG laser is also associated with a significant incidence of conjunctival perforation [11].

REVISION OF SCLEROSTOMY WITH LASER

Laser sclerostomy has recently attracted interest as a primary glaucoma filtering procedure because of its simplicity and less invasive manner. Both ab interno and ab externo techniques have been used to create a full-thickness opening of the sclera, using various wavelengths of laser. Similarly, the laser can be effective in reopening a failing trabeculectomy in a select small group of patients who have had initial success. Both argon and Nd:YAG lasers have been used either transconjunctivally or by gonioscopic internal approach with varying rates of success [4–10]. Patient selection is crucial to the success of this laser therapy. Patients who had well-established filtering blebs before the failure should be selected, and reopening should be attempted

TABLE 20-1	LASER SETTINGS FOR ARGON LASER SUTURE LYSIS	
Power		300–500 mW
Spot size		50 μm
Duration		0.1 s
Number of Applications		1–2

before subconjunctival scar tissue forms external to the filtration fistula.

Argon laser internal sclerostomy

The argon laser has been used by several investigators to reopen a failing trabeculectomy site via an internal approach [4,5]. Reopening of occluded filtering blebs was initially attempted by Ticho using an argon laser [4]. In his series, the time of occlusion of the fistula ranged from 2 weeks to 20 years with an average of 8 years after surgeries. Five out of 11 patients responded to argon laser treatment, with lowering of the average IOP from 34 mm Hg to 16 mm Hg and with increased size of filtering blebs. The IOP remained controlled during a follow-up period of over 1 to 2 years.

Similarly, Van Buskirk [5] described four failed filtration fistulas that reopened internally after argon laser applications. In all four cases, the fistula had become occluded internally by pigmented membrane after having remained patent for an extended period before occlusion.

Although 50% to 75% of the patients in these small series responded to treatment, the use of the argon laser is limited, because the target tissue must be pigmented to allow laser energy absorption.

Transconjunctival reopening of fistula

Transconjunctival reopening of fistula with argon or Nd:YAG lasers has been reported [6,7]. Kurata and coworkers [6] successfully reopened filtration fistula in three patients by using transconjunctival argon laser

photocoagulation. It should be noted, however, that all three patients had previously successful full-thickness filtering procedures. These patients later developed pigmented tissue blocking the external side of the fistula whereas the internal sclerostomy remained patent. Argon laser applications were delivered to pigment in the external region of the sclerostomy opening. This method may be considered in failed full-thickness procedures, but it would not be successful in failed trabeculectomy because the scleral flap scars over the external opening in the latter cases. The major disadvantage of this approach would be inadvertent perforation of the conjunctiva and poor visualization of the sclerostomy for laser application.

Yttrium aluminum garnet laser internal sclerostomy for failing bleb

The yttrium aluminum garnet (YAG) laser via the internal approach seems ideal to reopen occluded fistulas with minimal postoperative inflammation because of the laser's cutting ability even in the absence of pigmentation of the membrane. Several investigators have reported their case series of Nd:YAG laser treatment in reopening the closed fistula [8,9,10]. Their studies are summarized along with the results of previous works in Table 20-2.

Patient selection is crucial to the success of this therapy. Patients who had well-established filtering blebs before the failure should be selected and treated before subconjunctival scar tissue forms external to the filtration fistula. Careful gonioscopy should be performed to confirm internal obstruction of the sclerostomy.

TABLE 20-2	REVISION OF FAILING BLEB				
Series	**Method**	**Setting**	**Time since surgery**	**Success ratio**
Swan [2]	Gonio-incision with knife		1.5 mo–19 y	21/27
Yablonski	Ultrasound	10 kW/cm 2–4 applications	3 mo	15/20
Kurata and coworkers [6]	Argon laser, transconjunctival	0.3–1.0 W	4–8 y	3/3
Ticho and Ivry [4]	Argon laser, internal	1.0 W 200 applications 50 μm	9 y (2 wk–20 y)	5/11
Van Buskirk [5]	Argon laser, internal	0.8–1.0 W >15 applications 50 μm	3 mo–33 y	3/4
Cohn and Aron-Rosa [11]	Nd:YAG, internal	20 applications	3 mo	1/1
Praeger [10]	Nd:YAG, internal	3.5 mJ 300–500 applications	4–7 wk	4/4
Dailey and coworkers [8]	Nd:YAG, internal	0.7–8.5 mJ 30–70 applications	1 mo–26 y	5/9
Oh	Nd:YAG, internal	6.0–6.9 mJ	1 mo–22 y	6/10

Nd:YAG—neodymium-yttrium aluminum garnet.

Dailey and coworkers [8] used the mode-locked Nd:YAG laser to reopen filtration fistulas in nine eyes in which the fistula had become occluded internally. In five of the nine eyes, filtration was successfully reestablished, whereas in the remaining four eyes, filtration was not established because of external subconjunctival scarring of the bleb [8]. It was noted that the mean interval between filtration surgery and laser reopening was only 5 months for the failure group and was 5 years for the success group. Overall, the patients in whom filtration had been successfully established for at least 6 months responded much better [8].

However, Praeger [9] reported successful reopening of filtering blebs with early failure. Four eyes developed closure of the filtering bleb within the 6th postoperative week in his series. After 300 to 500 applications from the mode-locked Nd:YAG laser delivered at 3.5 mJ were directed to a membrane at the internal sclerostomy site, the bleb reformed in each case with significant reduction of IOP [9].

Our clinical series included 10 consecutive cases with an internal fistula that was noted to be closed with a membrane, pigment, or iris tissue. All patients had undergone trabeculectomy with well-established filtering blebs postoperatively, which lasted 3 weeks to 12 years before they abruptly began to fail. The average time interval between the YAG laser for reopening

of the fistula and the previous trabeculectomy was 36 months. The Nd:YAG laser was used with a gonioprism in all patients to reopen the internal fistula. The laser power was set at 6.0 to 6.9 mJ, aiming at the radial edge of the internal sclerostomy, which was thought to be the predominant filtration site before closing (Fig. 20-3). A total of 16 to 50 applications of YAG laser at the average power setting at 6.4 mJ was required to reopen the fistula (Table 20-3). The end point was bubble formation at the target site. When failing blebs are reopened with the YAG laser, successful treatment can be indicated by: 1) deepening of the sclerostomy, 2) pigment flowing through the sclerostomy, 3) elevation of the bleb, and 4) reduction of the IOP. Ocular massage was applied immediately after treatment to encourage filtration. The mean IOP was reduced from 29.4 mm Hg to 10.4 mm Hg immediately after the reopening of the fistula with successful control of IOP at 21 mm Hg or lower in six of the 10 eyes. Although a single treatment is usually enough to reopen the fistula, the procedure may need to be repeated, especially in patients with indocorneal endothelial syndrome syndrome with regrowth of the endothelial membrane over the fistula.

No complications from the Nd:YAG laser were noted in our series. Yet hemorrhage can theoretically be one of the possible complications. Pretreatment with argon laser is advised if large blood vessels are noted at the target site. Prywes [13] reported one case with ciliary body detachment and hypotony after attempted YAG laser repair of a failed bleb.

DISCUSSION

The equipment for laser procedures has become widely available, and the cost of surgical intervention is lower. The simplicity of these procedures also allows an advantage as they can be performed in the clinic rather than in an operating room.

When determining whether an attempt should be made to reopen the fistula, one should consider whether significant subconjunctival scarring has occurred. Either laser suture lysis or laser internal sclerostomy would be ineffective in reversing the course once external fibrosis of the fistula has developed.

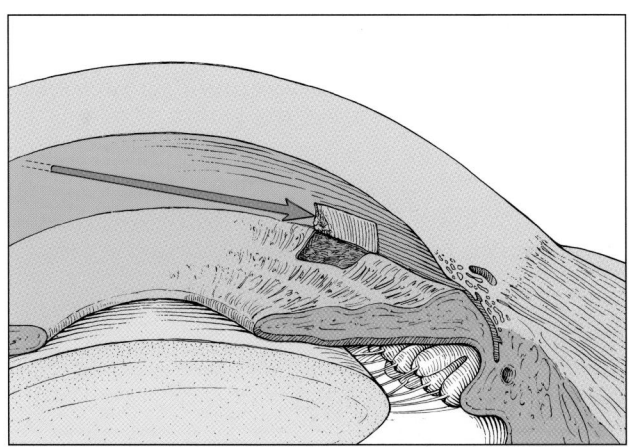

FIGURE 20-3 Revision of failing filtering bleb with argon or neodymium-yttrium aluminum garnet laser. A laser beam is aimed at the radial edge of the internal sclerostomy.

TABLE 20-3   REVISION OF INTERNAL SCLEROSTOMY

Laser	Power	Duration	Spot size	Number of applications
Argon	1000 mW	5.0 s	50 μm	50–200
Nd:YAG	6.0–7.0 mJ			20–50

Nd:YAG—neodymium-yttrium aluminum garnet.

Argon laser suture lysis enhances filtration in the early postoperative period after trabeculectomy. The most substantial effects occur during the first 2 postoperative weeks, and rarely after the 4th postoperative week unless antimetabolites are used in conjunction with glaucoma filtering surgery [11]. The use of antimetabolites usually prolongs the period for effective suture lysis up to several months. However, if there are signs of early subconjunctival fibrosis with elevated IOP, laser suture lysis should be performed earlier even if antimetabolites have been used. The complications of laser suture lysis can be minimized by proper timing of the procedure, the lowest possible setting of laser, and selecting a right type of laser for each case.

The advantage of the Nd:YAG laser over the previous methods is that the laser can be applied to nonpigmented tissue to cause a nonthermal vaporization of tissue at the target site. As demonstrated in several series, filtration was reestablished by the YAG or argon laser treatment in eyes that once had well-established filtration blebs for several months to years before the fistula became occluded. This finding suggests the subconjunctival space is still open and would allow aqueous flow if the sclerostomy is reopened. Those eyes that never developed good bleb function after the original glaucoma filtering surgery do not respond to laser reopening. The proposed indications for laser treatment for reopening of the fistula include 1) a previously well-established filtration bleb, 2) the site of bleb failure at the level of the sclerostomy with an identifiable membrane occluding the fistula, 3) clear media for the unobscured view of the sclerostomy site, and 4) absence of any significant inflammation. These criteria unfortunately apply to only a small select group of patients whose bleb function fails following glaucoma filtering surgery. However, this select group should be identified so that a relatively simple laser procedure may be attempted before repeating filtering surgery.

REFERENCES AND RECOMMENDED READING

Recently published papers of particular interest have been highlighted as:
• Of interest
•• Of outstanding interest

1.   Maumenee AE: External filtering operations for glaucoma: the mechanism of function and failure. *Tr Am Ophthalmol Soc* 1960, 58:319–328.

2.   Swan KC: Reopening of nonfunctioning filters-simplified surgical technique. *Tr Am Acad Ophthalmol Otorar* 1975, 79:342–348.

3.   Sugar HS: Complications, repair and reoperation of antiglaucoma filtering blebs. *Am J Ophthalmol* 1967, 63:825–833.

4.   Ticho U, Ivry M: Reopening of occluded filtering blebs by argon laser photocoagulation. *Am J Ophthalmol* 1977, 84:413–418.

5.   Van Buskirk EM: Reopening filtration fistulas with the argon laser. *Am J Ophthalmol* 1982, 94:1–3.

6.   Kurata F, Krupin T, Kolker AE: Reopening filtration fistulas with transconjunctival argon laser photocoagulation. *Am J Ophthalmol* 1984, 98:340–343.

7.   Van Rens GHMB: Transconjunctival reopening of an occluded filtration fistula with the Q-switched Nd:YAG laser. *Doc Ophthalmologica* 1988, 70:205–208.

8.   Dailey RA, Samples JR, Van Buskirk MV: Reopening filtration fistulas with the neodymium-YAG laser. *Am J Ophthalmol* 1986, 102:491–495.

9.   Praeger DL: The reopening of closed filtering blebs using the neodymium:YAG laser. *Ophthalmology* 1984, 91:373–377.

10. Cohn HC, Aron-Rosa D: Reopening blocked trabeculectomy sites with the YAG laser. *Am J Ophthal* 1983, 95:593–594.

11. Savage JA, Condon GP, Lytle RA, *et al.*:Laser suture lysis after trabeculectomy. *Ophthalmology* 1988, 95:1631–1638.

12. Pappa KS, Derick RJ, Weber PA, *et al.*: Late argon laser suture lysis after mitomycin C trabeculectomy. *Ophthalmology* 1993, 100:1268–1271.

13. Prywes AS, Lopinto RJ: Temporary visual loss of ciliary body detachment and hypotony after attempted YAG laser repair of failed filtering surgery. *Am J Ophthalmol* 1986, 101:305–307.

SELECT BIBLIOGRAPHY

Katz LJ: Blockage of the internal sclerostomy. In *Complications of Glaucoma Therapy*. Edited by Sherwood MB and Spaeth GL. Thorofare, NJ: Slack; 1990:227.

Oh Y, Katz LJ: Indications and technique for reopening closed filtering blebs using the Nd:YAG laser—a review a case series. Ophthalmic Surg 1993, 24:617–622.

Index

FREE POSTAGE! No stamp required if you live in the following countries:

AUSTRALIA, BELGIUM, BERMUDA, CYPRUS, DENMARK, FINLAND, FRANCE, GERMANY, HONG KONG, ICELAND, ISRAEL, ITALY, LUXEMBOURG, MONACO, THE NETHERLANDS, NEW ZEALAND, NORWAY, PORTUGAL, REPUBLIC OF IRELAND, SINGAPORE, SPAIN, SWEDEN, SWITZERLAND, THE UNITED ARAB EMIRATES, UNITED KINGDOM, UNITED STATES.

NO POSTAGE
NECESSARY
IF MAILED
IN THE
UNITED STATES

BUSINESS REPLY MAIL

FIRST CLASS MAIL PERMIT NO. 33925 PHILADELPHIA, PA

Postage Will Be Paid By Addressee

CURRENT SCIENCE
SUBSCRIPTIONS
20 N THIRD ST
PHILADELPHIA,   PA   19106-9815

By air mail
Par avion

IBRS/CCRI NUMBER: PHQ-D/453/W

NE PAS AFFRANCHIR

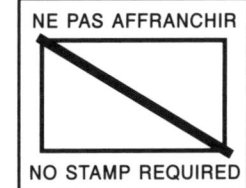

NO STAMP REQUIRED

**REPONSE PAYEE
GRANDE-BRETAGNE**

CURRENT SCIENCE
34-42 CLEVELAND STREET
LONDON   W1E 4QZ
GREAT BRITAIN

NO POSTAGE
NECESSARY
IF MAILED
IN THE
UNITED STATES

BUSINESS REPLY MAIL

FIRST CLASS PERMIT NO. 33925 PHILADELPHIA, PA

Postage Will Be Paid By Addressee

CURRENT SCIENCE
SUBSCRIPTIONS
20 N THIRD ST
PHILADELPHIA,   PA   19106-9815

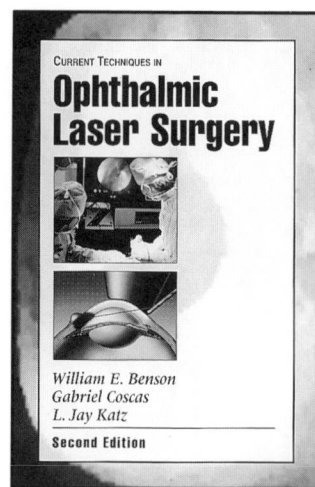